The AutPlay⌣
Therapy Handbook

The AutPlay® Therapy Handbook provides a thorough explanation and understanding of AutPlay® Therapy (an integrative family play therapy framework) and details how to effectively implement AutPlay® Therapy for addressing the mental health needs of autistic and neurodivergent children and their families.

This handbook guides the mental health therapist working with children and adolescents through their natural language of play. Opening with an extensive review of the neurodiversity paradigm and ableism, the chapters cover AutPlay® Therapy protocol, phases of therapy, assessment strategies, and common need areas along with understanding neurodiversity affirming processes. Additional chapters highlight the therapeutic powers of play, integrative play therapy approaches, understanding co-occurring conditions, working with high support needs, and using AutPlay® Therapy to address regulation, sensory, social/emotional, and other mental health concerns that neurodivergent children may be experiencing.

The handbook serves as a thorough guide for play therapists, child therapists, and family therapists who work with neurodivergent children and their families.

Dr. Robert Jason Grant is a licensed professional counselor, national board certified counselor, and registered play therapist-supervisor based in Missouri, USA.

The AutPlay® Therapy Handbook

Integrative Family Play Therapy with Neurodivergent Children

By Robert Jason Grant

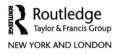
Routledge
Taylor & Francis Group

NEW YORK AND LONDON

Designed cover image: Getty Image

First published 2023
by Routledge
605 Third Avenue, New York, NY 10158

and by Routledge
4 Park Square, Milton Park, Abingdon, Oxon, OX14 4RN

Routledge is an imprint of the Taylor & Francis Group, an informa business

© 2023 Robert Jason Grant

Library of Congress Cataloging-in-Publication Data
Names: Grant, Robert Jason, 1971– author.
Title: The Autplay® therapy handbook: integrative family play therapy with
neurodivergent children / by Robert Jason Grant.
Description: First edition. | New York, NY: Routledge, 2023. |
Includes bibliographical references and index.
Identifiers: LCCN 2022027819 (print) | LCCN 2022027820 (ebook) |
ISBN 9781032075495 (hbk) | ISBN 9781032075488 (pbk) |
ISBN 9781003207610 (ebk)
Subjects: LCSH: Play therapy. | Developmentally disabled
children—Treatment. | Play assessment (Child psychology)
Classification: LCC RJ505.P6 G733 2023 (print) | LCC RJ505.P6 (ebook) |
DDC 618.92/891653—dc23/eng/20220802
LC record available at https://lccn.loc.gov/2022027819
LC ebook record available at https://lccn.loc.gov/2022027820

ISBN: 978-1-032-07549-5 (hbk)
ISBN: 978-1-032-07548-8 (pbk)
ISBN: 978-1-003-20761-0 (ebk)

DOI: 10.4324/9781003207610

Typeset in Goudy
by codeMantra

Contents

Foreword

The AutPlay® Therapy Handbook:
Integrative Family Play Therapy with Neurodivergent Children

Connection

Dr. Robert Jason Grant and I met through the play therapy community. We were both invited to a week-long, international meeting for play therapists. I was immediately drawn to Dr. Grant and his vast knowledge regarding the neurodivergent population. Having worked in therapeutic settings since 1991, I had provided services to a number of clients who were neurodivergent by the time I met Dr. Grant. The topic of neurodiversity in general, along with specific considerations, identification, understanding, and therapy was not a prominent part of my graduate school training. Meeting Dr. Grant and learning from him allowed me to greatly expand my repertoire beyond the piecemeal education and research I had pursued to date. I attended his trainings, read his books, and became a Certified AutPlay Therapy Provider. Along the way, it was my pleasure to know him better. We have since collaborated on a number of projects such as the AutPlay Expansion Pack for the Virtual Sandtray App©, multiple presentations, and publications such as *Play Therapy Theory and Perspectives: A Collection of Thoughts in the Field* and *Implementing Play Therapy with Groups: Contemporary Issues in Practice* (both of these texts were co-edited with Clair Mellenthin). Dr. Grant's contribution to my knowledge and scope of practice has been invaluable. I am certain it will be the same for you.

Challenging the Traditional Neurodivergence View

In March 2020, Drs. JÂcqûelyn Fede and Amy Laurent challenged people to Level Up! their knowledge base regarding neurodivergence. This team of professionals includes both neurodivergent and neurotypical members, with a philosophy which includes beliefs that "through education, accessible resources, practical strategies and a commitment to consistently incorporating the experiences and perspectives of autistic people, we can support the leveling up of society when it comes to autism and neurodiversity" (Fede & Laurent, 2020, para 46). A key aim of this article is to challenge the traditional view of "deficit and disorder" regarding neurodiversity (para 6).

Fede and Laurent proposed that simple awareness is not enough, particularly regarding autism. We must be aware and strive toward advocacy, with acceptance, appreciation, and empowerment along the path (Fede & Laurent, 2020). It is a process of recognizing where you are currently, looking inward and performing a self-evaluation of biases and belief systems, and then taking the next steps toward greater understanding, learning, and active involvement. These are some of the critical components of increasing everyone's understanding of the realities of neurodiversity and autism (Fede & Laurent, 2020).

The AutPlay® Therapy Handbook

The AutPlay® Therapy Handbook encompasses the philosophies of Autism Level Up. Building upon a quickly growing set of Dr. Grant's authored resources, the addition of the AutPlay® Therapy Handbook presents neurodivergence as an inclusion of differences which are "normal, natural variations in the human genome." The shift in conceptualization from pathology to normalcy is very powerful and sets the stage for many ways to work with individuals in mental health settings utilizing the approaches, goals, and interventions outlined in this book.

Grounded in the acknowledgement of each individual as unique and encompassing a multitude of ideologies, Dr. Grant has provided the reader with a critical foundation. This foundation springs into 18 additional chapters, each geared toward understanding and working with neurodivergent clients and their families. Neurodiversity, Grant explains, is not a belief, a political position, paradigm, perspective, or approach – "it is a fact"; it is a "the variance of human neurotypes."

Of particular interest to me is Chapter 10. Important works by Dr. Eliana Gil (1994, 2015) and Dr. Kay Trotter (2013) are referenced for further understanding of family play therapy. Grant describes a "synergetic effect" regarding the complementary relationship between play therapy and family therapy when integrated. This is a powerful statement; inviting the reader to learn more about the integration, synergy, and impact that utilizing the tenets of AutPlay® Therapy will have on the family therapy process. This chapter of the AutPlay® Therapy Handbook informs us about important concepts such as "parents might find play challenging, parents should follow their child's lead, parents need to play within their child's zone of proximal development..." and so much more. These are skills and conceptualizations that will be powerful with both the neurodivergent and neurotypical populations!

Importance of Understanding the Realities

Returning to the importance of the above challenge posed by Fede and Laurent, and the importance of increasing our understanding of the realities of neurodiversity and autism, we can see that Dr. Grant works to guide the reader toward achieving this goal. Chapters 1–4 are defining key foundational concepts regarding neurodiversity and setting the stage for the rest of the book. Chapters 5–9 introduce and discuss the key components of play therapy, an integrative approach, and AutPlay Therapy. Chapters 10–17, Conclusion present a number of interventions and examples to fill the play therapist's toolbox and illustrate the concepts. Easy to follow and use handouts, inventories, and forms are provided for smooth integration of the concepts.

This text is certain to contribute valuable foundations, understandings, concepts, interventions, and more to your professional development and offerings. We can all work toward the challenge to Level Up! and the AutPlay® Therapy Handbook provides a number of concepts and tools to rise to the challenge. Here we go!

Jessica Stone, Ph.D., RPT-S

Affiliate, East Carolina University Neurocognition Science Lab

Certified AutPlay Therapy Provider

Author, Digital Play Therapy

References

Fede, J. & Laurent, A. (2020). So, you want to Autism Level UP!? Game on! https://neuroclastic.com/so-you-want-to-autism-level-up-game-on/

Gil, E. (1994). *Play in family therapy*. Guilford Press.

Gil, E. (2015). *Play in family therapy* (2nd ed.). Guilford Press.

Trotter, K. (2013). Family play therapy. In N. R. Bowers (Ed.). *Play therapy with families*. Jason Aronson.

Acknowledgements

This book has been a great labor of love for me that has span almost a year and half of consistent focus and writing. I want to thank my family for their support and all those who kept me motivated. I also want to thank Routledge publishing for believing is this Handbook concept and committing to this high-volume book.

I want to acknowledge so many wonderful people who contributed to this book. I want to thank each of you who shared a case example and shared your own personal lived experience stories. Jennifer Gerlach, Boontarika Sripom, Rebekah Brown, Spencer Beard, Sarah Moran, Patricia Lomando, Elaine Hutchinson, Jen Taylor, Lily Wake, Daysi B. Onstad, Canace Yee, and Jaya Ramesh – you all made this handbook much more dynamic, and I appreciate your efforts and support.

Thank you to the play therapy and neurodivergent communities. I have learned so much and continue to learn much from you. So many influencers, leaders, advocates, and authors have inspired my own journey and helped me understand and grow. Lastly, thank you to Dr. Jessica Stone for writing the foreword to this book and thank you to Dr. Linda Homeyer, Jackie Flynn, and Lisa Dion who took the time to write reviews for this book.

My hope is that the result of this project helps provide awareness, acceptance, much better affirming processes to the mental health care of neurodivergent children.

Robert Jason Grant

Introduction

Introduction

Macy was 9 years old when I first met her. She was sitting with her mother in my office. It was their first session to see me, her mother was bringing her to therapy to help with regulation needs. Macy was autistic and gifted. She was being home schooled due to regulation struggles in the mainstream school. Macy would regularly crawl under desks and refuse to come out. Her mother described her regulation struggles to be frequent and lasted for long periods of time. Macy struggled with becoming dysregulated in most events she navigated including in her own home. She currently stayed mostly at home, did not participate in any activities outside the home, and rarely left the house to complete errands with her mother.

Sitting in my office in this first session it was clear Macy felt uncomfortable. I could see her anxiety and a child who was likely "one more thing" away from a dysregulated meltdown. Luckily this was not my first experience with a child such as Macy. I knew the process would be vital and that process must be supportive, affirming, and focused on building relationship with Macy that nurtured safety and familiarity. I also knew the therapeutic key to helping Macy existed in the transformative process I had seen over and over again from child to child – the child's own natural language of play.

The AutPlay Therapy framework was on full display in my time working with Macy. There was a central focus on building relationship, identifying and valuing her play preference of movement play which greatly helped regulate her system, assessing her strengths, discovering her talents with humor, and providing her space to shine in her strength at each play therapy session. It was also important to include her mother in the therapy process and the three of us working together as partners to help Macy improve her regulation needs, value her identity as a neurodivergent child, improve her self-worth,

DOI: 10.4324/9781003207610-1

and amplifying Macy's voice in the therapeutic process – empowerment in her own growth.

A neurodiversity affirming foundation and play therapy framework provided the platform for Macy to process and grow at her pace and achieve her therapy goals. The child I met, who could hardly leave her home and was crawling under tables in a state of dysregulation started attending a private school, created a self-advocacy program for students in the private school, began to develop her strength with humor and starting entering comedy competitions, began leaving the house without consideration for all types of activities, and at last check-in, was performing in a main role in her second community theater musical. We could call my experience with Macy the current me. The me who can easily define the neurodiversity paradigm and being neurodiversity affirming. The me who understands the therapeutic powers of play and how affirming integrative play therapy can be a wonderful mental health approach for neurodivergent children. The me who understands my own lived experience and is fully engaged in advocacy and the neurodiversity movement. But this hasn't always been me.

What is neurodivergence? What is play therapy? How do the two intertwine in a rhythmic fashion where the neurodivergent child finds their therapeutic outlet that is not only affirming but provides the natural means to address a whole host of needs. At the same time, how does play therapy find its child, the opportunity to shine in what it does best – bringing its therapeutic powers to a historically discarded population working in an empowering and healing radiance. My neurodivergent and play therapy journeys have intertwined on many levels and ultimately combined to form what is known as AutPlay Therapy. The road to this handbook has been a progression which began several decades ago with my own childhood.

I knew I was different as a child. I was bright and fairly perceptive. I could see that I navigated things differently from most of the other children. I was aware that things seemed to bother me, or I would have struggles where other children seemed non-affected. The only diagnosis I received (which was somewhat haphazard) was social anxiety. It would not be until I was an adult that I would understand my sensory processing challenges and my own neurodivergence. It did not take me long to figure out that many environments were dysregulating for me. The social challenges, the sensory issues, the lack of understanding my own system and the confusion and awkwardness that many environments held for me began to create high levels of anxiety. A great deal of my childhood (mostly anything outside of my home) is a reflection of survival. I would plan, plot, strategize, and lie to get myself through various social situations as smoothly and less dysregulating as possible. I made up illnesses, faked being sick, and would even go to the doctor with one of my "sicknesses" to avoid going to school – which was a nightmare for my neurodivergent self. I would pretend to go to school but instead hide in empty homes in my neighborhood all day until I got caught. I would also pretend to be sick at school and spend hours sitting in the nurse's office. Lying, seeing a doctor for no reason, and hanging out in empty homes all day were a relief compared to the bombardment my system would take trying to get through a day of school.

Eventually I stopped attending public school. My parents realized the anxiety levels and that it had become impossible for me to attend. They found an alternative education setting for me which worked fairly well and enabled me to complete my high school education. For the most part, my parents did not understand what was happening with me nor did they provide much support. An affirming presence was a complete absence in my childhood. The concept of being neurodivergent was not known and I doubt anyone had even heard of sensory processing challenges. We lived in a rural environment and my childhood was at a time when different was viewed as problematic. I think my parents likely did the best they could for me with the knowledge they possessed.

Many environments were a struggle, but I was able to regularly avoid most of them and spent a great deal of time at home. I spent a lot of time alone and I liked it that way – alone was peaceful. By the time I graduated, I had a bit better sense of myself. Meeting a couple of affirming individuals late into my teen years helped me begin to understand a stronger self-worth instead of viewing my differences as negative. This led to the motivation to go to college. My adult life proved to be far more productive than my childhood. It was full-speed ahead in discovery and growth. I finally learned about my sensory processing differences, began to understand and appreciate my neurodivergence, and begin to heal from the devaluing messages and struggles of my childhood.

By the time I became a play therapy therapist, things navigated much more successfully for me. My process of growth took a certain protectory. First, I began to understand myself and my sensory system. I stopped judging and taking in negative cognitions about being different. I learned to appreciate myself and the way I navigated. Second, once I understood myself better, I was able to learn strategies, techniques, tips, etc. for things that helped me navigate specific situations better. I also began to understand how to advocate for myself. Lastly, I realized my control. As an adult I was able to greatly control how I lived. I could enter or avoid environments mostly based on my choice. I realized as this time the great divide between my neurodivergent adult self and my neurodivergent child self. As a child I had little to no control, as an adult I have control and that control gives me options to better navigate a greater society that still falls short in appreciating and supporting neurodivergent individuals.

I was a neurodivergent child and I am a neurodivergent adult. Neurodivergence isn't something that goes away. My issues and struggles have never been about being neurodivergent. I say to clients and parents often that the reality is a neurodivergent person will be a neurodivergent person throughout their life. How they feel and what they believe about their neurodivergence will have a massive impact on their overall mental health. I have reflected many times that I would have loved having an affirming play therapist in my life as a child. It would have uplifted me and helped me gain a healthy perspective. I know it would have provided me a greater peace within the storm.

This is my goal in creating AutPlay Therapy and writing this book – that play therapists across communities can be that safe, affirming space for neurodivergent children. As you navigate through this handbook, I hope you will clearly understand what is neurodivergence, what is play therapy, and how the therapeutic powers of play in the atmosphere of an affirming play therapist can be a powerfully supportive and growth producing experience for the neurodivergent child.

1

Neurodiversity, Ableism, and Being Neurodiversity Affirming

Neurodiversity

What is diversity? Queensborough College (2021) defines the concept of diversity as encompassing acceptance and respect. It means understanding that each individual is unique and recognizing our individual differences. These can be along the dimensions of race, ethnicity, gender, sexual orientation, socio-economic status, age, physical abilities, religious beliefs, political beliefs, or other ideologies. Diversity is a reality created by individuals and groups from a broad spectrum of demographic and philosophical differences. It is extremely important to support and protect diversity because by valuing individuals and groups free from prejudice and by fostering a climate where equity and mutual respect are intrinsic, we will create a success-oriented, cooperative, and caring community that draws intellectual strength and produces innovative solutions from the synergy of its people.

Popular definitions of diversity include the state of being diverse; variety, the practice or quality of including or involving people from a range of different social and ethnic backgrounds and of different genders, sexual orientations, etc., the quality or state of having many different forms, types, ideas, etc., and an instance of being composed of differing elements or qualities: an instance of being diverse. Much has been written about diversity, and much diversity information can be discovered in a quick resource search. A slightly further exploration will produce a wide variety of offering on specific diversity needs within specific populations such as race or sexual orientation. But what about neurodiversity? What about the population – neurodiverse? Neurodiversity and more specifically, the diversity needs of neurodivergent individuals, can be conceptualized within the greater diversity awareness paradigm. Indeed, an understanding of racism, discrimination, prejudice, bigotry, etc. provides for a greater understating of what neurodiversity means

DOI: 10.4324/9781003207610-2

and how neurodivergent people and their allies are leading efforts in the neurodiversity movement to help improve acceptance and inclusion in societies that have historically lacked neurodivergent affirming constructs.

The term "neurodiversity" appears to have first been seen publicly in 1998 when journalist Harvey Blume published an article in the *Atlantic*. He stated that "Neurodiversity may be every bit as crucial for the human race as biodiversity is for life in general. Who can say what form of wiring will prove best at any given moment?" Judy Singer, an Australian sociologist, is widely credited with coining the term "neurodiversity." It is reported that Singer and Blume corresponded about the topic and Singer wrote about neurodiversity in her thesis in 1998. It was in 1999 that she furthered her work in neurodiversity while writing a chapter "Why Can't You be Normal for Once in Your Life?" based on her thesis which was published in the UK. Since its origins, the term has grown immensely with additional understanding and research support.

Walker (2021) stated that neurodiversity is the diversity of human minds, the infinite variation in neurocognitive functioning within our species. Neurodiversity is a biological fact. It's not a perspective, an approach, a belief, a political position, or a paradigm. There exists a great deal of scientific evidence that shows clearly that there's considerable variation among human brains. Neurodiversity can be thought of as the variance of human neurotype.

Robinson (2013) proposed that neurodiversity is the idea that neurological differences like autism and attention-deficit hyperactive disorder (ADHD) are the result of normal, natural variation in the human genome. Science suggests that conditions like autism have a stable prevalence in human society as far back as we can measure. There is awareness that autism, ADHD, sensory differences, and other conditions emerge through a combination of genetic predisposition and environmental interaction; they are not the result of disease or injury. This represents a new and fundamentally different way of looking at conditions that were traditionally pathologized. For neurodivergent individuals, talk of "cure" feels like an attack on their very being. They detest those words for the same reason other groups detest talk of "curing gayness" or "passing for white," and they perceive the accommodation of neurological differences as a similarly charged civil rights issue. If their diversity is part of their makeup, they believe it's their right to be accepted and supported "as is." They should not be made into something else – especially against their will – to fit some imagined societal ideal.

Silberman (2015) shared that one way to understand neurodiversity is to think in terms of human operating systems instead of diagnostic labels such as dyslexia and ADHD. The brain is, above all, a marvelous adaptive organism, adept at maximizing its chance of success even in the face of limitations. Just because a computer is not running windows, does not mean it's broken. Not all features of a neurodivergent operating system are bugs. Different is just different, it does not have to be pathologized.

The term "neurodiversity" has descriptive appeal as it reflects both the difficulties that neurodiverse people face as well as the positive dimensions of their lives. Neurodiversity is not an attempt to disregard the suffering undergone by neurodivergent people or to romanticize what many still consider significant needs. Rather, neurodiversity seeks to acknowledge the richness and complexity of human nature and of the human brain (Armstrong, 2010).

As we understand neurodiversity to represent the diversity of neurotype that exists in humans, we can begin to value this diversity in children. Realizing that children do not have to all funnel into a one-way, narrow look. Providing real experiences that support diverse neurotypes, begins to show awareness of neurodiversity in application. Armstrong (2010) put forth that:

> Neurodiversity provides a more balanced perspective. Instead of regarding traditionally pathologized populations as disabled or disordered, the emphasis in neurodiversity is placed on differences. Dyslexics often have minds that visualize clearly in three dimensions. People with ADHD have a different, more diffused, attention style. Autistic individuals relate better to objects than people. This is not, as some people might suspect, merely a new form of political correctness. Instead, research from brain science and evolutionary psychology, as well as from anthropology, sociology, and the humanities, demonstrates that these differences are real and deserve serious consideration.
>
> (pp. 5–6)

A true understanding of neurodiversity requires an understanding of several terms related to neurodiversity. Walker (2021) defined the following constructs related to neurodiversity. *Neurotypical* – often abbreviated as NT, means having a style of neurocognitive functioning that falls within the dominant societal standards of "normal."

Neurodivergent – sometimes abbreviated as ND, means having a mind that functions in ways which diverge significantly from the dominant societal standards of "normal." Autism, ADHD, sensory differences, and learning disorders are examples of innate forms of neurodivergence.

The neurodiversity movement – a social justice movement that seeks civil rights, equality, respect, and full societal inclusion for the neurodivergent.

The neurodiversity paradigm – a specific perspective on neurodiversity – a perspective or approach that boils down to these fundamental principles:

1 Neurodiversity is a natural and valuable form of human diversity.
2 The idea that there is one "normal" or "healthy" type of brain or mind, or one "right" style of neurocognitive functioning, is a culturally constructed fiction, no more valid (and no more conducive to a healthy society or to the overall well-being of humanity) than the idea that there is one "normal" or "right" ethnicity, gender, or culture.
3 The social dynamics that manifest in regard to neurodiversity are similar to the social dynamics that manifest in regard to other forms of human diversity (e.g., diversity of ethnicity, gender, or culture). These dynamics include the dynamics of social power inequalities, and also the dynamics by which diversity, when embraced, acts as a source of creative potential.

(pp. 34–46)

Ableism

Understanding neurodiversity, the neurodivergent child, and being neurodiversity affirming must include a thorough awareness of ableism. The term "ableism" is often defined as discrimination and social prejudice against people with disabilities or who are perceived to have disabilities. Ableism characterizes persons as defined by their disabilities and as inferior to the non-disabled. On this basis, people are assigned or denied certain perceived abilities, skills, or character orientations. Ableism can take the form of ideas and assumptions, stereotypes, attitudes and practices, physical barriers in the environment, or larger scale oppression. It is oftentimes unintentional, and most people are completely unaware of the impact of their words or actions (Urban Dictionary, 2021).

Pulrang (2020) stated that there seem to be two main schools of ableist belief. One is that disabled people are unfortunate but innocent victims of circumstance who should be loved, cared for, and shielded from harm. The other is that disabled people are naturally inferior, disagreeable, and at the same time beneficiaries of unfair and unjustified generosity and social protection. Neither belief is true, and both beliefs are limiting and poison relationships between disabled and non-disabled people, and sometimes between disabled people themselves. He identified three points for evaluation of possessing personal ableism:

1 Feeling instinctively uncomfortable around disabled people, or anyone who seems "strange" in ways that might be connected to a disability of some kind. This manifests in hundreds of ways, and can include:

- Being nervous, clumsy, and awkward around people in wheelchairs.
- Being viscerally disgusted by people whose bodies appear to be very different or "deformed."
- Avoiding talking to disabled people in order to avoid some kind of feared embarrassment.

2 Holding stereotypical views about disabled people in general, or about certain sub-groups of disabled people. For example:

- Assuming that disabled people's personalities fit into just a few main categories, like sad and pitiful, cheerful and innocent, or bitter and complaining.
- Associating specific stereotypes with particular conditions. For example, that people with Down syndrome are happy, friendly, and naive, mentally ill people are unpredictable and dangerous, or autistic people are cold, tactless, and unknowable.
- Placing different disabilities in a hierarchy of "severity" or relative value. A prime example of this is the widely held belief, even among disabled people, that physical disability isn't so bad because at least there's "nothing wrong with your mind."

3 Resenting disabled people for advantages or privileges you think they have as a group. This is one of the main flip sides of condescension and sentimentality toward disabled people. It's driven by a combination of petty everyday resentments and false, dark, and quasi-political convictions, such as:

- Disabled people get good parking spaces, discounts, and all kinds of other little unearned favors.
- Unlike other "minorities," everyone likes and supports disabled people. They aren't oppressed, they are coddled.
- Disabled people don't have to work and get government benefits for life.

(para. 8)

Scuro (2018) described ableism as a harmful bias, which is often trivialized but can be very damaging. The embeddedness in cultural conditioning and

Table 1.1 What Can Ableism Look Like?

Lack of compliance with disability rights laws like the ADA
Segregating students with disabilities into separate schools
Punishing a disability
Segregating adults and children with disabilities in institutions
Failing to incorporate accessibility into building design plans
Buildings without braille on signs, elevator buttons, etc.
Talking to, interacting with, and treating a person with a disability like they have no cognitive ability.
Framing disability as either tragic or inspirational in news stories, movies, and other popular forms of media
The assumption that people with disabilities want or need to be 'fixed'
Using disability as a punchline, or mocking people with disabilities
Refusing to provide reasonable accommodations
Talking to a person with a disability like they are a child, talking about them instead of directly to them, or speaking for them
Questioning if someone is 'actually' disabled, or 'how much' they are disabled

---

societal system is widespread and somewhat menacing. Often ableist constructs are put forth (without awareness) by well-intended and even established, respected, individuals and institutions. Consider the accepted (well-conditioned) ableist language that permeates society. That is, they are, you are retarded. That's crazy. The short bus, special needs, idiot, the blind leading the blind, and even symbols such as the autism puzzle piece designed to imply that there is something "missing" with this child, and we have to figure it out. Table 1.1 further highlights what ableism can look like.

The writings of play therapist Lyles (2022) illustrate the realness of ableism and its processes, especially by those who experience it.

> Ableism – Keeping the world most convenient for people whose bodies and minds operate like yours, fueled by the fear that your own body and mind will inevitably change in ways you like to pretend isn't real.

> Ableist Microaggressions – Subtly insulting words and actions regardless of intention, that let those with culturally sanctioned "strengths" feel superior while chipping away at the dignity of those not possessing or demonstrating so-called normative abilities.

> Inspiration Porn – Borrowing from the pain-laced survivalism of a weary soul (pain to which you may have even contributed) by just scraping off

the top layer of feel good while ignoring the intense lived experience of distress informing that "inspirational" strength.

Ableism and ableist practices can manifest (and often do) in any system or setting including mental health care and play therapy. Reeve (2000) identified ableism in counseling practice where counselors employ a predominantly medical model of disability that risks discounting alternative relational understandings. In counseling/therapy, disability is constructed in relation to the normal. Disability is always understood as a problematic deviation from the normal, as an imperfection when judged against what is considered normative. There is a risk of needing to "fix" or "cure" something that is actually a part of or who the person identifies as. This can manifest through the therapist attitude, approach, and microaggressions such as treatment goals.

Medical Model of Disability

Many organizations, groups, and agencies have historically viewed neurodivergence through a medical model heavily influenced by the American Psychiatric Association's Diagnostic and Statistical Manual (DSM). This manual has served as the guide in the United States (and other countries) for providing a formal diagnosis of autism, ADHD, learning disorders, etc. Typically, the process of a formal psychological evaluation diagnosis uses the protocol outlined in the DSM and thus works out of a medical model, which views neurodivergence as problematic, highlighting deficits and struggles and the need to cure or correct deficits. The medical model looks at neurodivergence as something that should not be happening regarding "normal" development and must be addressed to help the child become more neurotypical. Under the medical model, diagnosis is given so impairments or differences can be "fixed/cured" or changed by medical and other treatments, even when the impairment or difference does not cause pain or illness. The medical model looks at what is "wrong" with the person, instead of strengths or what that person needs and does not consider the concept of neurodiversity or neurodivergent as identity.

It is essential to understand that the current mental health system supports a neurodivergent-related diagnosis typically being given through a psychological evaluation conducted by a trained psychologist, which would be a medical diagnosis. This diagnosis would be based on the DSM and thus be influenced in the medical model view. Schools may also implement testing to diagnose for autism and other neurodivergent-related diagnosis, which would be an educational diagnosis. Psychiatrists, neurologists, and medical doctors can provide a medical diagnosis. The psychological evaluation process typically includes several assessment/evaluation inventories, can take anywhere from three hours to two days to complete, and is based on the DSM criteria and process.

Many services, programs, and therapies that may be helpful for a neurodivergent child require a formal diagnosis. The AutPlay therapist will need to help children and parents understand how the medical model works and ensure that families do not receive this information as the totality of their understanding of the diagnosis or neurodivergence. Therapists will need to provide additional reading, resources, and have conversations to help families be aware of neurodiversity and a non-pathologizing view of neurodivergence.

Although we could highlight and deconstruct multiple neurodivergent DSM diagnoses, for conceptualization purposes we will focus on autism. The following will present a synopsis of the American Psychiatric Association's DSM 5th Edition (2013) criteria for receiving an autism spectrum disorder diagnosis followed by information providing a non-pathologizing, affirming view of autism.

A   Persistent deficits in social communication and social interaction across multiple contexts, as manifested by the following, currently or by history:

1   Deficits in social-emotional reciprocity; for example, abnormal social approach and failure of normal back-and-forth conversation; reduced sharing of interests, emotions, or affect; and failure to initiate or respond to social interactions.

2   Deficits in nonverbal communicative behaviors used for social interaction; for example, poorly integrated verbal and nonverbal communication; abnormalities in eye contact and body language or deficits in understanding and use of gestures; and a total lack of facial expressions and nonverbal communication.

3   Deficits in developing, maintaining, and understanding relationships; for example, difficulties adjusting behavior to suit various social contexts; difficulties in sharing imaginative play or in making friends; and absence of interest in peers.

B   Restricted, repetitive patterns of behavior, interests, or activities, as manifested by at least two of the following, currently or by history:

1   Stereotyped or repetitive motor movements, use of objects, or speech.

2   Insistence on sameness, inflexible adherence to routines, or ritualized patterns of verbal or nonverbal behavior.

3   Highly restricted, fixated interests that are abnormal in intensity or focus.
4   Hyper- or hyporeactivity to sensory input or unusual interests in sensory aspects of the environment.

There are three levels in the DSM-5:

Level 3: Requiring Very Substantial Support
Severe deficits in verbal and nonverbal social communication skills cause severe impairments in functioning; very limited initiation of social interactions; minimal response to social overtures from others. Inflexibility of behavior, extreme difficulty coping with change, or other restricted/repetitive behaviors markedly interfere with functioning in all spheres.
Level 2: Requiring Substantial Support
Marked deficits in verbal and nonverbal social communication skills; social impairments apparent even with supports in place; limited initiation of social interactions; and reduced or abnormal responses to social overtures from others. Inflexibility of behavior, difficulty coping with change, or other restricted/repetitive behaviors appear frequently enough to be obvious to the casual observer and interfere with functioning in a variety of contexts.
Level 1: Requiring Support
Without supports in place, deficits in social communication cause noticeable impairments; difficulty initiating social interactions and clear examples of atypical or unsuccessful responses to social overtures of others; may appear to have decreased interest in social interactions. Inflexibility of behavior causes significant interference with functioning in one or more contexts.

(pp. 50–59)

A Non-Pathology Affirming Perspective

The neurodiversity movement, which maintains that autism can be a positive practical identity, is an attempt to eliminate the harm of pathologizing autism and neurodivergence. An initiative at the center of the neurodiversity movement is that neurological diversity is a fact that should not be identified with psychiatric problems. It is unfair to treat the neurodiversity movement as a monolith. It should be focused on from a social perspective. Their needs to be an emphasis on the idea that aspects that make life challenging for neurodivergent individuals are not intrinsically linked to individual flaws, but to a mismatch between the individual and the environment, and a lack of support (Bervoets & Hesn, 2020).

Lowry (2021), an autistic psychologist, developed a reframe of DSM autistic traits from a strengths-based (Strength-Based Autism Diagnostic Criteria) rather than a deficits-based perspective. He presents the following strength-based view of diagnosing autism:

I To meet diagnostic criteria for autism according to DSM-5, a child must have persistent differences in each of three areas of social communication and interaction (see A1–A3 below) plus at least two of four types of repetitive behaviors (see B1–B4 below).

   A Different social communication and interaction as evidenced by the following:

      1 Differences in communication – tendency to go off on tangents, tendency to talk passionately about special interests, and tendency to not engage in small talk.

      2 Differences in nonverbal communication, including stimming while talking, looking at something else while talking, and being bored with conversations.

      3 Due to the above differences in communication, autistic people tend to be shunned by neurotypicals and, therefore, are conditioned to believe that they are somehow less social.

   B Repetitive behavior or interests as evidenced by at least two of the following:

      1 Stimming or engaging in echolalia.

      2 Security in routines. Autistic people do not have a sensory filter, so the world is perceived as a constant state of chaos. Routines and expectations give comfort to overwhelmed autistic people.

      3 Special Interests (SPINS). Due to hyperconnected brains, autistic people feel more passionately about what they love, so when they have a special interest, they tend to fawn over and fixate on it.

      4 Hyper- or hyporeactivity to stimuli. Again, due to hyperconnections, they feel emotions more intensely. Sometimes, they feel emotions less intensely because they tune them out in favor of other stimuli.

II Autistic people are born with these traits but learn how to mask them. Sometimes, the traits show up only when they are stressed and let down their guards.

III These traits cause other people distress. Note the DSM ONLY indicates impairment when it affects other people or jobs, but not when it is a daily issue that the autistic person learns to live with.

IV Autism is not due to intellectual disability.

The Autism Self Advocacy Network (ASAN) (2021) is an organization operated by and for autistic people. ASAN was created to serve as a national grassroots disability rights organization for the autistic community. The organization seeks to advance the principles of the disability rights movement regarding autism. ASAN defines autism as the following:

> Autism is a developmental disability that affects how we experience the world around us. Autistic people are an important part of the world. Autism is a normal part of life and makes us who we are.
>
> Autism has always existed. Autistic people are born autistic, and we will be autistic our whole lives. Autism can be diagnosed by a doctor, but you can be autistic even if you don't have a formal diagnosis. Because of myths about autism, it can be harder for autistic adults, autistic girls, and autistic people of color to get a diagnosis. But anyone can be autistic, regardless of race, gender, or age.
>
> Autistic people are in every community, and we always have been. Autistic people are people of color. Autistic people are immigrants. Autistic people are a part of every religion, every income level, and every age group. Autistic people are women. Autistic people are queer, and autistic people are trans. Autistic people are often many of these things at once. The communities we are a part of and the ways we are treated shape what autism is like for us.
>
> There is no one way to be autistic. Some autistic people can speak, and some autistic people need to communicate in other ways. Some autistic people also have intellectual disabilities, and some autistic people don't. Some people need a lot of help in their day-to-day lives, and some autistic people only need a little help. All of these people are autistic, because there is no right or wrong way to be autistic. All of us experience autism differently, but we all contribute to the world in meaningful ways

(para. 1–4)

ASAN (2021) further explains that autistic people deserve understanding and acceptance. Every autistic person experiences autism differently, but there are some things that many have in common. Autistic individuals think differently, process senses differently, move differently, communicate differently, socialize differently, and might need help with daily living

Within the AutPlay Therapy process, therapists have the ability to implement an autism screening process from a strength-based perspective. The AutPlay autism screening process serves as a tool for therapists to observe and assess a child to identify if there appears to be a need for further evaluation or referral regarding a possible diagnosis. Autism screenings are not a diagnostic process; they provide a simpler protocol to screen for the need for further evaluation. Although there are many options open to a therapist when conducting an autism screening, the following highlights the screening process in AutPlay Therapy that is designed from a strength-based perspective.

1 The entire process should take two to three hours that can be implemented in one setting or across sessions.
2 Parents are given the AutPlay Autism Checklist Revised (located in the appendix of this book) to complete on their child. Parents can also give the inventory to other adults who know the child well so multiple individuals can complete the inventory regarding the child.
3 Therapists can give additional inventories if they are familiar with other screening tools that are strength-based. All inventories are given to parents or caregivers to complete and return to the therapist for scoring and review.
4 The therapist will conduct an observation with the child in a playroom. This observation typically lasts 30–45 minutes. The therapist can use the Child Observation form located in the appendix section of this book. The therapist then conducts an observation of the parent and child playing together in a playroom. This observation lasts approximately 30 minutes. The therapist can use the Parent/Child Observation form located in the appendix section of this book. Observations should have a relational focus with the therapist staying attuned to the child in observing their play preferences and interests. The therapist will also observe the child's communication, interaction, and basic play style. Any strengths observed should be noted.
5 Once the AutPlay Autism Checklist Revised and observations have been completed, the therapist and parent discuss the process and results to identify if there is a need for further evaluation. If there are any significant indicators, the therapist should refer the family for a full psychological evaluation. If a referral for a full evaluation is made, the therapist will want to spend time talking with the parent about affirming ideas related to autism. The therapist can explain the medical model perspective and help prepare the family for what they will experience during the evaluation process. This might be an appropriate time to provide the family with additional affirming information about autism. One such resource

would be the Autism Self Advocacy Network's parent guide "Start Here: A Guide for Parents of Autistic Kids." This guide is affirming and covers many topics such as what is autism, what parents should do next, where parents can learn more, what good services look like, and topics such as self-advocacy, communication, and presuming competence.

Although autism was highlighted as a specific example of the medal model perspective versus a non-pathologizing and affirming perceptive, the same process can apply to any area of neurodivergence. All neurodivergence will be pathologized in the medical model perspective. Likewise, all neurodivergence can be viewed through an affirming lens, looking at the whole child. This certainly includes recognizing issues or needs but it does not stop there, it also looks at strengths, identity, and a healthy understanding and view of self. Consider the discourse offered by Dr. Nick Walker (2021)

> At the root of the pathology paradigm is the assumption that there is one "right" style of human neurocognitive functioning. Variations in neurocognitive functioning that diverge substantially from socially constructed standards of "normal"– including the variations that constitute autism – are framed within this paradigm as medical pathologies, as deficits, damage, or "disorders."

> Through the lens of the neurodiversity paradigm, the pathology paradigm's medicalized framing of autism and various other constellations of neurological, cognitive, and behavioral characteristics as "disorders" or "conditions" can be seen for what it is: a social construction rooted in cultural norms and social power inequalities, rather than a "scientifically objective" description of reality.

> The choice to frame the minds, bodies, and lives of autistic people (or any other neurological minority group) in terms of pathology does not represent an inevitable and objective scientific conclusion but is merely a cultural value judgment. Similar pathologizing frameworks have been used time and again to lend an aura of scientific legitimacy to all manner of other bigotry, and to the oppression of women, indigenous peoples, people of color, and queer people, among others.

> (pp. 18–20)

Social Model of Disability

In contrast to the medical model is the social model of disability. It was not designed to be a perfect theory of disability but an explanation of disabled people's experience in society and, equally importantly, a tool for creating social change. What is powerful and liberating about the social model is that it does reflect disabled people's real life experience and puts forward a radical and practical approach to ending disabled people's exclusion and oppression that does not require disabled people to change who they are in order to be deemed to be entitled to the same rights and opportunities as non-disabled people (Inclusion London, 2021).

The social model of disability maintains that disability is caused by the way society is organized. It identifies systemic barriers, negative attitudes, and exclusion by society (purposely or inadvertently) that mean society is the main contributory factor in disabling people. A social model perspective does not deny the reality of impairment nor its impact on the individual. However, it does challenge the physical, attitudinal, communication, and social environment to accommodate impairment as an expected incident of human diversity. The social model seeks to change society in order to accommodate people living with impairment; it does not seek to change persons with impairment to accommodate society (People with Disability Australia, 2021).

Goering (2015) stated that the social model of disability focuses attention on the attitudinal obstacles faced by people with non-standard bodies. Other people's expectations about quality of life and ability to work for a person with a disability not only affect the ways in which physical structures and institutional norms are made and sustained (based on presumptions about inability to perform), but also can create additional disability by making it harder for such individuals to feel good about themselves. The social model reminds us to be careful about what we presume to be irremediable through social change and to question the ways in which we currently understand disability. Challenging standard definitions of disability and impairment will require listening carefully to the experiences of people living with those impairments and thinking creatively about possibilities for inclusion, accommodation, and accessibility.

Inclusion London (2021) stated that barriers "disable" individuals by creating exclusion, discrimination, and disadvantage for people with impairments. The social model, in highlighting the barriers, often simultaneously can identify solutions. There are three types of barriers common within the social model of disability.

1   Attitudinal barriers – These are social and cultural attitudes and assumptions about people who are neurodiverse or have a disability that explain, justify, and perpetuate prejudice, discrimination, and exclusion in society; for example, assumptions that people with certain impairments

can't work, can't be independent, can't have sex, shouldn't have children, need protecting, are "child-like", are " dangerous", should not be seen because they are upsetting, are unpredictable, etc.

2 Physical barriers – These are barriers linked to the physical and built environment and cover a huge range of barriers that prevent equal access, such as stairs/ steps, narrow corridors and doorways, curbs, inaccessible toilets, inaccessible housing, poor lighting, poor seating, broken elevators, or poorly managed streets and public spaces.

3 Information/Communication Barriers – These are barriers linked to information and communication, such as lack of Sign Language interpreters for Deaf people, lack of provision of hearing induction loops, lack of information in different accessible formats such as Easy Read, plain English, and large font, lack of sensory accommodations, and lack of understanding there are more ways to communicate than verbally.

(para. 15–17)

Consider this simple but clear example of the social model of disability: the case of Adam, an autistic teen who was attending a public high school. As a freshman in high school, Adam was testing at a 3rd grade level in math (which he had been testing at since 3rd grade). Adam's mother sought tutoring services outside of the school to help Adam increase his math skills. Upon participation with special tutors, it was discovered that if Adam could use a calculator to complete his math work, he scored at a 9th grade level in math – five grade levels higher than he was scoring in public school testing processes. It was further discovered that some of Adam's school teachers had recognized that Adam could do more advanced math when he used a calculator versus pencil-and-paper equation operations, but they felt he needed to learn how to do math the way they were teaching it and did/would not allow him to use a calculator. Adam continued to struggle until his parents removed him from the public school he was attending and placed him in a private school that was more accommodating of Adam's specific learning styles, which included being able to use a calculator to perform math equations. Due to being behind in grade levels, Adam spent an extra semester in high school but graduated on grade level in all his subjects (including math). In summary, Adam did not have a math disorder. He could comprehend and perform math equations at grade level when allowed to use a calculator. It was his environment (societal perspective that using a calculator was invalid) that was disabling him from advancing in math ability.

It is important to note the neurodiverse advocates (those that highlight the social model of disability) do not say that disabled people don't have problems, needs, or struggles, that is invalidation. That is not what the so-cial model of disability communicates. The central idea of the social model is that needs and differences (no matter how difficult or distressing) do not make neurodivergent individuals any less worthy of access to society than others.

Neurodivergence is not a disorder, but neurodivergent individuals may have needs such as executive dysfunction, regulation struggles, trauma responses, and extreme sensory differences. There is no treatment or cure for neuro-divergence, but a neurodivergent individual may need accommodations or therapies. The social model promotes a society where neurodivergent needs (any needs) are accommodated and where disabled people are able to enjoy full access to society.

Being Neurodiversity Affirming

Neurodiversity affirming is an action. It is a set of multiple processes that col-late from a neurodiversity informed understanding. The neurodiversity af-firming play therapist has a thorough understanding of neurodiversity which includes the neurodiversity movement and paradigm, ableism, the medical and social models of disability, and the history of non-affirming/ableist ther-apy approaches initiated with neurodivergent children. It is this knowledge that translates into (guides) affirming awareness and approaches in therapy practice.

When working with neurodivergent children, it is critical for therapists to assess and conceptualize each individual child in order to fully understand the child's strengths and needs. Although there may be some commonali-ties, each neurodivergent child will present their uniqueness. Therapists are encouraged to develop a process to help them build a relationship with the child, get to know the individual child, more accurately identify the child's strengths and needs, and understand any particulars a child might be expe-riencing related to being neurodivergent. In AutPlay Therapy, this process (outlined in later chapters) can be accomplished through parent-completed inventories, background information from the child's parents, therapist play observations, and simply talking, spending time, being attuned, and building relationship with the child.

Any type of therapy, support, care, or education process with a neurodi-vergent child or teen should be grounded in valuing the child's identity. Therapists will want to conceptualize how their interactions with the child promote value and acceptance and avoid ableist concepts. Lambert (2018) stated that non-autistic disability advocates often neglect to apply the social model when they talk about autism and proposed five suggestions for valuing autistic individuals. Although specifically talking about autistic individuals, these principles apply across neurodivergent representation:

1 Nothing About Us, Without Us: A popular adage with disability advocates – and it's still relevant. You can't talk about autism if you're ignoring autistic people and what they have to say. All those people advocating for a cure. Most of them aren't autistic.

2 You Don't Know Me: Much of the information out there about autism isn't accurate to the real experiences of autistic people. It's nice to hear that you're interested in autistic issues, but don't assume you know more about autism than an autistic person does. In fact, it's sometimes best to assume that you don't know anything about autism at all.

3 Educate Yourself: So maybe you don't know anything about autism. It's time to learn – from autistics. Read what autistic activists write about their experiences – not only the voices that are easy to find, but also those that are often quieter. Autistic women, autistic people of color, queer and trans autistic people, and poor autistic people all have stories to tell.

4 This Space Is Our Space: Your disability-centered social circles, articles, and theories aren't always accessible to autistic people. If you don't make any efforts to make easy-read materials, sensory-friendly environments, or spaces where people can communicate in the ways that are most comfortable for them, you aren't including autistic people.

5 Who Are You Speaking To?: Many autistic advocates prefer identity-first language ("autistic person" instead of "person with autism"). An autistic person's disability is part of them, and they don't want to dance around it. And please – don't call them high functioning or low functioning. If you don't respect their language, you don't respect them.

(para. 6–10)

Grant (2021) proposes a guideline for being neurodivergent informed that includes several philosophical points neurotypical individuals can implement to provide value and affirming practices for neurodivergent children:

1 Do not assume neurodivergent children have limitations. Some are gifted, some have strengths in a variety of areas. Some do not need any therapies. A neurodivergent child is not in therapy because they are neurodivergent.

2 Ask the child about themselves, allow their voice in the therapy process, and listen to what they say.
3 Remember that processing speed, communication, and other executive skills might be different from your own and differences are valued as okay.
4 Remember social interactions may look differently and the neurodivergent child may have preferences that differ from the typical society standard. This is not negative; it is different but not a lesser way of doing things.
5 Do not rely on verbal or nonverbal messages or body language to communicate with neurodivergent children. The child may have a variety of ways of communicating. Remember that play is the natural language of all children, and all children play. Commit to learning about the neurodivergent child's play preferences and interests.
6 Respect the child's right to decide how they want or do not want to talk about themselves and how they want their neurodivergence referenced.
7 Provide space for neurodivergent children to share what they are thinking and feeling; do not assume based on a diagnosis or how you would think or feel.
8 Be willing to use visual supports (schedules, pictures), technology, and any other communication/learning accommodations that best fit the child.
9 Do not judge behavior that is different from your own. Consistently check your interaction, approach, and process for ableist constructs.
10 Look for the strengths the neurodivergent child possesses and try to build upon those strengths.
11 See the world from the child's viewpoint. How are they experiencing what is happening?
12 Do not try to force the child to be like, look like, and act like you. Respect and learn about the neurodiversity paradigm.

(p. 31)

A Focus on Strengths

How disability is conceptualized will often depends on who is viewing it. Those working from the outside (let's say neurotypical individuals) may view disability as an impairment, deficit, or problem. Those with the disability (let's say neurodivergent individuals) will likely view the social factors they encounter as the real impairment or problem. This view that neurodivergence is the disability and thus the problem, completely eliminates the truth or even the consideration of the strengths a neurodivergent child possesses.

A key component of being neurodiversity affirming is taking a strength-based approach when implementing therapy. Focusing on the strengths a child possesses, building upon their strengths, and using them to address therapy needs can be an effective and neurodiversity affirming approach for helping neurodivergent children. Stoerkel (2021) proposed that a strength-based approach is successful because the client is the agent of change by providing the right environment for controlling change. This approach is highly dependent on the thought process and emotional and information processing of the individual. It allows for open communication and thought process for individuals to identify value and assemble their strengths and capacities in the course of change. A strength-based approach allows for habitable conditions for a child to see themselves at their best, to see the value they bring, by just being themselves.

Pattoni (2012) described a strength-based practice as a collaborative process between the person supported by services and those supporting them (the therapist and the child), allowing them to work together to determine an outcome that draws on the child's strengths and assets. In therapeutic settings, it focuses principally on the quality of the relationship that develops between the therapist and the child, as well as the already developed resources the child brings to the process. Working in a collaborative way promotes the opportunity for children to be participants in creating support rather than being directed by the therapist. Strength-based approaches concentrate on the inherent strengths of children, families, groups, and organizations, deploying personal strengths to aid growth and healing. In essence, to focus on health and well-being is to embrace an asset-based approach where the goal is to promote the positive. Strength-based approaches value the capacity, skills, knowledge, connections, and potential in children.

Rapp, Saleebey, and Sullivan (2008) suggested six standards for determining a strength-based approach. If in agreement, therapists can use the following list when considering the method they will use when practicing the strength-based approach:

1 Goal orientation: It is crucial and vital for the person to set goals.
2 Strengths assessment: The person finds and assesses their strengths and inherent resources.
3 Resources from the environment: Connect resources in the person's environment that can be useful or enable the person to create links to these resources. The resources could be individuals, associations, institutions, or groups.

4 Different methods are used first for different situations: Clients will determine goals first and then strengths that can be used. In strength-based
   case management, individuals determine their strengths by first using an
   assessment.
5 The relationship is hope-inducing: By finding strengths and linking to
   connections (with other people, communities, or culture), the client
   finds hope.
6 Meaningful choice: Each person is an expert on their strengths, resources, and hopes. It is the practitioner's duty to improve upon choices
   the person makes and encourage making informed decisions.

(pp. 81–82)

Bronfenbrenner (1994) defines childhood as a beautiful time where children
are learning how to do things, and what they like. When using the strength-
based approach in early childhood practice you would implement the same
aspects you would for an adult. This would include paying attention to what
the child likes and offer a variety of ways for the child to learn, grow, and
heal. A great way for children to develop their strengths is to live expres-
sively. Children can express themselves in all sorts of ways (their play preferences and interests), and this can lend well to understanding what someone
truly enjoys and is good at.

A strength-based approach not only examines the child but also the child's
environment. For example, it looks at how systems are set up, especially
where power can be out of balance between a system or service and the child
it is supposed to serve. In addition, strength-based approaches identify any
constraints that might be holding back a child's growth. These constraints
can be when the child must deal with social, personal, and/or cultural issues
in environments that cannot be balanced fairly (Stoerkel, 2021).

Taylor (2019) describes a strength-based approach as the therapist is no
longer the expert, the child is. The therapist approaches the child with curiosity and interests in terms of how the child perceives the problems or
needs and solutions. The therapist no longer views the child through a certain therapeutic philosophy, that, in turn, shifts and perhaps distorts how
the child is viewed. Rather, the therapist works with the child, ready to be
informed by the child regarding how the child views their needs. For neurodivergent children, it means not viewing the child as a diagnosis and the
diagnosis is the need.

Solution-focused play therapy highlights the process of implementing a
strength-based approach when working with neurodivergent children. In

solution-focused therapy, the focus on strengths counters the negative focus that others often have on weaknesses, deficits, and disabilities. Focusing on strengths increases the child's feelings of self-efficacy and hope in the face of personal challenges. Strengths focus also increases the child's attention to resources that may be employed to compensate for challenges (Taylor, 2019). Solution-focused play therapy has been shown to be relevant for working with children and adjustments can be easily made from child to child according to the child's developmental level (Nims, 2007). The play involved in solution-focused play therapy can involve a variety of type and respects the child's play preferences such as art, sandtray, puppets, gamming, toys, movement, etc.

Focusing on strengths and implementing a strength-based approach does not mean ignoring challenges or needs the child might have or suggesting that struggles are strengths. Therapists working from a strength approach will need to work with the child in collaboration – helping them to implement their strengths to successfully address their challenges or needs. In this way, children become co-change agents (partners) in their therapy goals. Consider the following in the practical application of looking at and utilizing strengths:

- What does the child do well (dresses themself, is kind to others, plays independently)?
- What has the child accomplished (beat several video games, learned how to use a tablet, built an original LEGO creation)?
- How can you assess strengths (inventories, observations, play techniques, asking the child)?
- What can you observe about strengths the child has (plays reciprocally and alone, follows rules, helps clean the playroom)?

These considerations begin to inform the therapist about the child's strengths and conceptualizing how the strengths can be used to address therapy needs. It also helps the child recognize they are much more than their therapy needs. Consider the following play therapy interventions designed to help the child and therapist recognize the child's strengths.

Look at My Strengths

Therapy Needs: Strengths and self-worth

Level: Child and adolescent

Materials: Construction paper (various colors), tape, scissors, and a pen

Modality: Individual, group, and family

Instructions:

1 The therapist collects construction paper, scissors, tape, and a pen or pencil to use in this intervention. The therapist explains to the child they are going to use the construction paper to help learn about the child's strengths.
2 The therapist instructs the child to think about things they are good at, things they do well, things they can achieve, etc. Some children may have a difficult time with this, especially if their self-worth is low. The therapist may use language like "What do you like to do?" "What do you like to play with?" "How would you spend your day if you could do whatever you wanted?" Children may be able to better answer these types of questions and typically they will communicate answers that indicate their strengths.
3 The therapist instructs the child to cut out different shapes from the construction paper. The child can cut out as many shapes as they want and in any color they want. Each shape will have one of the child's strengths written on it.
4 Once the child has cut out the shapes, the child (and therapist if needed) will write a strength the child has identified on each cut-out shape.
5 The child will then put a piece of tape on the back of each shape and tape them to their chest, stomach, and/or arms.
6 Once the shapes have been taped onto the child, the therapist and the child will look in a mirror and read each shape and discuss each strength further if necessary. The therapist will help point out all the strengths the child identified and the importance of having and knowing one's strengths.
7 The therapist or the child's parent can take a picture of the child with their strengths and have it at home to reference.
8 The therapist can contribute strengths if they know of strengths the child possesses. The therapist can cut out shapes and share them with the child. This intervention helps the child recognize they do have strengths. Many neurodivergent children spend much of their time hearing about what they do wrong from adults in the various environments they navigate. It is important that children understand and recognize the strengths they possess. This play intervention also helps the therapist recognize some of the child's strengths and the therapist can begin to conceptualize how to use those strengths to help address therapy needs.

LEGO Build (Strengths)

Therapy Needs: Strengths and self-worth

Level: Child and adolescent

Materials: LEGO bricks

Modality: Individual, group, and family

Instructions:

1 The therapist explains that they are going to build some things using LEGO bricks.
2 The therapist displays several bricks to use in the intervention.
3 The therapist states that the child is going to build something with the bricks that describes or represents a strength they have. The therapist may need to explain the concept of a strength. It might be helpful to phrase it as something you are good at or something you do well.
4 The child can build anything they want in any way they want. The only guide is that must represent a strength.
5 The therapist should also do a strength build.
6 Once the therapist and child have both completed their builds, they can take turns sharing what they built and what strength it describes.
7 If the child wants, they can complete another build describing another strength.

Strengths Plate

Therapy Needs: Strengths and self-worth

Level: Child and adolescent

Materials: Paper plate and a pen

Modality: Individual, group, and family

Instructions:

1 The therapist explains to the child that they are going to do an activity talking about the child's strengths (things they do well).
2 The therapist gets a paper plate and draws a line down the middle (one half for the child and one half for the therapist).
3 The therapist writes their name at the top of the plate on their side and the child writes their name on the top of the plate on their side.

4 On the far-left side of the paper plate the therapist and child will write all the strengths they can think of that a person might have. The therapist will want to make sure that several different types of strengths get listed, especially some they know the child has.

5 Once the list of strengths is complete, the child and therapist will take turns putting a check mark under their name that corresponds with any of the strengths listed that they believe is a strength they possess.

6 Once both the therapist and child have finished their checks, they look at the plate, share, and compare what they put checkmarks beside.

7 The therapist can talk about how everyone has different strengths. The therapist can also talk about how the child has strengths the therapist does not have and vice versa. Everybody has strengths and it is important to focus on your strengths.

8 The child can keep the paper plate strengths to remind them of the strengths they possess.

Nims (2007) describes the solution focused strength-based play intervention *Wows and Hows*, which uses statements that begin with the words wow and how. They are designed to affirm children's positive conclusions about their lives in spite of what has happened to them – the "wow" – and asking them how they knew their behavior was the right thing to do under these circumstances – the "how." This helps them to discover their own capabilities and feel encouraged to use these skills in the future. Examples of this technique are "Wow, you were able to control your anger that time and stay calm. I wonder how you knew to do that?" "Wow, you did your homework that day. I wonder how you did that? There have been so many times you didn't do your homework. What was different that time?"

Mottron (2017) concluded that child therapies should allow the child to achieve an abstract level of happiness, personal accomplishment, access to cultural material, and social integration, an essential human right, regardless of the way in which this is achieved and the form that it takes. An acceptance of autistic and neurodivergent humanity begins by changing targets, methods, and efficiency variables of the processes offered to autistic and neurodivergent children, in favor of strength-informed and affirming approaches.

Essentially, the basic concept of valuing a child is not complicated. The play therapist may simply reflect on how they would want to be treated by a professional they might be seeing. Would they want to be heard, be listened to, have a say in what happens to them, be able to freely share and ask questions, make decisions concerning what happens to them, etc.? In most cases, adults would answer yes to all the above questions and desire this type of value. We should do no less for the children and adolescents we work with and serve. Being affirming empowers, and empowerment can achieve and heal as this becomes the meaningful pursuit in our work with neurodivergent children and their families.

References

American Psychiatric Association. (2013). *Diagnostic and statistical manual of mental disorders* (5th ed.). American Psychiatric Association.

Armstrong, T. (2010). *Neurodiversity: Discovering the extraordinary gifts of autism, ADHD, dyslexia, and other brain differences.* Da Capo Press.

Autistic Self Advocacy Network. (2021). About autism. https://autisticadvocacy.org/aboutasan/about-autism/

Bervoets, J., & Hens, K. (2020). Going beyond the catch-22 of autism diagnosis and research. The moral implications of (not) asking "What is autism?". *Frontiers in Psychology, 10.* https://doi.org/10.3389/fpsyg.2020.529193

Bronfenbrenner, U. (1994). Ecological models of human development. In *International encyclopedia of education* (Vol. 3, 2nd ed.). Elsevier.

Goering, S. (2015). Rethinking disability: The social model of disability and chronic disease. *Current Reviews in Musculoskeletal Medicine, 8*(2), 134–138. https://doi.org/10.1007/s12178-015-9273-z

Grant, R. J. (2021). *Understanding autism: A neurodiversity affirming guidebook for children and teens.* AutPlay Publishing.

Inclusion London. (2021). The social model of disability. https://www.inclusion-london.org.uk/disability-in-london/social-model/the-social-model-of-disability-and-the-cultural-model-of-deafness/

Lambert, M. (2018). *What the social model of disability can tell us about autism.* The American Association of People with Disabilities. https://www.aapd.com/what-the-social-model-of-disability-can-tell-us-about-autism/

Lowry, M. (2021). *Strengths-based autism diagnostic criteria.* Child & Adolescent Psychological Evaluations, LLC. https://www.mattlowrylpp.com/meme-gallery

Lyles, M. (2022). Ableism. https://www.marshalllyles.com/poetry.html

Mottron, L. (2017). Should we change targets and methods of early intervention in autism, in favor of a strengths-based education? *European Child & Adolescent Psychiatry, 26,* 815–825. https://doi.org/10.1007/s00787-017-0955-5

Nims. (2007). Integrating play therapy techniques into solution-focused brief therapy. *International Journal of Play Therapy, 16*(1), 54–68.

Pattoni, L. (2012). Strengths-based approach working with individuals. *Iriss.* Retrieved from https://www.iriss.org.uk/resources/insights/strengths-based-approaches-working-individuals

People with Disability Australia. (2021). Social model of disability. https://pwd.org.au/resources/disability-info/social-model-of-disability/

Pulrang, A. (2020). Words matter, and it's time to explore the meaning of "ableism." *Forbes*. https://www.forbes.com/sites/andrewpulrang/2020/10/25/words-matter-and-its-time-to-explore-the-meaning-of-ableism/?sh=1369771c7162

Queensborough Community College. (2021). Definition of diversity. https://www.qcc.cuny.edu/diversity/definition.html

Rapp, C., Saleebey, D., & Sullivan, P. W. (2008). The future of strengths-based social work practice. *Advances in Social Work*, 6(1), 79–90.

Reeve, D. (2000). Oppression within the counselling room. *Disability & Society*, 15(4), 669–682.

Robinson, J. E. (2013). What is neurodiversity? Neurodiversity means many things to people. Here's my first-person definition. *Psychology Today*. https://www.psychologytoday.com/us/blog/my-life-aspergers/201310/what-is-neurodiversity

Scuro, J. (2018). *Addressing ableism: Philosophical questions via disability studies*. Lexington Books.

Silberman, S. (2015). *Neurotribes: The legacy of autism and how to think smarter about people who think differently*. Allen & Unwin.

Stoerkel, E. (2021). What is a strength-based approach? *Positive Psychology*. https://positivepsychology.com/strengths-based-interventions/

Taylor, E. R. (2019). *Solution-focused therapy with children and adolescents: Creative and play based approaches*. Routledge.

Urban Dictionary. (2022). Ableism. https://www.urbandictionary.com/search.php

Walker, N. (2021). *Neuroqueer heresies: Notes on the neurodiversity paradigm, autistic empowerment, and postnormal possibilities*. Autonomous Press.

2

The Neurodivergent Child

Who Is a Neurodivergent Child?

Neurodiversity or being neurodiverse refers to all humans. We are all neurodiverse (different neurotypes) and thus neurodiversity exits. Underneath the "umbrella" of neurodiversity, there currently exits two primary categories of people – neurodivergent and neurotypical – to understand the definition of one is to understand the definition of the other. Children may be neurotypical or they may be neurodivergent, but all children are neurodiverse. Basically, even in the neurotypical category there is still neurodiversity as no two neurotypical brains are exactly alike.

Neurodivergent refers to an individual who has a less typical (societal considered "normal") cognitive variation such as autism, ADHD, dyslexia, dyspraxia, dyscalculia, sensory differences, Obsessive Compulsive Disorder (OCD), Tourette's Syndrome, etc. Although not exhaustive, Table 2.1 displays the range of who is neurodivergent. "Neurodivergence" is the term for people whose brains function differently in one or more ways than is considered standard or typical. Neurodivergence refers to any structured, consistent way that brains work differently for a group of people than they do for the majority of others.

It is estimated that over 1.2 billion people identify as neurodivergent. "Neuro" refers to neurology, or the study of nerves and the nervous system, which includes the brain. "Divergent" recognizes that these cognitive profiles diverge from what is considered to be a "typical" cognitive profile. In a binary framework, those who aren't neurodivergent are neurotypical. Neurodivergence can also be referred to as neurotypes, differences, and variances, highlighting that while some brains are unlike what is considered more the norm, all are natural.

DOI: 10.4324/9781003207610-3

Table 2.1 Who Is the Neurodivergent Child?

Examples by Diagnosis		
Autistic	Highly sensitive person (HSP)	Sensory processing disorder (differences)
Dyslexia	Dyspraxia	Dyscalculia
Tourette's syndrome	Developmental disabilities	Intellectual developmental disorder (IDD)
Obsessive compulsive disorder (OCD)	Gifted/twice exceptional	Attention deficit hyperactive disorder (ADHD)

"Neurotypical" describes individuals who display a society-defined typical intellectual and cognitive development. Human beings are social animals that band together for survival. As we have formed societies, we have also formed ways of teaching our new generations skills like reading, math, and the overt and subtle forms of interaction with one another. These individuals acquire physical, verbal, intellectual, and social processes proceeding at a specific pace and meeting standardly accepted milestones for development. Neurotypical people may also display commonly expected physical behaviors such as being able to easily modulate their volume when speaking based on the situation, and they don't find it distressing to maintain eye contact. Individuals who are described as neurotypical can generally meet the societally expected presentation of navigating social situations, producing communication, establishing social connections like friendships, and can function in distracting or stimulating settings without becoming overloaded by stimuli (Weathington, 2020). Systems and environments have operated and continue to operate with a conditioned belief and thus performance that the neurotypical "look" is the look that everyone needs to strive for and sets the standard of accomplishment. The neurodivergent child is then often seen as missing the mark and needing help to become more like the standard.

It would be impossible to write a couple of paragraphs or create a list or table that solidly identify the neurodivergent child. Likely it has become clear that being neurodivergent can and does have many looks or presentations. There may be some similarities across neurodivergence but there are many differences. Many of the neurodivergent children I have worked with present with some level of rejection, being misunderstood, feeling confused, anxious, feeling devalued, having poor self-worth, and being regularly disabled by society and systems. It an attempt to bring some perspective in working with neuro-divergent children in general, the following five dichotomous constructs are reviewed regarding the neurodivergent child experience.

Inclusion vs Seclusion – Inclusion is defined as the practice or policy of pro-viding equal access to opportunities and resources for people who might otherwise be excluded or marginalized, such as those who have physical or mental disabilities. Seclusion is defined as the state of being private and away from other people. Unfortunately, many neurodivergent children experience seclusion in many of the systems and environments they navigate. I have witnessed many examples of children begin secluded in an educational set-ting, being asked not to return to a church, being secluded to a "special" extracurricular activity set up for "special" kids. The rejection and message of "not being good enough" is an easy internalization when inclusion is not respected, and the message being delivered to the child is they do not belong with everyone else.

Acceptance vs Ableism – Am I okay being myself? Am I okay just being who I am? The message of acceptance of self and feeling accepted by others is a powerful healing and change agent. Acceptance means the child values themselves (self-acceptance) and feels accepted by others instead of feeling like they are less than and not as good as others. Ableism is the discrimina-tion of and social prejudice against people with disabilities based on the be-lief that typical abilities are superior. Ableism in application is the opposite of acceptance. Many instances of ableism are likely not intentional, but the message received by the neurodivergent child is one of not being accepted. Many neurodivergent children struggle with believing they are accepted and okay as people. Often this is due to many messages communicated to the child that the child, as they are, is not accepted and needs to change to gain acceptance. Gabor Mate, a Hungarian Canadian physician is credited with the statement "when authenticity threatens attachment… the attach-ment will trump the authenticity." A powerful and accurate statement that so many neurodivergent children understand too well. The desire for accept-ance will painfully create an internalized hate of self and empty striving to please others who are perceived to grant acceptance.

Value vs Devaluing – Value has been described as seeing, feeling, knowing, and understanding the beauty and worth of every human being and to give love with the power of our soul, subconscious, conscience, and conscious-ness. How many neurodivergent children feel valued sitting in a classroom at their school, within their family, participating in society? Many neurodi-vergent children enter play therapy in a state of not only feeling devalued but having had real experience that devalue them. The understanding and active practice of valuing often becomes a primary therapy goal in the family play therapy process in AutPlay.

Identity freedom vs Masking – Identity is defined as the fact of being who or what a person or thing is. Identity freedom is the uninhibited or unrestricted path to explore, embrace, and celebrate one's identity. Masking involves hiding aspects of yourself or pretending to be like someone else, pretending to be someone you are not. Masking in neurodivergence is not manipulative, it is implemented out of a survival response, an inability to feel that being yourself is acceptable. Masking is the antagonist to identity freedom, yet many neurodivergent adults share about their experiences with masking and the harmful effects it created on their mental health and view of self. Masking is such a common issue with neurodivergent individuals that it has become almost synonymous with being neurodivergent. Unfortunately, non-affirming systems and societies continue to send a strong message to neurodivergent children that identity freedom is not supported or encouraged.

Empowerment vs Trauma – Being empowered means to make (someone) stronger and more confident, especially in controlling their life and claiming their rights. Many neurodivergent children will surely travel one of two roads. They will embrace and feel empowered by their neurodivergence, or they will experience a shame, rejection spiral that ends in a trauma response. The therapeutic goal becomes developing and increasing empowerment and ideally avoiding a trauma response. Unfortunately, many children find their way to therapy with a trauma response already established. At this point, the therapeutic approach shifts to addressing the trauma issues while trying to empower the child. A guiding truth to remember is that a neurodivergent individual will be a neurodivergent individual the totality of their life. How they feel about and what they believe about their neurodivergence will have a massive impact on their overall mental health.

Anastasia Phelps is an 18-year-old spoken word autistic artist. Among her many activities, she dedicates herself to advocating for others through public speaking, writing, and expressive arts. In an excerpt from her writing *My Life with Autism*, she shares her perspective and experiences about being an autistic child.

> Unhealthy comparison has always been an issue of mine. The best example I can think of was when I was in the second grade. I often went out into the playground and sat with my notebook and markers; scribbling

away while the other kids played. My hand only broke its rhythm when my eyes strayed, with much longing, over to my joyfully playing peers.

Over the past 18 years, I felt like an inadequate weirdo who was always striving too far, only to never get anywhere. On top of that, my medications always seemed to complicate my emotions and play with my perception, which really didn't help me much.

Over the years, I had developed such harsh views of myself. Not only that... I have also become so attached to the thoughts and opinions of others. It is a very unhealthy addiction for me – about as harmful to my mind as excessive amounts of drugs or alcohol might be to any individual.

I do not possess telepathic abilities... I cannot tell what you see in me. I can only take a guess. So, I like it when people talk to me like I am another human being like anyone else. I like it when they give me a chance instead of writing me off as a weirdo.

Just like anyone else, I want acceptance, and I want to be listened to.

Kayla Smith describes some of her thoughts as experiences as a young autistic person in the book *Sincerely, Your Autistic Child* by Ballou, daVanport, and Onaiwu (2021).

> Once I knew about my diagnosis, I didn't mind telling people that I am autistic. But all people would do is say, "Okay," or "I don't know anything about autism at all." I started getting bullied more, quite a bit, and I kind of started to hate myself for being different. I remember asking myself "Why me?" and wishing I didn't have it. I became ashamed of myself. Then I remembered what my mom said when I was ten years old: "Don't let autism define you." So, as a teenager, I got hard on myself and tried to be perfect at everything. I developed a mentality that I could "beat" autism and that I was an autism warrior (it wasn't until later I found out that is offensive and filled with internalized ableism).
>
> I tried to fight it. I spent most of my life trying to "prove" to people that I didn't let autism "define me" and that I could do the same things as everybody else. I struggled with my identity and how I saw myself in the world. For years, I tried to be somebody that I was not, and I was not happy. I felt like I was living a lie every day of my life. Sadly, in my teenage years, I was so unhappy that I thought about committing suicide, but I never had the guts to do it, so I did not try to commit suicide even though deep inside I wanted to.
>
> Now, I regret all those years I did not accept who I am. I want to tell the younger generation, "You were born right the first time, and don't be ashamed of it."
>
> (p. 97)

Autistic author Naoki Higashida in his book *The Reason I Jump* (2013) writes about being asked if he would like to be "normal." The following response from his book highlights the stigmatization and ableist views that so often impede the autistic individual's advancement through their life journey.

Question: Would you like to be "normal?"

Response: What would we do if there was some way that we could be "normal"? Well, I bet the people around us – our parents and teachers – would be ecstatic with joy and say, "Hallelujah! We'll change them back to normal right now!" And for ages and ages I badly wanted to be normal, too. Living with special needs is so depressing and so relentless; I used to think it would be the best thing if I could just live my life like a normal person by now, even if somebody developed a medicine to cure autism, I might well choose to stay as I am. Why have I come around to thinking this way?

To give the short version, I've learned that every human being, with or without, needs to strive to do their best, and by striving for happiness you will arrive at happiness. For us, you see, having autism is normal— see we can't know for sure what your "normal" is even like. But so long as we can learn to love ourselves, I'm not sure how much it matters whether we're normal or autistic.

(p. 45)

Life as a neurodivergent person does not have a singular look, feel, or experience. Just as the spectrum manifests many different looks of autism, so life as a neurodivergent person can look many ways. Autistic author Dr. Stephen Shore has famously coined "If you have met one child with autism, then you have met one child with autism." The following is a summary of several constructs that have challenged many of the neurodivergent children I have worked with over the past two decades. These are important for therapists to consider in their work with neurodivergent children and their families.

A *systemic issue*: Ableist practices and non-affirming processes regarding neurodivergent children is a systemic issue. The myriad of ways that a neurodivergent child can be negatively affected weave throughout home life, extended family, school environment, community, extracurricular activities, policies, and laws. When working with neurodivergent children, it is critical to remember how encompassing daily life can become. Everywhere the child goes, whether it be school, interacting with their family, or participating in a community event—they are likely to encounter environments that are not supportive, not affirming, and do not understand their neurodivergence.

School challenge: From the very beginnings of daycare and preschool and throughout college completion, neurodivergent individuals face an uphill battle in most educational settings. The school setting can present some of the greatest challenges to a neurodivergent child. The social and communication demands, rigid learning expectations, processing requirements, and sensory experiences present in every school day can create great dysregulation for neurodivergent children. Many schools find themselves in inadequate positions or are unwilling to provide resources and support that neurodivergent children need to be their most successful. Therapists can be beneficial in helping to educate school personnel about neurodivergence and providing suggestions for services and resources to facilitate a more successful learning experience.

Neurodivergence in the family: A neurodivergence-related diagnosis influences the whole family. The immediate and extended family can be either a great support or create problems for the neurodivergent child. Many of my neurodivergent clients have reported some of their biggest challenges have resulted from judgmental and unaware family members. Parents can help their family by informing extended family about their neurodivergent child and highlighting strengths and affirming approaches.

Therapies and interventions: The intensity and duration of therapy and interventions that a neurodivergent person participates in will vary, but it is likely that most individuals will participate in some form of therapy or intervention sometime during their lifetime. Some individuals may enter and exit therapies and interventions as needed and some may never be involved in therapy. Therapies and interventions may cover a variety of needs depending on the individual. Unfortunately, therapies can create overload for the neurodivergent child (especially if participating in several at once). Further, some therapies have been harmful for neurodivergent children and have created a trauma response due to the focus being on changing the child to be more neurotypical. Listening to adult neurodivergent voices is critical in evaluating and navigating affirming therapy practices.

Self-acceptance: Neurodivergent individuals may be in a continuous process of understanding themselves, their diagnosis, how it impacts the world around them, and how the world around them can create support or barriers. Gaining self-awareness of these issues will be critical for the neurodivergent individual to live their most healthy and content life. Children around the late elementary and pre-teen years can begin to learn more about their diagnosis and their identity. As they grow and mature, they should master self-advocacy skills and become the best expert on themselves. Therapists can be instrumental in introducing neurodivergence to children and assisting them in the self-awareness journey.

Educating others: Neurodivergent individuals may find much of their time spent educating others about their neurodivergence. Although education and awareness initiatives continue to increase, there still exists much inaccurate information, ignorance, and stereotypes regarding neurodivergence. Unfortunately, some neurodivergent individuals have found it easier to not disclose to others they are neurodivergent because of the mislabeling and stigmatization that can occur. Inevitably, neurodivergent people will find themselves in situations where it will be necessary to educate those around them. Resources found in the appendix of this book are a good place to begin to help children learn about neurodivergence, which will increase their ability to better educate others. There are also many neurodivergent adults who are writing, teaching, presenting, and sharing information that can be helpful in educating others. Resources by actual neurodivergent adults can be found in the appendix section of this book.

Listening to Neurodivergent Voices

The Neurodivergent Child – by Jennifer Gerlach

I was a weird kid. In preschool I hid from the sounds of the washroom dryer and chose to pace while eating my lunch. My teacher flagged me as someone who could be autistic, however, the school psychologist felt my diagnosis was not autism but ADHD. My language skills were good. I grew up in the early 1990s as a hyper-verbal female. I received a prescription for ADHD medication before beginning Kindergarten.

Then, I was a weird kid on ADHD medication. I remember my grandmother pulling up the words and telling me what they meant. "Attention, because you don't pay attention well" "Definite (deficit), because we are definitely sure you have it (I later learned it stands for deficit but I guess my grandmother thought I would not have known what that meant)" "Hyperactivity, you have literally tried to climb the walls" and "Disorder" something that could be used to describe my life then and now in multiple ways. I appreciated that description, it helped me be kinder to myself. I did not like the medication though. It made me sad and muted me. It felt as though for me to be acceptable I had to be quiet and sort of drugged for everyone's benefit.

I desperately wanted to be what I considered to be a "good" kid. As I got older, I remember copying down the class rules as soon as I got them. Somehow my name seemed permanently etched on the blackboard. My most common offenses were "talking" and "not following instructions." My third-grade teacher wrote on my report card "Jennifer seems to lack common sense." I would say that is also a decent description of me today.

I had small twitches since I could remember, but in fifth grade they got worse. I also began to make sounds. One of those sounds seemed a lot like laughing and another like a bark. I tried to use humor saying things like "I'm a dog" to explain something I did not understand and scared me. It didn't work. I seemed to get into some kind of trouble most days but luckily never any big trouble. I had no friends and sensed that I did not fully fit in with my somewhat rural, conservative cultured school and town.

Playing trumpet in band proved to be an exception from my problems. For some reason when I really concentrated on playing music my twitches and sounds would quiet. One year, I found my name marked on a solo and to my surprise there was no notes written for me. I learned about improvisation. You make it up yourself – on the spot – it does not have to be the same every time. I loved that. A freedom from rules which I seemed to fail so often at following.

Around this time my mind started to get stuck – especially on themes of death and cancer. My uncle had gotten lymphoma and died. I watched my mother grieve and I felt powerless. I worried constantly about losing people and took to rituals to try to prevent these bad things from happening. Many of these rituals were religious. I believed myself to be a bad person who God would punish severely if I did not punish myself first. I did not know other people had these kinds of thoughts and kept them to themselves. I became increasingly quiet, spending my time worrying and thinking by myself.

It seemed like it was my mouth that always got me in trouble, and I worried about the many sins that involved words – bragging, gossiping, etc. In middle school, I shut down. I went from a hyper-verbal female to a kid who didn't talk much at all. The school intervened. I went through testing, meetings with psychiatrists, neurologists, social workers, and counselors. I participated in social skills groups, intensive outpatient sessions, and hospitalizations. My diagnosis changed to "Asperger's Syndrome." Then "Obsessive Compulsive Disorder," then "psychosis," "Major Depressive Disorder," "Bipolar Disorder," "Oppositional Defiant Disorder," and then "Pervasive Developmental Disorder." One practitioner told my parents I would be the youngest person they had met who almost certainly had schizophrenia, but they had never diagnosed schizophrenia under the age of 18. At some point, I also learned I have Tourette's Syndrome, which of all the labels I was given, I found most helpful. Nonetheless, I began to dislike diagnosis.

I also began to hate the assumptions that came with them. I remember once attending a psychiatrist appointment where my parent complained about my inconsiderate behaviors. A psychiatrist told her in front of me "Jennifer has Asperger's Syndrome, which means that she cannot put herself in other people's shoes or have real empathy." That hurt. I wondered if she had empathy for how hearing that felt to a 13-year-old desperately trying to "be good," who feared she was so "bad" that even God would not love her and who worried intensely about how she affected others and all the negative things others had to say about her.

Isolation followed. I became aware that I freaked people out. On school nights, my worries made my physically sick. I cried myself to sleep and cried first thing each morning. I went days without talking in fear of saying the "wrong" things. I read volumes on rules of etiquette, and wrote lists of rules for myself, trying to be "better." Eventually, I stopped going to school.

I missed 30 days of school and begged my parents to homeschool me. My family did not have the resources for that. Luckily, I had an IEP. Instead of no school, I would go to a therapeutic school. Initially, being sent to a therapeutic school felt to me like being finally exiled from the small town I grew up in (the school was 45 minutes away in another state). Accurate or not, I felt at the time (and to some extent I still do) that this was how the school district kept us 'weird' kids from contaminating what was known to be a "good" school district in a town where differences were not tolerated. Looking back, I can see that I had never really been accepted there. I missed out on dances, band concerts, knowing my neighbors – things I thought were important parts of growing up. Still, sending me to this new school made a major difference for me. It is something in which I will be forever grateful.

For once, I did not feel weird compared to everyone else. Everyone there had something going on. Rather than placing me in slower paced classes because of special education, I was upgraded from middle school to high school a year early. The project-based learning gave me space to channel my special interests. The therapists and teachers showed me extreme patience as I worked toward navigating school again. I remember on one occasion a therapist sitting with me in the lobby as I was panicking and asking repeatedly to go home. They actually gave me the choice to go home, and I found this empowering. After they walked around the halls with me and we talked, I didn't want to leave. I felt I could do things again.

Sophomore year I was given another opportunity – to be a mentor to a younger student. I learned a love for connecting and I wanted to help others to feel comfortable being themselves, the way the school had done this for me.

Receiving quality psychotherapy to assist with my obsessions/compulsions and self-worth also helped immensely – especially group therapy where my fears were met with kindness and support from other teens. Taking a philosophy class and reading on my own an ethics text that I borrowed from the library gave me a new perspective. Utilitarianism, Kantian ethics, religious perspectives of all kinds. I stopped seeing both ethics and myself in black and white. It is okay to come across as awkward sometimes AND I can live by my values. I began to consider a career in the helping professions.

Each year I would meet in an IEP meeting with my public school district, and I would advocate to return to my mainstream school. After two years in the special therapeutic school, I believed I could succeed in a mainstream class. My grades were almost all As. I had not gotten in trouble since coming to the new school and by sophomore year attendance was hardly an issue. Although I would advocate, each year I was turned down. The end of my junior year I was offered to return to the mainstream public school my senior year in what would be an entirely self-contained classroom. I advocated as best I could for myself that I felt I would do well in all mainstream classes – expressing a goal to go to college and graduate school and not feeling that this would give me a chance to get the classes I would need to do that.

My voice was overshadowed by that of a school psychologist who I only met in these IEP meetings. He met my IEP before he met me. "Autism." "Serious Emotional Disturbance." Those words were on the first page of my IEP. He shared a story about having another "special needs" student in calculus and it being a nightmare. He did not think I would be able to do mainstream classes. I wondered if he knew that I was not that student, or that he did not know me at all. I did not have time to prove myself to him and began to accept this was not going to be possible. I graduated from the therapeutic school.

I began the next year in a mainstream university! A few years later, I found myself in graduate school and a few years after that opened my own practice as a psychotherapist. I still carry a list of diagnoses although I do not like to think of myself in those categories. I prefer the term "neurodivergent." I consider myself a neurodivergent person in mental health recovery.

My office has a swing for clients who prefer to move while we talk, we discuss social connection rather than social skills, and I work from a neurodiversity affirming perspective. I consider my clients the experts on their own situations and have yet to meet one who I would say lacked empathy or could not put self in another's shoes. Often, I find it is the adults around the youth I work with who struggle most with relating to the child's perspective. This makes sense because when two people are running on a different neurological setup, those two people will see things differently. A neurodivergent person is at an advantage in ways in that they are likely to have more experience syncing their own experience to understand another's. This is a concept I now know as the "double empathy paradox."

I have found curiosity to be key in relating to people in general and especially other neurodivergent people. I see diagnosis as an imperfect tool and stay away from diagnosis-based assumptions. I have come to see traditional social skills training as a sort of "neurotypical communication 101" rather than skills that neurodivergent people lack and need. I am looking forward to the day when neurotypical students are offered "neurodivergent communication 101" in the form of instruction on inclusion, acceptance, and celebration of differences. The people I wish most to take such a course are the adults who interface with neurodivergent youth.

Improvisation also remains a key piece of my practice. In communication, rarely is there a 'right' or 'wrong' – it's about context, openness, and willingness to adapt. This is something I integrate into my personal life each day and which I also seek to share with anyone willing to learn. I also integrate into my work evidence-based practices – most often Acceptance Commitment Therapy and Radically-Open DBT. I have found both of these approaches to help provide the neurodiversity affirming process I am striving to implement.

The Neurodivergent Child – by Boontarika Sripom

I recently participated on a panel at San Diego Comic-Con Special Edition with some colleagues in education and mental health. It's been a dream to speak, share, and build community with fellow geeks and divergent thinkers, and I finally did it! I spoke on representation in pop culture, archetypes, and heroism through the lens of comic books. I felt like I was speaking for my younger self; the little girl who sat alone between the buildings in elementary school, afraid of something, many things, other people. I spoke for the "lonely" girl who walked around on the blacktop by herself. I spoke for the girl who didn't speak English and desperately wanted to understand a confusing world.

Before the panel, I called my mom to wish her happy birthday, and to share my joy of having this dream come true. She cried on the phone, and I clearly remember her words. "I thought you were going to be a doctor. You were so good at biology. If your grandpa was still alive, he would at least be proud of your cousins in medicine." I listened to the worry through her words. Although I understood from an immigrant parent's perspective the worry for the financial success of a child, I also felt the pain, disappointment, and lack of support from her words.

My mother's comments took me back to a time when I was a "promising" child. Learning was my play. Books were my toys. Puzzles and word problems were my friends. I had potential that manifested into perpetual disappointment to my elders. I was born premature with my twin brother. At 28 weeks, we were small enough to fit in the palms of someone's hands. I was in NICU for six weeks and my parents visited me every day. In preschool my brother and I were separated because we spoke to each other in Thai. The school wanted us to learn English, so we were not allowed to play together. My mom once told me that I have "always been independent" and played alone.

Whenever we went to school, I did not engage with peers or adults. I went straight to building toys called Octons to visually stim with. The colors and translucent plastic calmed me while giving me something to build. Thinking about the colors of the toys now fills me with warmth, a feeling like I had a companion during times of isolation. I was seen as a sick and weak child. The doctors emphasized the hardships premature babies and children faced, so my parents were bound by fear and duty to help their sick child.

Hoping I would gain weight, my family forced me to sit at the dining table for countless hours from the ages of 3 to 6. I watched my siblings play as I sat. I used to hide food in the sofa cushions, throw food under the table, and hide in the bathroom until everyone went to bed. I spent so many hours in the bathroom just being alone. In kindergarten and first grade, my parents threatened me with the police or coming to my school to make sure I ate. They told me I was always being watched. As an adult, my aunts and parents still ask me, "Why did you do that? Why didn't you eat?" My 6-year-old self remembers thinking, "I'm not hungry. Why are they doing this to me?"

I experienced three near drownings as a child (likely due to my lungs being weaker as a preemie) and remember thinking, "No one will protect me. I'm alone." The themes of not being seen, heard, or having bodily autonomy would permeate my childhood and into my adulthood and interpersonal re-lationships. In second grade I hid between the buildings during recess and lunch. My twin brother visited me and asked why I was there, and I didn't have an answer. I couldn't speak or understand English very well and I felt afraid. It felt safer to be in small spaces. Occasionally, some kind children would pull me out from between the buildings to walk around the playground. Despite the kindness of others, I still isolated myself and was often alone.

I tried once to make a friend by kicking a boy at the lunch tables. He picked me up, slammed me against the table, then walked away. I stopped trying to make friends or initiate conversations at school for several years after that. I preferred playing in the dirt and looking at flowers alone.

My fifth-grade report card had a comment from Mrs. Short, "Boontarika is a kind and lonely girl." I keep this report card nearby as a reminder of where I have come from and all the personal work I've done. I was kind to others because I remember what it felt like to receive kindness and the unkindness of others. My siblings had playdates and visited friends' homes, but it was not something I wanted or thought about. I rarely had birthday parties. The only times I wanted one was at 6 and 17 years old. I was an observer and followed along my siblings' outings. When my parents asked about friends, I did not answer successfully. I wanted to talk about the ocean's depth and the sky's vastness, vocabulary words I learned, plants, and my confusion with why people hurt one another. Why did we have world hunger? Where did these rocks come from? These conversations were often met with silence or ridicule by siblings, so I talked to myself, my stuffed animals, and my sketchbook.

I enjoyed puzzles and learning trivia. I wrote math problems in the air and erased them when written incorrectly. Whenever possible, I stayed home and watched Batman movies on repeat. *Batman* and *Batman Returns* were my escape and comfort. I wished so badly to be a hero and fight for others. I wished for miracles that life could be different, even though I wasn't sure what it could be. When alone, I ritually organized items in groupings of ten. I'd take books or clothes out of shelves and reorganize them again and again. I also seemed to be blunt with how disorganized or dirty someone's home was. My dad laughed when sharing how I'd tell people, "Your house is so dirty," as a 4-year-old. I even started organizing or cleaning other people's things if it bothered me enough. It was quirky and endearing to do this as a child.

Another quirky and endearing trait to have as a child is to be clumsy. I tripped often, dropped electronics down the stairs, and many times fell down while standing still. I broke my nose, sprained knees and ankles from tripping over things that I knew were there. A few noteworthy times include being in high school at a family friend's home, I missed six steps and fell on my knee. I slipped down a mountain because I walked wrong (my dad thought I broke my neck that time). As I walked my bike up a hill, I paused to rest and very slowly fell onto a cactus. My sister loves reenacting that scene for people who need illustrations of how clumsy I am. I had and have bruises on my body from hitting the corners of the wall, and hitting my head with cabinet doors.

When it came to peer relationships and maintaining friendships, I had a few dear friends who taught me crucial life skills like conflict resolution and identifying unhealthy behaviors. While this was a gift, I had a skewed perspective of what I offered as a friend. I did not have enough guidance or experience with different types of friendships as a teen. I thought I provided value if I could help people answer their homework questions. I stayed up late waiting for the phone to ring so I could teach people how to solve biology questions the night before assignments were due. I stayed up until 1 or 2 am doing this. I thought it was a way to socialize with others. Looking back, I realize how one-sided and sad it looked from the outside. After observing cliques and peer behaviors, I thought I wanted to belong. The only way I thought I could contribute was to offer knowledge. Since information was always a friend to me, I thought it was something others would also see as a form of friendship.

While my social/emotional needs were not met, my family greatly provided for physical and financial needs, and I am grateful. It is an honor to be my parents' child. There have been times when I asked myself should I carry the emotional pain of unnurtured social/emotional needs in silence to honor my family, or speak up and dishonor them? I chose to carry my pain alone. I accepted isolation for not eating. I accepted isolation and being silenced for speaking my native tongue. I accepted being alone and not trusting others after many near drownings. I accepted a message that this world is an unsafe place after falling often. Many messages compounded to create an even more isolated young person who grew up to be an adult who continues to isolate.

Does the experience of constantly being "othered" and seen as the perpetual foreigner add another layer of never truly belonging, never deserving to be seen? I think about being a "Model Minority" student who excelled academically, yet one teacher saw a lonely girl who walked by herself on the blacktop. I think about how grades do not always reflect the whole child, yet many institutions go for numbers and "hard data" to confirm the curriculum works. I was a meek Asian girl who earned good grades. That fits the stereotype, so there was no need to explore. I think I was overlooked because I could function in a way that pleased those who wanted to see certain results, because this archaic education system still aims to create cogs in a machine. If I didn't challenge the system, it was equated to the system having no flaws. It means something on a personal level when you fail the children you're supposed to protect, teach, and uplift, and sometimes we don't see what's right before us.

Having the gift of time and applied knowledge now offers me the opportunity to share in a way that does not retraumatize, rather, validates and empowers. There can be healing from intergenerational systemic challenges. Part of intergenerational healing can come from cultivated perspective and compassion. My parents have never said they loved me. It's a very Westernized way of communicating. In Collectivist families, we ask, "Have you eaten?" We offer a warm meal, seconds, and cut of fruit for you. I know that my parents loved me. They tried very hard in the ways they understood to show love to a child they did not fully understand; a sick child who was not growing.

A main theme I see in many of my childhood snippets is isolation. I want to note that although I was alone often, I do not remember feeling lonely. I think people on the outside may feel pity or discomfort when they hear a child did not have strong bonds or friendships with peers. I had Batman with me the entire time and I had words and definitions to comfort me and felt very connected to the world around me through ideas. I was never truly alone. There are skills that I needed to develop like understanding healthy relationship dynamics and strengthening my proprioception. I am curious how I would have answered the questions, "Do you want friends? What do you think friends do for one another?" I believe my younger self would have loved meeting other children who read comic books (especially Batman) and played video games. My younger self would also have appreciated having an Occupational Therapist and/or other professionals to speak with. Someone who validated the messages or skills knowledge that honored a different definition of interpersonal connection, validated different journeys, and helped to connect with likeminded people. Just as we seek heroism and possibility through the myths we resonate with, we can very much instill ourselves with hope and mirroring of humanity when we see the struggles and triumphs of those who live similar life paths. It is like a kindred walking alongside you, and sometimes it takes a series of others stories to hit home.

I want to emphasize the shame that manifests when writing about my childhood experiences. As a child, I often did not question things as they happened. There was a perceived strength in not questioning things, and to stand out was to cause conflict. When I try to share my story with others, these early struggle experiences are often dismissed because I can present myself as very gregarious and social. I learned to mask in high school. I still mask and I do it very well. I also sometimes receive the backhanded compliment of, "You have empathy, so you're not Autistic."

I have not always felt I had permission to belong to the neurodivergent community because I have rarely experienced myself spoken to in this way. So, this is a bridge that will hopefully connect others to realms of healing and having truths witnessed. It's a rippling effect that can create community and waves of change. The following are affirming messages that I hope bring empowerment and comfort to others.

– You are welcome here. Come at your own pace, on your own time.
– The world can be a safe place, and we can learn to find and create these places together.
– The way you choose to spend time is valid. Parallel play can be a way to spend quality time with someone.
– Your body is yours. You have the power to speak for what it needs and wants.
– Books, words, and your geekdoms can be your best friends. Even if other people do not understand fully – you do not have to change to please them, they can try to explore your world with you.
– There is no need to provide answers or things for others to accept you. You are worthy as you are.
– Coming from an immigrant family means you have a foundation of perseverance and accomplished dreams. You are part of a legacy and can now redefine what it means to live a good life. You get to define it how you want, and it's okay for this to change over time.

The Neurodivergent Child – by Spencer Beard

There was a time in my life where I would never shut up. I was a kid, and I used to talk all the time to people I knew well. I loved talking about my thoughts and the things that really kept my interest. I thought a lot about people and animals and whatever came across my mind in the moment. Reflecting back, there were two reasons why I enjoyed talking so much. One is that I felt like I had to advocate for myself since I felt so different from everyone else. Ever since I can remember having legible thoughts and could study other people, I noted that I was different in various ways. What those ways were, I couldn't exactly tell. They were obvious in the sense that everyone, aside from me, seemed comfortable about each other and themselves. Everyone, even in the middle of arguments, in the middle of fights, in the middle of emotional outbursts, seemed to understand each other beyond a conscious level, but I could not. I could understand that they talk to each other using sounds and words, but it was like their movement of their bodies, their face could reveal something about themselves to others. I didn't understand what body language was, and I had a hard time understanding faces.

It was much later in life that I realized that the second reason I enjoyed talking so much was because, at the time, I didn't know that I was an autistic child. The issue wasn't being autistic but that I had to advocate for myself with those needs in mind, and I didn't know that when I was diagnosed. To advocate for themselves, autistic people need to embrace their autism as a unique part of themselves, and they shouldn't believe themselves to be a biological mistake, which is something that I did not fully understand as a child.

When I was 13 years old, I was diagnosed with Asperger's Syndrome. It was all a very bizarre ordeal as I remember that I was taken out of town to see a doctor. I wasn't told what it was for; all I was told was that I needed to get checked for "something important." At the time, I wondered if I was going to receive the news that I was going to die; I had ten months to live. Instead, I was told in medical terms that I was never actually normal. However, it's not the diagnosis itself that really changed me. As I said, I always knew that there was something off with everyone and that I was left out for some reason. What really changed me was what I was told to do with this information. Simply put, I was told to never mention it. I was told that I should never mention the trip and especially never mention the diagnosis. I was told by my parents that if I did talk to anyone about it, I would never be able to hold down a job or a place of my own, and it would be doubtful that I could start a family of my own.

Usually, when a movie or a show has a character discover something about themselves, even when it's something of a secret, they feel enlightened or empowered to do whatever they would like. That was absolutely not the case for me. Over time, I was increasingly confused and horrified. For all I understood, all the stuff that I felt that was off with the world wasn't because there was something wrong with the world. It was wrong with me, and I was inherently wrong. I always wanted to be "normal." I wanted to be like everyone else and I didn't want to think that I was wrong. But, according to the professional who diagnosed me, that wasn't the case. I am medically and essentially abnormal, a twisted caricature of the everyday human being.

I truly hated myself, and I hated myself more and more. For every fault that I saw, the more I blamed my Asperger's. Since the Asperger's was a part of me that I couldn't get rid of, I saw myself in all of my failures. Without going into too much detail about my social failures, I had very few friends and even fewer people I could confide my most inner thoughts to. Even the good moments I had were infested with doubts. Was the guy laughing with me or actually laughing at me? Was the lady that I was trying to hit on talking to me out of some pity or courtesy? Did everyone know me just as "that weird guy who makes weird faces and movements?" I was haunted by the very real fears that may have not existed in the first place because I knew that I was always terrible at hiding my autism and hiding is what I wanted.

As I was never talking about my autism to people, I never had conversations on how to talk to people as an autistic person, and I never was told what to expect from neurotypical people as an autistic person. It wasn't until late in my life that my family would even acknowledge my autism beyond the initial diagnosis. I wasn't told about how my condition would affect me with my romantic relationships. I don't know if it was because my parents assumed I would get it on my own or if it was because I was, in some way, a lost cause. I never thought they didn't love me, but I always wondered if they ever wished they had a more "normal" first born son.

The doubts about the positives in my life extended beyond awkward interactions at school but I was somewhat comforted by being surrounded by a familiar social environment and, despite all the issues I mentioned, a rather loving home. Then, I graduated from high school and went to a college in a different town. Not only was I starting anew, but I also had to start creating a future for myself. One of the vital things I learned about college over the years was the importance of the social connections a person makes in college. Out of everything in my life, it was the opportunity that I wasted the most. I was afraid of the world around me, and I was too afraid to approach anyone. Every opportunity to socialize with peers was deliberately avoided. I was afraid to open myself to conversation as I was embarrassed that I had barely any social life in high school. I much preferred the predictability of video games and online discussions where I never had to be honest about myself and never exposed myself to anything truly new. Of course, as time went on, I became even more afraid to talk to people as I was embarrassed over my lack of a college social life.

It was in my junior year of college that I truly considered suicide. It had somewhat surfaced in the past, but it was at this point in college that I realized that I was about three days away from finishing myself off. I called my parents and told them that I was going to hurt myself, and I needed counseling. As I called them and talked to their voicemail, I was distressed and horrified. However, what I didn't expect was that it was also relieving to finally get my thoughts out in the open, to be authentic and not bottling them up anymore. It was relieving, it was the first time in forever that I felt like I could just drift off to sleep. Usually I would need sleeping medication, but this time, I found myself growing more and more tired, and I went to bed expecting to contemplate all of my thoughts more in the morning. However, I was awakened by my resident hall assistant who informed me that my parents were trying to contact me. They were worried sick after hearing that message with such a dark tone that they were ready to drive up to my college to see if I was okay despite it being late at night.

In a way, this proved my fear about socializing. I literally called my parents asking for psychiatry help or I might hurt myself (anyone would be worried about a message like that), and as I talked to them about my issues, all I could think about was that even my attempts at help were confronted with social failure. Nevertheless, my dad asked me if I wanted a counselor who focuses on autistic people, and I told him that would be for the best. It's strange thinking about that question now. I didn't realize it at the time, but that was the first time in almost a decade that either of my parents acknowledged me as an autistic person. This would become the turning point for me and the beginning of the true journey of healthy exploration of being autistic.

Obviously, I never did kill myself. There are many people that I thank for moving me off that course. I thank my parents for listening. I thank my counselor for helping me with my needs. But ultimately, if I have to thank someone more than anyone else and place the full responsibility on for changing the course of my life – I would have to thank myself. If I hadn't opened myself up for the possibility of help, I do believe I would be dead now. Something that I wish I had known and believed in my youth was that for autistic people to advocate for themselves, they shouldn't see themselves as biological mistakes, and they need to embrace their autism as a unique part of themselves. It's ironic in a way. When I was younger, I could never shut up. It was because I was told my autism was bad that I shut myself down. I was told that I should never talk about me being an autistic person – this was the great fallacy. Now I fully understand that the only way that I got the help I did, obtained the growth I needed, and found the happiness I have now was because I advocated for my needs as an autistic person.

The Neurodivergent Child – by Rebekah Brown

Even from the time that I was little, I knew there was something different about me. I gave it many names as I grew up: bad, shy, nervous. Nothing ever explained all the quirks until I was diagnosed with autism spectrum disorder (Asperger's at that time) at the age of 15. I am currently 33 years old, and I live in a small town in the western tip of North Carolina. I am relatively independent but do still need support in some areas. I do live with my mom. I own a car and have a part time job in the box office of a performing arts center (live theater and concerts, not a movie cinema), and I have an extensive garage workshop where I make and sell art pieces made out of eggshell, wood, stone, and metal. In public, I am often able to mask the fact that I am autistic.

As an infant, my mom worried that I rarely made eye contact, even when nursing. I had a harder time with noises and smells than my siblings. As a young child the effectiveness of disciplinary methods correlated to my divergence; the confinement of "time-out" was significantly more painful than a spanking due to my disregard for pain. I was initially diagnosed at the age of 7 with ADHD and sensory integration problems by a developmental pediatrician. However, these diagnoses did not explain several of my other traits, including my knack for taking things literally.

My mom tells a story about when I was around 6 years old when my older sister had a high fever, and she made the comment, "Her forehead is so hot you could cook an egg on it." Hearing this, I immediately started walking to the kitchen to get an egg to attempt said cooking. As a 7 or 8 year old, I was at a store with my dad one time and picked out a Sprite bottle (back when they had rewards under the cap). As we checked out, I took the cap off, and read "Please try again." I immediately walked back to the soda case to get another bottle to "try again," before my dad, chuckling to himself, told me you had to wait to "try again" until you wanted to buy another bottle.

ADHD also did not explain my aversion to change and need for a rigid routine. My mom said when I was little, I often viewed the world with dispassionate clinical interest like a little scientist. When I was in elementary school, we had a lady visit us from India for a few days. I grew up in a very small town in Western NC and the diversity at that time was minimal. As I watched the visitor getting out of the car and greeting people, I saw that she had clothing I'd never seen before, a red dot on her forehead, and was a skin color I had never seen up close. In my mind the routine was broken, and I turned around and went inside and proceeded to hide behind a small trampoline behind the couch. Soon the adults realized I was gone, and everyone started looking for me. Even knowing people were looking for me I stayed hidden. This new person was different from what I'd ever seen, the clothes were strange, and in a risk versus reward analysis it was not worth it to expose myself.

As I reached my middle and high school years, I had an increasingly difficult time with social interactions and a positive self-perception. I remember in high school sitting holding the phone, crying and terrified, because I wanted to call a friend to have lunch but didn't know how to say the right things.

When I wrote in journals I often wrote about stressful experiences (getting in trouble, discipline, consequences) and often included the phrase "I am bad, I must be just bad."

I constantly misunderstood social interactions, and as a result, they became confirmation of how I thought about myself. I didn't know how to control my temper, and meltdowns included several hours afterwards of crying. I felt shame, guilt, and despair for my lack of ability to control myself. I sometimes felt that I must be stupid as well, and even the environment of homeschooling was at times difficult due to sensory overload. Once in a Sunday school class, I kept asking the teacher to repeat herself because I was having a hard time distinguishing her words due to ambient noises in the room. After the third time, she looked at me and said in front of everyone, "Rebekah, how can you look so smart and act so dumb." Immediately I felt ashamed and "dumb" and decided then that I would never ask for clarification again if it gave the appearance of being dumb. I believe this event eventually led to me having a hard time in college classes with asking for clarification or help on a subject, for fear of appearing dumb. As an adult, I now realize that I was having a hard time distinguishing that Sunday School teacher's words because I wasn't just hearing her voice. I was hearing my dress rustle, the lights buzzing, the little wood chairs creaking, my classmates giggling or whispering, people walking by outside the closed door, the sound of shoes scuffing under the table, and the list goes on. I never went back to that Sunday school class.

Social interaction and internal monolog did not begin to improve until I was formally diagnosed with Asperger's. Initially, there was a sense of sadness, and I didn't want my siblings to know about the diagnosis. However, there was also a sense of relief. I was not "bad," and there was a real reason that I had such a difficult time with social situations and emotional regulation. My mom quickly found resources and we started to work on my areas of difficulty. My ability to make and have friends improved, as well as my understanding of sensory overload and how to dissipate overstimulation.

I did have a fantastic support growing up with my mom. After my diagnosis at 15, my mom immediately found resources for addressing my needs. We would sit and literally practice all the parts of a conversation, the "rules" for different scenarios. She taught me how to be more comfortable with initial greetings and meeting people. She also explicitly taught me that when first talking to someone you have met you can ask them about their work, hobbies, and family, and that once you bring one of these topics up, the other person will likely start talking while you can think of other relevant things to say. I needed training on how my peers interacted with each other naturally and with ease. When do you say "Hello, how are you" versus "Hey girl, whatcha up to?" How long does a conversation have to run for small talk? How do you lead up to saying goodbye? Do you constantly face the person, half the time, a quarter? These were things that helped decrease my anxieties and gave me some sense of social pleasure.

Being neurodivergent has had its ups and downs. Some of the hard things for me were relating to peers, need for "recharge" time (which my counterparts didn't seem to find necessary), overwhelmed senses, and a general feeling of being "different." However, since the diagnosis, I have been able to change the way I think about and value myself. I wish I could have understood my neurodivergence earlier. However, I am content with having found out at 15, and I know of several friends that didn't find out until well into adult years. Having been able to participate in neurodiversity affirming therapies would have been great as well. Things like how to deal with overstimulation of my sensory system, how to head off a dysregulation meltdown, social navigation, anger management, instilling a positive view of my personhood, and how my brain worked (as opposed to the many times I thought that I was simply "bad" or "dumb").

In many ways, my neurodivergence has felt like a superpower instead of a disorder. I feel a great deal of contentment in my adult life. I am happily working at my part time job at a theater, where neurodiversity is quite common, and celebrated. I have a service dog, Faramond, who is specifically trained to help me with anxiety attacks and meltdowns. I have an awesome workshop that I have worked to add tools to for many years, and making things seems to scratch an itch in my brain that nothing else has. I play several local sports, including street hockey (goalie) as well as slow-pitch softball (I played fast-pitch in college for two years). I enjoy participating in local theater productions, and I believe that starting theater in my 20s was a crucial part of me learning to be truly comfortable in public settings. I understand figures of speech and metaphors far better and am quick to make pun jokes with my friends. Making people laugh is something near and dear to my heart (look at that figure of speech I used correctly). I am still learning and processing, but I am feeling quite comfortable in my neurodivergent self.

The Neurodivergent Child – by Sarah Moran

I was diagnosed with ADHD, combined type, when I was 22. I often reflect on my experiences as an undiagnosed neurodivergent child with the knowledge I have now and identify with many of the struggles my clients (particularly middle-school girls with ADHD) present with. I was an emotional child. I remember getting "worked up" about small things and it took a long time to calm down. I found pleasure in being outdoors, making art, and experimenting with cooking and baking. I needed to be hands-on, with sensory input, to really dive deep into something that was fulfilling. Cooking forced me to live in the moment and be present with myself, which is why I think I was so good at this skill from a young age. In hindsight, I was failing academically and at the same time I was mastering lemon bars and creme brulee – it turns out the world doesn't value the later successes when you're a fourth grader.

I have memories of spending hours in the Museum of Natural History, with my face pressed up against one window, absorbing all the details in hyperfocus. I would make sure the people around me were also seeing all the small things I saw, and I remember my mom moving on to the next thing, with me pulling her back, "Look at this! Did you see that!" Now I can hyperfixate on a 1, 000 piece puzzle and lose track of time and space, often completing it in one to two sittings.

I skipped preschool and went right into kindergarten when I was 4 years old. I am told this was because I could already read independently. I didn't really mind being the youngest in my class in those early years, or more likely I didn't notice. A norm for my family was to be enrolled in small private schools throughout childhood. While I see this as a benefit in a lot of ways, school is still the place where my undiagnosed ADHD received the most negative feedback. I have distinct memories of 3rd and 4th grade where my age difference started to have a social impact. I know I was gullible, and I know now it's because I couldn't read social cues like sarcasm. I remember trusting peers with secrets, only to have them shared with the class time and time again. I didn't understand what was happening, and I didn't see this repetition as a pattern or part of a bigger social construct. I also lied often.

I started to really struggle academically in 3rd grade, but my teacher was patient and kind with me. Then came 4th grade. I had an older teacher who wasn't patient and really wasn't kind. I don't have many memories of her or the class that year. I repeated the 4th grade. I remember my parents providing me with the choice to do so at my same school and watch my friends move up, or to switch schools. I chose to change schools, and I appreciated being offered that choice. From all accounts, it sounds like when my family went to tour my new school, all were pleased by the emphasis on art and music, the less rigid class structure, the ability to have snacks while in class, and everyone sitting at group tables or on the floor, rather than at individual desks. Everyone agreed "This is the place for Sarah" and 4th grade round two was much better. I felt supported by my teacher and enjoyed being with peers who were now closer to my age and started to do better socially. I remember reading more for enjoyment around that time and hating math a little bit less. I stayed at that new school from 4th grade through 12th, so those peers became my family.

By 5th grade I wasn't turning in my homework because I wasn't doing my homework, at least not to completion. One assignment that I hated in 5th grade was memorizing poems. You could pick any poem of a certain number of lines, and if you memorized a poem that was twice the required length, that got you off the hook for a week. I tried that once, but I ended up missing a few lines, and I felt humiliated. I learned that if I did it wrong, I would be publicly shamed, and if I didn't do it then the worst thing that would happen was that I had to go sit in front of the principal. So, I stopped memorizing poems, and I stopped doing homework. I would walk into my 5th grade classroom every day and be asked "Did you do your homework?" And I would say "Nope" and spin on my heel to walk myself to the principal's office.

The first time I attended a school meeting with my parents was in 5th grade. My teacher called me "passive aggressive," and the school psychologist addressed the homework issue as being "disobedient and disrespectful to the school." If labels were given out at the time, I am certain I wouldn't have been recognized as unorganized and scattered ADHD, I would have been seen as an oppositional and defiant child. My mother remembers thinking around that time, "I don't understand how she is wired."

There was a study skills class along the way, where we talked about organizing our binders and sucking on a mint to help us study. I remember thinking, yes, I can do this! And getting excited about organizing, but the follow through was lacking when I was left to my own devices. This has stayed common over time. I have multiple journals and planners, that all started with good intention… and then one or two days off routine leads to an end in utilizing that tool. I started doing my homework at the kitchen table while my siblings watched TV and I played music in the background. If not in this process, I would become easily distracted by things happening around me (namely, whatever my three younger siblings, dog, or cat was up to). The combination of sounds confused and annoyed my parents, but I think they saw it worked best to get me to focus on the task at hand, so they allowed it.

One paradox of having ADHD is being distracted by noise but also needing noise to focus. As an adult (as I write this paper) I need soft, yet familiar lyrics blaring in my ears via headphones. This is the only way I can block out everything around me and give myself the best chance of focusing on the correct task. It is easy for me to jump from task to task, and then become frustrated by my lack of progress on the initial assignment. Hence, why my emails are often answered, my schedule is organized, and my paperwork piles up into an overwhelming mountain.

I remember middle-school history class, where we had an open book test and I failed it. My history teacher yelled at me, making me feel awful for failing because I could look at my book. All I thought about during that test was that I couldn't remember exactly where I had read the fact I was looking for, so I frantically flipped back and forth between pages and ran out of time before my essay was complete. I remember feeling like something was wrong with me. My first encounter with therapy was in 8th grade, which was prompted by my parents' divorce. Like so many children, my ADHD was hidden under a layer of trauma. My actions were explained as a result of my unsteady home life, rather than because of my own brain's doing. This reframe didn't stop me from feeling like everyone around me was swimming with life vests on and I was trying not to drown with a rock tied to my ankle.

The second time I attended a school meeting with my parents was at the end of 8th grade. The dean of academics told us my private school contract was being threatened due to my grades. He told me that I wasn't going to pass physics, which was a 9th grade requirement. I cried in that meeting and was told I was being "dramatic." Turns out 9th grade physics wasn't so bad. I had a wonderful teacher. After a failed test, he asked me to meet with him. I remember anxiously biting all my nails in anticipation. I remember this interaction like it was yesterday. This little old man, my physics teacher, put his hand on my shoulder and said, "Sarah, do you want to be a physicist?" No. "Sarah, do you want to be a scientist?" No. "Ok then. We don't have to master physics. We just have to pass this class." That was the first time since 4th grade (part two) that I felt a teacher really saw me. He really understood that I was trying my hardest and I was on the brink of failing because the topic didn't interest me. I was seen, and then I excelled. I not only passed physics, but I aced it. I qualified for honors biology. I had never once qualified for an honors level course; I was so excited. I got to be in class with my friends, who were almost exclusively good students.

It should be noted that my high school was a college preparatory school, meaning it is more challenging than a typical high school curriculum. I was surrounded by intelligent and driven peers, who had aspirations to become doctors, dentists, surgeons, lawyers, and the like. I did not know this at the time, I was just going through the motions and moving up in grade levels with all my friends. I had a wonderful group of smart and driven friends in high school. They were academically competitive and didn't study, and I was academically challenged and didn't study. We were acting in the same way, but with different outcomes. I remember studying hard for a test, and everyone around me saying they didn't study at all and feeling that internal blame and shame. But I had mastered the art of masking by then, a term I only learned after my diagnosis. I was socially savvy enough to fit in, even if my grades were collectively unacceptable to all of my peers.

I participated in several extracurricular activities throughout high school, including drama, volleyball, and photography. I poured myself into volleyball. I played competitively three out of four seasons in the year. I sought novelty and I wanted to improve this skill, because at my school, you were either academically gifted and/or athletically gifted. I was not either, but I knew I wasn't the former, so I tried to be the latter. When you're tall and clumsy, and easily distracted, and bad at school, you do what you can to fly under the radar. I felt that if I could just be good at one thing, that would take the pressure off my back. I jumped through the hoops of requirements to play a musical instrument, jumping from one thing to the next without demonstrating any passion for instrument playing. I kept taking drama classes and never landed big speaking parts. I didn't have the self confidence in my body or my brain.

All three of my siblings are musical and artistic. I could feel that they had found their interests and completely submerged into them, while I was always trying something new and trying my best to blend in and present as average. My mom worried that if I did not find my interest, as my siblings did, I would become aimless and lean into drugs and alcohol. Which is a valid fear, as statistics show that undiagnosed ADHD girls are at a higher risk for partaking in high-risk activities. I was primarily shielded from this by being at a highly competitive school. I dated the class valedictorian, and he wasn't drinking, so neither was I. I was surrounded by squares, and I was socially masking as one.

There were some highs but a lot of lows. It was 10th grade history and we were allowed to bring a notecard to our exam. While other people wrote bullet points and dates to spark their memory, I spent hours the night before flipping through my textbook and writing a tiny essay on an index card so that I could copy it word for word in my exam. Passed it. It was 10th grade in honors biology class and we were doing the experiment with an egg in vinegar. I remember looking at it with fascination as it became rubbery in its beaker on the front counter. I remember wanting to touch it, and then picking up the first item in my view, which happened to be a pencil – I popped it. It happened so fast. I was yelled at for acting on my impulse. I felt humiliated. Turns out I wasn't cut out for honors biology at a college preparatory school. I went in on a high and came crashing down. I can see now, where my self-esteem was taking a hit. I didn't qualify for honors chemistry; I think I barely passed through to land in regular chemistry. The dean of academics, the one who had told me that I wouldn't pass physics, said to me in passing at the start of 11th grade, "It looks like you're back where you belong."

By the start of 11th grade my eyes were on the prize of graduating from high school. I did everything I could to jump through the hoops in front of me. I started cheating in most of my classes. Granted, I was cheating for Cs, not for As. All I had to do was pass my classes. I was in survival mode. By 12th grade, I had signed up for the bare minimum requirements and all electives. What a classic ADHD move.

Shortly after I learned how to drive, I started noticing that I was forgetful, disorganized, and getting lost easily (a prime example of executive functioning skills). I blamed this on a poor sense of direction at first, but the more it happened, the more shame I felt because I thought I was just bad at driving. There was that time I was driving my Volvo back from youth group with my high school boyfriend in the car, and I turned around because I was sure I missed my intersection. My boyfriend kept telling me I hadn't, and I drove an extra 15 minutes just to discover I was backtracking and I had gone the right way the first time. There was a time that I took the wrong exit ramp on the way home from my grandma's house, with my brother in the car. We were on the northbound highway, instead of south. We didn't notice my error until we came across a sign for a town we recognized. We searched and searched my car but could not find my cell phone (because I had forgotten it at my grandma's). We found just enough change in the car to use a payphone to frantically call our mom to express our distress and write down detailed instructions to come home.

I remember taking the train with a friend, who pointed out that I was very anxious about missing my stop. She was concerned about my observable level of panic, standing up two stops ahead. In hindsight I can see that I was just desperately avoiding messing up a step in my plan because it would be a whole planning organizing time consuming mess to reroute myself. Instead, I was hyper-prepared to get off at the right stop. I wish I could have had a name for that then, the executive functioning challenges. Executive functioning challenges really troubled me when I was a new driver. High school driving for me came in the era of Mapquest, and I remember needing to print off the instructions in both directions of my destination – one for the way to the aquarium, and one for the way home. I could not organize my thoughts to read the instructions backwards to make the same paperwork twice. While driving home from familiar places, I often needed play by play instructions from my mom on the phone. My mother reports that when she explained this to her therapist at the time, that therapist stated, "It sounds like she has ADHD."

That was not the first time ADHD came up as a possibility, but no action was taken. My mom has reported suspicions that something was off over time. The primary reason there was no action toward diagnosis was due to lack of support. No support from my father, who told my mom she was making excuses for my behavior. No support from my grandparents, who were worried about me being labeled. The pressure to attend college right after high school was high in my world. I went to culinary school, because I couldn't fathom the idea of putting myself through more academics. College was the mento in my already shaken up bottle of soda; I burst. I left home heartbroken and reluctant to attend college. I fell into the trap of being an undiagnosed ADHD brain, removed from my routine and structure, and left to my own devices with no coping skills to manage. I acted on every impulse and harmed myself and my relationships by my actions. I was forgetful, I blamed my roommates for stealing things I had lost or misplaced. I drank too much, and I got caught stealing. Ultimately, I dropped out, and impulsively took an international nanny job.

I would say I took the long way around, eventually finding my way back to school. When I started college the second time, I loved it. I was motivated to stay there. I realized I needed to figure out why the amount of studying I was doing did not equal the grades I expected. Something was wrong, but instead of shutting down like I had in the past, my more mature brain was determined to figure out why. I was tested by a psychologist in my hometown. She diagnosed me with ADHD and prescribed me medication. Even my mom, who had the insight that I was wired differently, didn't know how to approach this new information. It was confirming, but we didn't know what to do next.

When I went back to college, now medicated, I noticed my grades started to reflect the work I was putting in. I could sit and study or write in the library for hours on end without needing a break. I could retain what I read, without having to reread. I was less forgetful, less emotionally reactive, less impulsive, and was more mindful of my routines and my need for them. It turns out I got in trouble a lot less when my impulses had a pause button. I have learned about ADHD on my own and in my career with the clients I see. So many children and teens feel trapped in a world where they are expected to exceed expectations, but they struggle to stay afloat like I once did. I validate their experiences by sharing some of my stories to support their own acceptance that there is a reason they are acting the way they are.

It is important for ADHD brains to feel seen and heard because no one really sees what they can do. In general, most adults are focused only on what they can't do. It is exhausting. I strive to help ADHD brains find ways to work with their brains, rather than against them, and I encourage all the exploration of novel experiences. I strive to remember and share, something I was once told – ADHD brains are glittery brains, a very apt metaphor in describing disorganization, creativity, the need for novelty, and trying new things.

The Neurodivergent Child – by Patricia Lomando

As a child in elementary school, I don't remember hearing anything about ADHD or autism. Looking back, I don't think diagnoses were as sought out as they are today. While I was evaluated for gifted placement in school, I didn't receive a diagnosis for ADHD until I was around 20 years old. Nonetheless, school was almost a caricature of ADHD experiences. As early as second grade, I recall sitting at my desk and a large three walled cardboard box being brought down over my head. I still remember the surprise of my teacher lowering it in front of me, the way it covered the front and the sides of my desk, so that it was boxed in like a cubicle. There were little rectangle cutouts on the sides of the box she called "windows." I remember hearing something like, "maybe now I can focus, if I have nothing to look at." It was confusing. I recall looking around and I was the only one with this contraption. No-one had ever spoken to me about attention. I wasn't receiving poor grades, but I would stare off into the distance and struggled to get started or finished with work.

I was a visual learner that had passing grades and was demonstrating the need for advanced levels. I recall in elementary school, my family being told that my reading level surpassed the 6th grade books they had in classrooms so I could be by myself or join a group. I don't recall that I warranted much attention, but there were situations. At one point, two teachers were sharing my large classroom and I needed to shift between them for different classes, I lived in a state of perpetual anxiety over this switching. Looking back, I realize I couldn't keep track of when I needed to shift classes, even though it had been explained. I had no sense of time or sequence and would get lost in whatever work I was doing, oblivious to class changes. I could also become hyper focused on when the classes would change and too distracted by that preoccupation to get any work done. It felt hopeless and I couldn't understand why I was the only one who seemed to panic and mess up. I recall that being a fairly common confusion and frustration; why couldn't I do what others seemed to have no struggle with?

Homework was an all-night process. I was asked to sit at the dining table to complete my work because I was told I would do better where I was visible and had space. In reality, I would sit and adults and/or animals would walk around, and I was drawn to their movement. All of the sounds that were made as people would get food/drinks, talk to each other, do anything at all, focused my attention. I wouldn't get up, but I would work until after midnight. I recall my father's pacing and frustration, saying I was getting too much homework, but I "knew" it shouldn't be taking me that long. That attention to sounds and smells never wavered. I remain just as focused on facial expressions, body language, and the changes of intonation when someone speaks. Pauses, the way people change their breathing, and differences in patterns with the way someone moves are all things that catch my focus and I believe are part of what help me to "see" clients as a clinician today. In a crowded room, in traffic, or on a deadline however, those same qualities can become overwhelming.

Although socially I had friends, I often felt awkward and isolated. In class, I was impulsive or quiet. I recall feeling incapable of answering questions for teachers because they insisted I raise my hand first, and I couldn't handle the combination of the anxiety between raising my hand and answering a question in the spotlight unless I blurted it out to get past those feelings. I stopped contributing unless I was so excited about the topic that the impulsive desire to speak overruled any concern for rules. It was precisely those many rules, both formal and informal, that made me feel uncomfortable in social settings.

Whether at school or in public, I did not enjoy crowds. It was too much to process, too many social rules and expectations that seemed to be "common sense," but to me felt restrictive. I "felt" people as though they were each screaming through a bullhorn, and I was so sensitive to sound, touch, and smells. I remember barely making it through one day of Brownies (the young version of girl scouts). I didn't feel comfortable speaking with strangers and wouldn't complete activities because there were too many people involved, keeping me from focusing in on any one task. I despised new social environments that came with new social structures and assumptions. I still laugh when I recall a day that a teacher told my mother I had never arrived at "aftercare," because I'd slipped underneath a desk (pretending it was my personal cave) to get away from all the students and noise. That may have been my last day at aftercare! As an adolescent, I befriended others who struggled to "fit" social norms, often as a kind of ringleader, but I was the one to generally be found outside by myself (with books or pets) at any social gathering.

The support I received back then was mostly to "just do this or just do that." I hated phrases about "common sense." Everything was considered to be so easy for me and any struggle was considered oppositional. Neither box fit me. I became self-conscious early on about how others would communicate and view "my process" for things. I didn't like being told how to do things, because it felt like that spotlight shining on everything I couldn't get right. The more spotlight that was focused on me, the more of a mess I felt like. I walked around with the heaviest book bag of my classmates because I carried ALL books, folders, and papers around with me in a spectacular disaster. By the time I thought of unpacking, it was time to leave. I was repeatedly told I would "break my back," but I was also compensating. I always had everything with me I needed, and packing and unpacking were additional steps that threw off my rhythm. These were the little strategies I used to make things easier for myself. I would be completely overwhelmed by trying to clean a room for instance, but sequenced steps worked for me (e.g., I recall a book I was given which broke cleaning down into categorized boxes and I still use that "format" today). I would read anything I was given as a child. I realize now that a lot of strategies I used to adapt were in areas of executive functioning.

Observing without the expectation of performance also helped. I was a perfectionist. Any new experience resulted in dysregulation. I didn't want to try new experiences I wasn't able to figure out. I preferred to watch how things were done. If I could observe from the outside until I understood how something was handled, I had a better chance of creating a rhythm for how to do it in my head. I would say I didn't want to do things even if I did, in the hopes I would be able to watch until I felt comfortable to join in. Sometimes, "grown-ups" would say if I wasn't going to join, I couldn't watch. I'm sure the attempt was motivation, but it didn't work that way. It was when I knew what was going to happen, what would be expected of me, and what actions ended in success that I felt safe enough to join activities.

I believe it is so important for awareness and understanding that some people struggle with holding back and aren't interrupting or blurting to be rude, but because it's the only way the flow comes out. I think a recognition from teachers and adults that children try to adapt in their own ways, and that not everything is attempted disrespect could have been helpful for me. I was alright with working on interruptions, but to this day when people ask me to raise my hand, I just let the others respond. Allowing me to observe first and jumping in when ready versus assuming that would enabling or rewarding inappropriate behaviors would have been affirming. Even respecting whatever is easiest for everyone to participate in activities could have made a huge difference in feelings of self-worth, acceptance, and the ability to participate equally, not only for me as a child, but for all kinds of learners.

For the most part accommodations were not coming from the "grown-ups" around me. I do remember the way an art teacher and a creative writing teacher embodied affirming experiences. They were the coolest! They both heard my words; they didn't criticize my need to move and even allowed me to have "hall passes" to accommodate my struggles with "waiting" for others to complete their work. Interestingly, I remember both of them asking me to write or draw about my hallway experiences and those were the teachers that showed me acceptance, interest, and the freedom to be.

As an adolescent, it felt that everywhere the message was that emotions caused discomfort for others. I remember being asked to "calm down," because my hands would flap, my eyes would get wide, and I would get excited about ideas. I was "supposed to" fake it and say everything was fine, regardless of how I felt. I had spent years being most accepted when I was quiet and invisible. Being quiet and invisible meant well-behaved, but I was more than that. As a teenager, it had been too much time being told to suck it up, calm down, and to present as more appropriate. I pursued poets who railed against repression of emotion. I gravitated toward peers who felt similarly, who echoed and heightened my own voice of societal rebellion. I embodied rebel musicians, superheroes, all that highlighted alienation as strength. I railed against the concept of mental health disorders and internalized the belief that society wanted to quiet the masses. Institutionalization seemed the only avenue for intense or depressed teens when I was young. Therapy wasn't really spoken about as an option. I was convinced if I went into therapy, they'd never let me escape. I wouldn't pass a sanity test, not because I wasn't sane, but because I wouldn't be able to fit their mold under a spotlight, and I didn't even know what that mold looked like.

As I have raised my own autistic son, I have heard other "professionals" instructing children to look at them, what to say, how to stand, etc. I've listened to professionals tell me that they needed to hold children down, allow them to scream, etc. all while asking for my understanding. As I watched the actions "corrections," and attempted to explain to these individuals that I couldn't maintain eye contact, that I blurt, that I did all of the same things as a child, that these weren't things that required correction – I began to recall those old feelings and realize how much autistic children have become spotlighted.

I firmly believe that neurodivergent individuals of all flavors are the cathartic expression of community and should be cherished for their vibrant light in the same way others have said that theatric performances were the cathartic expression of an audience. These are the clients who I cherish today, those who feel so much, think so much, those who believe they are wrong, when the lens of right and wrong comes from the societal attempt to stifle that spirit under the guise of civilization.

I didn't have a diagnosis during my childhood, and I think that changed the way I experienced receiving one. I am me. I pretty much already knew I was "neurodivergent" by the time the ADHD diagnosis came along, but my childhood was one of being that kid who was invisible and "left of center." That identity is a part of me, and I embrace it. ADHDers are often seen as "lazy, lacking motivation, and not demonstrating effort," and I grew up in the midst of those stereotypes. It led me to understand that we lived in a society that could be intolerant, repressive, and judgmental. It also forged a passionate desire to be the opposite of those elements and to support those who were on the other end of it as well. I can be quirky, messy, loud, impulsive, organized, passionate, creative, and bright. I have time blindness and struggle to meet commitments unless I turn them into carefully orchestrated plans that don't come at me when I'm overwhelmed. I do not multitask, and I do not always act in ways considered appropriate and expected. I am authentic, compassionate, and encourage coloring outside the lines.

At times, I feel as though I'm a computer with zero connection to what I've been raised to believe I "should be feeling." As a child reading about Alexithymia (a condition of struggling with feeling emotions), I thought I had found myself. To understand things, I need facts and percentages – emotions distract me. Humor has always been a challenge because it doesn't make sense and I am fairly obsessed with understanding the origin of idioms and words in general. At other times, my energy can and has activated a room full of reluctant rescuers to pull and save eight dogs at once from a county shelter, a day I will never forget. That same energy can cause a room to treat me like a ticking time bomb that has to be brought down or can have me sitting on my hands, picking fingers, kicking, or doodling if feeling forced to keep it all inside. That energy or adrenaline isn't good or bad. So much of how it's received is related to how others understand it…and so much of handling it is being aware of it, and how it's channeled so that it doesn't eat me up inside. Research, art, journaling, projects, movement, sounds, flapping, playing – there are so many ways that neurodivergent individuals like myself are able to channel and regulate that energy when it's not obstructed or judged. That channeling is a need, whether it's ADHD, autism, depression, anxiety, etc. Working with other neurodivergent individuals has once again brought me face to face with society and families who, though well intentioned, encourage "masking" and the adaptation to the masses. But that is not where joy, purpose and self-fulfillment are found.

As the autistic community has continued to strengthen its voice (and along with it that of all neurodivergent populations), I have realized that by believing society was incapable of change because they were "the norm," that the majority didn't have the capacity for depth, tolerance, understanding, etc., I let them off the hook. The majority is accountable. There are concrete changes that can be made to the way we parent, educate, and offer therapeutic support that allow for neurodivergent connection, appreciation, support, collaborative skill building, acceptance, and self-worth.

If those changes are made for the neurodivergent community, they support everyone, because neurodivergent supports are those of flexibility, tolerance, and authentic acceptance. They are supports that help with executive functioning strategies, regulation, and being emotionally overwhelmed; strategies that help with restlessness, distraction, and anxiety. They support those at every developmental stage as well as those experiencing trauma, grief, anxiety, and depression. They support introverts who struggle with advocacy and fear as well as extroverts who have difficulty containing their excitement. These supports can be provided in the classroom, at home, and in the public arena. I have heard people say that they don't have the resources, finances, and specializations to work with neurodivergent populations. The truth is that as we support neurodivergent populations, we support everyone, including those who have yet to be diagnosed.

References

Ballou, E. P., daVanport, S., & Onaiwu, M. G. (2021). *Sincerely, your autistic child: What people on the autism spectrum with their parents knew about growing up, acceptance, and identity.* Beacon Press Books.

Higashida, N. (2013). *The reason I jump.* Random House.

Weathington, L. (2020). Neurotypical vs. neurodivergent: What's the difference? *Daivergent.* https://daivergent.com/blog/neurotypical-vs-neurodivergent

3
Neurodivergent Mental Health Needs

History of Addressing Mental Health Needs of Neurodivergent Children

Understanding the mental health history of autistic and neurodivergent children requires an understanding of the constructs of stigmatization and the movement toward being neurodiversity affirming and informed. Stigma is defined as the unwanted shadow of a person, produced when society disdains certain human differences. Stigmatized people are often seen as incompetent, blamed for their suffering, and socially marginalized in ways that we might now consider "ableist." Stigma comes from deep structural conditions, such as capitalism, ideologies of individualism and personal responsibility, and the complicated legacies of racism and colonialism. Our dynamic conceptions of mental illness ride on the waves of broader historical cultural changes (Grinker, 2020).

Grinker (2020) contended that although psychiatric disorders and developmental disabilities have become increasingly normalized over the past several decades, this is a stunning reversal of a shameful and stigmatized history that most autistic and neurodivergent individuals faced for a very long time. In 1944, for example, one of the most celebrated twentieth-century psychologists, Erik Erickson, sent his infant son Neil, born with Down syndrome, to a residential institution and told everyone, including his other children, that the baby had died at birth (Friedman, 1999). In the 1960s and 1970s, autistic children were often diagnosed with childhood schizophrenia or intellectual developmental disorder (mental retardation at the time), and schools and employers offered few opportunities. With no evidence to back up their accusations, clinicians commonly blamed autism on supposedly unloving "refrigerator mothers" (Bettelheim, 1972) and conceived of autism in the framework of psychotic disorders. In these historical contexts, few parents wanted to disclose that they had an autistic child (Grinker, 2020).

DOI: 10.4324/9781003207610-4

The historical struggles with mental health and neurodivergence can be best reviewed with a closer look at autism. Arguable, two individuals are responsible for recognizing and perpetuating what would become known as autism. First, Leo Kanner, following his seminal child psychiatry text in 1935, introduced the world to the condition known as autism. Kanner was an Austrian psychiatrist who wrote a paper describing the behavior he had observed in 11 children. Secondly, the work of Hans Asperger who was writing in parallel with Kanner and wrote about the characteristics of children in similar ways. Asperger was a German pediatrician who observed the behavior of four boys who he argued were showing challenges in forming friendships, displayed a general lack of empathy toward others, had clumsy movements, and had difficulties with communication (which he identified as autism). Although much has been learned and changed since their initial efforts, Kanner and Asperger laid a foundation for what would come under the medical model describing these children (O'Reilly, Lester, & Kiyimba, 2019).

O'Reilly, Lester, and Kiyimba (2019) stated that even in the historical present, the classification of autism as a mental health condition is controversial and contested. The ambition to 'fix' a disorder or disability is central to the medical model and pathologizing practices, and for many autistic and neurodivergent people, this provides a perspective that they are 'broken' in some way. Such ideas are co-constructed by the mental health profession and taken directly from medical, psychological, neurological, and developmental positions of autism and grounded in the criteria created through DSM-5. Importantly, neurodivergent individuals and advocates do not use the same knowledge spheres or frames of reference as some professionals, and their relationships with services can be stressful and, in some cases, conflicting.

O'Reilly, Lester, and Kiyimba (2019) proposed a significant historical event, the advent of the DSM-III in 1980 that recognized autism as a distinct conceptual category, almost 40 years after its inception by Kanner. It was this point in the twentieth century, with the inclusion of autism on the DSM-III that the work of Kanner and Asperger were revived by two British professionals who coined the notion of autistic spectrum disorder, and the triad of impairments became part of common clinical discourse. This triad consisted of three core characteristics attributed to autism.

1 Impairments in social interaction
2 Impairments in communication
3 Restrictive repetitive patterns of behavior

This was later reconfigured in the twenty-first century as a dyad of impairments and reconstructed as autism spectrum disorder, but the notion of the spectrum has been maintained. Much of what has been recognized and practiced in mental health care with neurodivergent children is a result of the labels and conceptualizations for the DSM. Iannelli (2020) put forth a historical timeline highlighting significant happenings in the course of autism's history.

1943: Leo Kanner publishes a paper describing 11 patients who were focused on or obsessed with objects and had a "resistance to (unexpected) change." He later named this condition "infantile autism."

1944: Austrian pediatrician Hans Asperger publishes a scientific study of autistic children, a case study describing four children ages 6–11. He notices parents of some of the children have similar personalities or eccentricities and regards this as evidence of a genetic link. He is also credited with describing a form of autism, later called Asperger's syndrome.

1952: In the first edition of the American Psychiatric Association's Diagnostic and Statistical Manual of Mental Disorders (DSM), children with symptoms of autism are labeled as having childhood schizophrenia.

1965: A group of parents of autistic children have the first meeting of the National Society of Autistic Children (now called the Autism Society of America).

1975: The Education for All Handicapped Children Act is enacted to help protect the rights and meet the needs of children with disabilities, most of whom were previously excluded from school.

1980: The third edition of the Diagnostic and Statistical Manual of Mental Disorders (DSM-III) includes criteria for a diagnosis of infantile autism for the first time.

1983: Throughout the 1970s and 1080s the social model of disability was emerging. In 1983 disabled academic Mike Oliver coined the phrase *social model of disability*.

1990: Autism is included as a disability category in the Individuals with Disabilities Education Act (IDEA), making it easier for autistic children to get special education services.

1994: Asperger's Syndrome is added to the DSM, expanding the autism spectrum to include milder cases in which individuals tend to be more "highly functioning."

1998: Harvey Blume and Judy Singer coined and defined the term neurodiversity.

2006: Ari Ne'eman establishes the Autistic Self Advocacy Network (ASAN).

2013: The DSM-5 combines autism, Asperger's, and childhood disintegrative disorder into autism spectrum disorder.

2013 to Present: The last couple of decades have seen the emergence of the neurodiversity paradigm and neurodiversity movement with an increase in advocacy and activism for the acceptance and affirming identity of neurodivergent individuals.

In the time since autism was first identified as a "mental illness," this diagnostic category has undergone remarkable changes. Once considered exceedingly rare and profoundly debilitating, it is now relatively common; once highly stigmatized, it is increasingly accepted under the banner of neurodiversity/neurodivergent put forth by autistic self-advocates in the United States, many of whom identify as part of the American disability rights movement. Indeed, one reason autistic self-advocates chose to represent themselves through the term "neurodiversity" was to claim ownership of and redefine the currently powerful brain-based model. The claiming of a new identity term – "neurodivergent" and its counterpart "neurotypical" – stands as an awakening of awareness and acceptance to disrupt the stigma long associated with "autism-as-mental-illness." Assigning this diagnosis as a positive social value resembles the strategy of LGBTQ+ theorists who subverted and disidentified with normative categories and definitions that have subjected them all to stigma for many decades (Grinker, 2020).

A core focus of the neurodiversity movement and paradigm is on the language we use around autism and other neurodivergent categories. This movement rejects pathologized negative concepts such as disorder, deficit, and 'impairment' and instead reconstitutes autism as a way of being. The neurodiversity movement therefore directly challenged framing autism in a medical model-pathologizing way. The popularity of neurodiversity as a movement arose mostly online in response to what was argued to be a marginalization of autistic people. Thus, this movement sought to establish a culture where autistic and neurodivergent people could have pride in their neurodivergent identity and provide mutual support in self-advocacy (O'Reilly, Lester, & Kiyimba, 2019).

An underpinning principle of neurodiversity was the foundational idea of a "differently wired brain." This movement has been instrumental in advocating strength-based discourses for autism and other neurodivergence. For autism, neurodiversity has two main claims as outlined by Jaarsma and Welin (2012):

1 That autism is simply a natural variation in humans, and being neurodivergent or neurotypical, reflect different ways of being human.

2 That neurodiversity connects to human rights, political issues, and non-discrimination of autistic people.

This paradigm and movement therefore became associated with the struggle for civil rights (known as the neurodiversity movement) for those individuals traditionally diagnosed with neurodevelopmental conditions and as such became a counterargument for the deficit (medical) model to prevent discrimination and stigmatization. This is important, as society tends to be organized around neurotypical values and by contrast autism and any neurodivergence is then positioned as a deficit. The history has been a "rocky" one at best. It has not been kind or very accurate. Fortunately, the neurodiversity movement is progressing forward with a goal of changing ableist systems to a more accurate, valuing, and equitable view of autism and all neurodivergence.

Neurodivergent Therapy Approaches

Historically, therapies focused on neurodivergent children were viewed as treatments, designed to address the disorder, and correct the child so they could live a healthy life. This was basically a code for implementing whatever treatment approach could be thought of that would take away the child's neurodivergence and make the child neurotypical. Further, most of these approaches were not mental health-based.

Currently there still exists a significant number of purported neurodivergent focused "treatments" mostly targeting autism. Many of the most recognized and/or evidence-based purported "treatments" consist of behavioral methods, social skills training, biomedical, existential, and developmental approaches, many of which are non-affirming. Actual autistics and neurodiversity affirming advocates resist the notion of "treatment" for autism and neurodivergence. There is no cure for autism or any neurodivergence, and neurodivergent people do not have a disease. The terms "therapy" or "support" are much preferred and more affirming than the term treatment. Further, the proposition that a neurodivergent child automatically needs a certain therapy because they are neurodivergent is an ableist concept and can be detrimental to the child's wellbeing. A neurodivergent child or adolescent does not enter a therapy because they are neurodivergent. They enter a therapy because they have a need that the therapy can help address.

Siri and Lyons (2010) suggested that since the etiology as well as the manifestations of neurodivergence are influenced by a variety of multiple factors, a one-size-fits-all approach to interventions is not the most beneficial approach. No two children will have the same therapy needs or respond to the same combination of therapies. Each child's therapy plan needs to be unique, taking into consideration the child's specific strengths, needs, culture, and family dynamics. Many autistic and neurodivergent children will participate in some type of program, therapy, or intervention. The variety and depth of the service can look different for each child.

It would be easy to produce a list of over 100 promoted and advertised therapies, or services focused on autistic and neurodivergent children. The variety of options include biomedical, behavioral, developmental, alternative, and difficult-to-categorize interventions. Unfortunately, many options are not neurodiversity informed or affirming. With the plethora of neurodivergent-focused services bombarding parents and considering the vulnerability issues, many parents struggle in wanting to provide beneficial supports for their child, it becomes essential to critically evaluate promoted services geared toward neurodivergent children and their families. The following guide can serve as a beginning protocol for evaluating services.

1 Is the therapy neurodiversity informed and affirming? Prizant (2015) stated that autism is not an illness. It's a different way of being human. Children with autism are not sick; they are progressing through developmental stages as we all do. To help them, we don't need to change them or fix them. We need to work to understand them, and then change what we do. The best way to help an autistic or neurodivergent child to change for the better is to change ourselves – our attitudes, our behavior, and the types of support we provide. Therapy services should have a clearly identified neurodiversity affirming focus. It should go beyond just a claim of being neurodiversity affirming and be able to show how an affirming process is implemented with the therapy approach.

2 What does the research say about the promoted service or therapy? Is there any research support? Does the service incorporate any evidence for addressing what it promotes? Remember that a therapy approach may be helpful even if it is not evidence-based or research-supported, but it is important to know what research has been presented on the approach. Also, remember that historically (and often still in present day), research specifically focused on autistic and neurodivergent children has been laden with ableist bias and thus may not be applicable for validating the therapy. For research specific to the neurodivergent population, it would be important to consider neurodiversity affirming research.

3 What are the potential risks of participating in the therapy? Are there any potentially dangerous side effects? Can any harm be done to the child or family? If a therapy approach contains possible harm or risk to the child, it should be highly scrutinized before beginning. There are plenty of therapies designed to help neurodivergent children with their mental health needs that do not cause harm. Anything that has the potential to cause any type of emotional or physical harm is a large red flag warning.

4 What is the cost of the therapy? How much money will the family have to pay out of pocket to receive the therapy? It is important to be aware that some therapies may exist to take advantage of families. The cost of the therapy should be within reason for the type of service that is being provided. A sad reality is that there exists special, new, or unique "therapies" advertised to help neurodivergent children that are money-making scams. If a "therapy" is costing a large amount of money and cannot be validated (for the cost) from other sources, this should be another large red flag warning.

5 Does the therapy promise to cure autism or take the autism/neurodivergence away? What are the proposed benefits of participating in the therapy? What are the therapy outcomes? Does the therapy make any promises? If so, what are the promises? Any therapy that promises to cure autism/neurodivergence or promises absolutes in gains should be avoided. Therapy should also have an evaluation component that can be explained to families so everyone can see how the therapy works and how the therapy is helping the child/family.

6 Does the therapy seem like a good fit for the child and the family considering financial demands, time demands, and therapy expectations/processes? Families should consider if the therapy approach is something the family can commit their time, finances, and energy to before beginning.

7 How is the therapy governed or monitored? Families should understand if there is any oversight for the therapy or the professional providing the therapy. Families should also understand if they can observe or be a part of the therapy in which their child is participating. If the therapy has no accountability and/or parents are not allowed to observe or participate, this may be a caution for families regarding the therapy.

8 How is the professional implementing the therapy considered a valid and reliable person to do so? Professionals or those implementing therapy should be able to communicate to families how they are qualified to implement the therapy. They should be able to produce education and/or training documents that demonstrates they are qualified to be offering the therapy service.

9 What do actual autistics/neurodivergent people say about certain therapies, especially therapies they have participated in as children? Why is the therapy beneficial for the child? What are the child's actual needs that align with the therapy?

10 How did you hear about or learn about the therapy or service? Does it seem like it has a reliable history? Has anyone else you know participated in the therapy and what did they think? And lastly, what is your first impression? Does it seem like something that your child would be empowered by, help them feel better about themselves? Often if your instinct is telling you something does not seem right, it's important to listen.

What Are the Mental Health Needs of Neurodivergent Children?

Understanding the mental health needs of neurodivergent children means understanding the role of mental health with neurodivergent children. In AutPlay Therapy, the role of mental health (play therapy) is not to fix, cure, or heal, a child from their neurodivergence. The AutPlay therapist does not view the process as a treatment for autism, neurodivergence, etc. The process is a therapy designed to help the child overcome, manage, process through, heal from, etc. any mental health issues which may be a current struggle.

It's an important distinction to make that neurodivergence may be different from other psychological disorders such as attachment disorders and trauma disorders. It's extremely common for symptoms of neurodivergent conditions and symptoms of mental illness to overlap. For example, people with ADHD are often misdiagnosed with depression or anxiety and treated for those conditions, instead of receiving help for the legitimate diagnosis. However, it's also not uncommon for people who have ADHD to experience depression and anxiety as difficulty with executive functioning in the brain can trigger those symptoms. Mental health challenges can impact anyone, but there is research to suggest that neurodivergent people have high rates of mental illness as a product of not being valued and accepted in a neurotypical society. The neurodivergent brain is often not naturally accommodated in many academic institutions and work environments, leaving many neurodivergent people to constantly "mask" their needs and identity ultimately creating unhealthy constructs for the neurodivergent person (Tricaso, 2021). The following highlights some common mental health needs that neurodivergent children experience and may result in them entering a play therapy process:

Anxiety – Perhaps one of the more common mental health issues for neurodivergent children is experiencing anxiety struggles. The anxiety levels of some children can produce debilitating results where daily struggles are difficult to accomplish. Social anxiety, agoraphobia, and other fears can also be present – creating challenges for the child and the child's family. Often anxiety struggles are misunderstood, and children may be labeled as defiant or stubborn. The child may not understand their own anxiety issues and may not be able to communicate their issues to others.

Depression – Neurodivergent children can experience rejection, social isolation, bullying, confusion, and being misunderstood. All of which can lead to feelings of depression. As most of the environments that neurodivergent children navigate are not neurodiversity affirming or friendly, many encounters can leave the child struggling with feelings of depressions. As with anxiety, children may not understand their feelings of depression, how to communicate what is happening with them, and how to process and manage depression. Issues such as anxiety, depression, and even trauma, which are not addressed, can lead to even more serious situations such as suicidal ideation and attempts.

Trauma – Abuse, sexual assault, violence, natural disasters, and wartime combat are all common causes of PTSD in the general population. Among autistic people, though, less extreme experiences – fire alarms, paperwork, the loss of a family pet, even a stranger's offhand comment – can also be destabilizing. They can also be traumatized by others' behavior toward them (Gravitz, 2018). Research indicates that autistic children reported a significantly higher level of exposure to neighborhood violence, parental divorce, traumatic loss, poverty, mental illness, and substance abuse in the family. These situational indicators of stress and trauma experienced by the family are called adverse childhood experiences (ACE) and the probability of reporting one or more of them was higher in autistic children compared to non-autistic children (Lobregt-van Buuren et al., 2021). Autistic and neurodivergent children appear more prone to experiencing trauma and thus presenting in therapy with unaddressed trauma issues. This may be due to experiencing a traumatic event or may be ongoing developmental trauma being experienced as a result of navigating as a neurodivergent child.

Poor self-worth – Many neurodivergent children find themselves entering a play therapy process after they have already been experiencing life as a neurodivergent child. Many enter play therapy with low self-esteem and worth. Much of this is influenced by the rejection they have had and continue to experience. As much of society is based on, accommodates, and values a more ideal neurotypical presentation, neurodivergent children find themselves on the outside, feeling devalued, and being excluded. Many children receive a constant message of "You are not right," "You need to change," and "There is something wrong with you being you." These messages, whether they are direct or more subtle, do a considerable amount of damage to the child's self-worth. Thus, working on building the child's self-image and self-esteem can become a primary goal in mental health care.

Identity struggles (self-acceptance, masking, code switching) – "Masking" is a popular term in the neurodivergent community that refers to minimizing or completely hiding symptoms to fit in with societal norms. Many neurodivergent people learn to mask as a survival technique as it is often more accepting to appear neurotypical. Masking can include suppressing symptoms and needs, mimicking behaviors someone who is neurotypical engages in, having go-to scripts for social interactions, and anything else that helps them camouflage within society.

Code switching involves adjusting one's style of speech, appearance, behavior, and expression in ways that will optimize the comfort of others in exchange for fair treatment, quality service, and employment opportunities. It has been widely understood within the BIPOC community but also applies to the neurodivergent people. Masking and code switching are two examples of neurodivergent struggles with self-acceptance and feeling like being themselves will not be acceptable in society. Continually denying self and "masking" to feel accepted can create a host of mental health struggles including depression, anxiety, anger, etc.

Peer issues (bullying, rejection, friends) – Research has well documented that neurodivergent children are highly susceptible to being bullied by peers; three to four times the rate of neurotypical children (Hoover, 2015). This can be compounded by experiencing social (peer) rejection, feeling isolated, and struggling to find friendships. The results can be devastating to a positive sense of self. Often children do not know how to address bullying and peer rejection and suffer in silence. This can become a critical therapy goal for many neurodivergent children.

Regulation struggles – Becoming dysregulated and needing help with regulating one's system is a common and highly misunderstood therapy need. Many neurodivergent children struggle with their system becoming overwhelmed (dysregulated) and this often leads to behaviors that can feel out of control and unsafe. The dysregulation can come from a variety of places (and often does). This might include sensory challenges, fears, anxiety, confusion, feeling unsafe, the unknown or unexpected, biomedical issues, etc. Often it is a combination of issues that has contributed to the child becoming dys-regulated. Understanding how to regulate one's system and the process of co-regulation can become important therapy goals.

Sensory needs – Autistic and other neurodivergent children often have co-occurring sensory processing needs/differences. Sensory needs can manifest in ways that create dysregulation, pain, and problematic behaviors. Under-standing and addressing sensory needs becomes a therapy goal when the child's sensory differences are creating struggles for the child. Sensory work may be a part of a larger focus on helping the child regulate their system. Sensory work may also be done in collaboration with other professionals such as an occupational therapist training in addressing sensory needs.

Emotion expression – Many of the children I have seen in play therapy ini-tially lack an awareness and conceptualization of their own emotions. Being able to label a feeling, understand feelings, why they are happening, how to identify them, how to express them, and how to manage them as part of an overall regulation ability can become therapy goals. It is important to note that neurodivergent children may recognize, express, and communicate feel-ings in their own unique ways. This work, as all work with neurodivergent children, requires the ability to understand neurodivergent presentation without the expectation that a neurodivergent child must express feelings the way a neurotypical child would or there is something wrong with the neurodivergent child. Therapists will want to take care to recognize and al-low for a neurodivergent understanding and expression of emotion that may be different from what the therapist is used to experiencing.

Social related needs – Social related needs can be vast and complex. The myr-iad of issues a child might be facing that involve some type of social situation or navigation can almost feel endless. It is not unusual for social needs to be creating other issues such as anxiety, depression, and low self-worth. Ther-apists will want to take care to thoroughly assess and understand the social needs of the child and ensure that social related goals are not supporting ableist ideas. Historically, "social skills" work has been implemented and de-signed in a way that autistic and neurodivergent children are trained to look and act neurotypical. This would not be an appropriate or affirming goal. Social needs are real and can certainly be addressed in play therapy, but any process that involves trying to change the child's identity is counterproduc-tive to improving a child's mental health.

Parent/child relationship – When working with children clients, it is not unu-sual to discover issues related to parent/child relationship strain. This can be due to many factors and if left unaddressed can interfere with advancement in other therapy goals and can create additional issues. Addressing parent/child relationship issues would require the therapist to implement a more family play therapy approach. This is something supported in AutPlay Therapy and other play therapy approaches such as Filial Therapy and Theraplay. Therapists should take care to gain training in family play therapy work and understand the dynamics of working with a family versus the individual child before attempting to involve the family in the play therapy process.

Life issues/transitions – Possibly one of the most important things about implementing mental health therapy with neurodivergent children is understanding the following construct – this child is not here because they are neurodivergent, they are here because they have a mental health need – in conjunction with – I need to be aware this is a neurodivergent child and whatever therapy goals we are working on need to be affirmative and individualized to support their neurotype. Neurodivergent children can enter play therapy with needs same as any child. They may be experiencing a parent's divorce, grief issues, physical or sexual abuse, attachment issues, or any life adjustment concern. What may be different, is the process of working on these needs. The therapist will want to understand the child's neurotype and take care to work on therapy goals in ways the child responds to and understands.

Rosa (2022) created a list to help those who aren't autistic themselves (or whose autistic traits differ from those of their child) to understand what may upset an autistic person, and cause distress. There hope is to highlight issues that may not be obvious to a bystander, and how you (parent, therapist, etc.) can help the autistic people in your life thrive, as much as possible. Although the creators focus their list on the autistic experience, much of what is communicated could apply to any neurodivergent child and should help highlight the play therapist's awareness and relationship in working with neurodivergent children. Rosa and Autistic Science Person's full list (the *Autism Checklist of Doom*) can be found in checklist form on the website "Thinking Person's Guide to Autism" – thinkingautismguide.com and includes the following important constructs:

- You treat meltdowns, and their triggers, as though they are tantrums and voluntary, when they are in reality involuntary, and in many cases can be avoided.
- You insist that they make eye contact with you or other people, even though eye contact can be painful or overwhelming for autistic people, and indeed in many cultures is considered an act of aggression.

- You ask them to name their feelings and get frustrated when they cannot, without considering that they may have alexithymia (difficulty perceiving or describing their own emotions) like so many autistic people do.
- They experience sensory discomforts that seem minor to you but are overwhelming to them: Clothes tags, tight clothes, dry skin, even individual acne blemishes, humming machines, loud sounds, sunlight, temperature, strong scents, low-key flickering lights.
- You don't believe in their sensory sensitivities or their perception of pain, and think they are ways of making excuses or getting out of events.
- You consider their passions to be "special interests" or disruptive, so they are not given time to delve into them to a satisfying degree – or even worse, those passions are gatekept to negotiate compliance. They are only allowed to talk about their special interest to you for a short period of time, and no effort is made from you to engage in the subject.
- They are overwhelmed by their emotions and can't express that distress any other way than a meltdown or shutdown.
- You do not allow them to stim or flap their hands at all because you think it looks weird, or worry what other people may think – even if you know they are happy.
- They are never given opportunities to succeed, or even to feel good about themselves. They are only criticized or made to feel deficient.
- They don't know they're autistic, and so they think they are a broken person because they aren't like other people.
- They know they're autistic, but everything they hear, see, or read about autism makes them feel like a burden or an alien.
- You just don't accept them for who they are, and they are depressed, anxious, and/or stressed.
- You know they are autistic, yet you keep expecting them to "just do things" like adapt to surprises without distress or interact socially like a non-autistic person, and are upset with them when they are not able to.

Affirming Therapies

Some common affirming therapies are listed below with a brief description. Therapists should be cautioned that at present, there is no one profession/ therapy/discipline that is completely neurodiversity affirming. Play therapy in general encapsulates the most neurodiversity affirming principles but still has some history and current protocols that can be ableist. Other professions and disciplines have some movement toward becoming more neurodiversity affirming but are not fully realized. It basically comes down to the individual provider within a certain discipline. Each individual therapist/provider needs to be reviewed for implementing affirming practices. Some simple questions to ask the professional could be:

- What is your view on neurodiversity?
- Do you implement neurodiversity affirming practices?
- How are you neurodiversity affirming?
- Can you explain what it means?
- Can you give me examples of how you implement a neurodiversity affirming approach?

Play Therapy – The Association for Play Therapy (2022) defines play therapy as the systematic use of a theoretical model to establish an interpersonal process wherein trained play therapists use the therapeutic powers of play to help clients prevent or resolve psychosocial difficulties and achieve optimal growth and development. There exist several affirming play therapy theories and approaches such as AutPlay Therapy, which is designed to address the mental health needs of autistic and neurodivergent children. Certified AutPlay Therapy Providers implement a variety of play therapy approaches and interventions to address needs such as regulation struggles, anxiety issues, trauma, and self-advocacy (Grant, 2017). Play therapy approaches such as Child Centered Play Therapy, Theraplay, Gestalt Play Therapy, Filial Therapy, and Synergetic Play Therapy also present affirming protocols and can be beneficial for neurodivergent children.

Speech Therapy – Speech-language pathologists are professionals who are educated to assess speech and language development and to treat speech and language disorders as well as swallowing disorders. These professionals may implement a variety of interventions to help neurodivergent children improve speech and language needs.

Occupational Therapy – Common occupational therapy interventions include helping neurodivergent children participate fully in school and social situations, address sensory struggles, and regain skills after injury. Occupational therapy services may include comprehensive evaluations of the client's home and other environments (e.g., workplace, school), recommendations for adaptive equipment and training in its use, and guidance and education for family members and caregivers. Occupational therapy practitioners have a holistic perspective, in which the focus is on adapting the environment to fit the person, and the person is an integral part of the therapy team (American Occupational Therapy Association, 2021).

Music Therapy – The American Music Therapy Association (2021) describes music therapy as the process in which music is used within a therapeutic relationship to address physical, emotional, cognitive, and social needs of individuals. After assessing the strengths and needs of each client, the qualified music therapist provides the indicated therapy including creating, singing, moving to, and/or listening to music. Through musical involvement in the therapeutic context, clients' abilities are strengthened and transferred to other areas of their lives. Music therapists work with autistic children to activate the whole brain and improve communication and interactions with others.

Neurodiversity Affirming Play Therapist Constructs

Presume Competence – A strength-based approach and philosophy that assumes neurodivergent children have abilities to learn, think, grow, and understand. Presuming competence means you believe that the neurodivergent child client has current ability and potential to develop their thinking, processing, and understanding. Jorgensen (2022) identified four reasons why presuming competence is important.

1 People's expectations matter. When therapists, parents, teachers, etc. expect children to do well, they do even better than expected.
2 Intelligence Quotient (I.Q.) and other tests that purport to measure human capacity are terribly flawed. They usually tell us what children can't do rather than what they might do if they had good instruction and high-quality supports. Basing a child's whole future on a test score just seems fraught with potential harm.
3 A growing body of research shows "unexpected" abilities in people who had been identified as intellectually disabled until they were provided with a means to communicate.
4 To presume incompetence could cause irreparable harm to children.
5 If we are wrong about presuming a student's ability to learn and to communicate in ways that are on par with their peers without disabilities, being wrong about that isn't as dangerous as the alternative.

Value Relationship as a Core Change Agent – Landreth (1991) stated that the relationship, not the utilization of toys, or interpretation of behavior, is the key to growth. Therefore, the relationship is always focused on the present, living experience. Axline (1947) outlined eight principles for therapeutic relationship with the child:

1 The therapist must develop a warm, friendly relationship with the child, in which good rapport is established as soon as possible.
2 The therapist accepts the child exactly as they are.
3 The therapist establishes a feeling of permissiveness in the relationship so that the child feels free to express their feelings completely.
4 The therapist is alert to recognize the feelings the child is expressing and reflects those feelings back to them in such a manner that they gain insight into their behavior.
5 The therapist maintains a deep respect for the child's ability to solve their own problems if given an opportunity to do so. The responsibility to make choices and to institute change is the child's.
6 The therapist does not attempt to direct the child's actions or conversation in any manner. The child leads the way; the therapist follows.
7 The therapist does not attempt to hurry the therapy along. It is a gradual process and is recognized as such by the therapist.
8 The therapist establishes only those limitations that are necessary to anchor the therapy to the world of reality and to make the child aware of their responsibilities in the relationship.

(pp. 73–74)

Value and Allow for Multiple ways of Communication – If a child is nonverbal it does not mean they are not communicating, and it does not mean they do not have anything to say. The play therapist will understand that children can communicate in many ways that are not verbal and these ways will be respected and valued. Some children may communicate through their play, use an augmentative and alternative communication device (AAC), body language, etc. Some children may be nonverbal, or they may be non-speaking. Whatever the child's communication presentation, the play therapist will make accommodation for the child and make every effort to allow the child's way of communicating to be expressed.

Value and Provide Space for the Child's Voice – Children (both neurotypical and neurodivergent) are arguably the most marginalized group of people across the planet. For the most part, children have no rights and are often completely under the control of their caregivers – sometimes this works for their benefit and sometimes it does not. In play therapy, the therapist should strive to provide space and opportunity for the neurodivergent child's voice to be heard. The child should be allowed to express their thoughts, feelings, and opinions about the play therapy process. In AutPlay Therapy, the child is considered a partner in the process with the therapist and parent. Many spaces eliminate the neurodivergent child's voice. In play therapy there is an active effort to amplify the child's voice.

Partner with Parent/Caregiver and the Child – There are multiple play therapy approaches that focus on working with the parent and child together (Filial Therapy, Theraplay, Child Parent Relationship Therapy). When working with neurodivergent children it is important to have parent/caregiver involvement and work with both the parent and child as partners in the process. Parents often have needs to address and require information about neurodiversity affirming processes. In AutPlay Therapy, the parent/caregiver plays an active role in learning about their child's play and learning play times and techniques to implement at home with their child. Parents are empowered and gain tools for parenting their child while improving their relationship with their child.

Use a Strength-Based Approach – An approach that focuses on identifying what works for the child instead of focusing on what is "wrong" with the child and on their supposed deficits. Instead of insisting the child participate in therapy one certain way, the therapy is individualized to algin with the strengths the child possesses. The strength-based approach is focusing on the positive attributes of a child, rather than the negative ones. Any play therapy theory or approach can incorporate a strength-based approach and should utilize this method when working with neurodivergent children.

Recognize the Child's Play Preferences and Interests – Many play therapists may find they are accustomed to seeing one or two types of play presented in play therapy sessions. Many neurotypical children display pretend and symbolic play and this may be what most play therapists are familiar with. Neurodivergent children will likely present a wide range of different types of play. Some of the many types of play are presented in Chapter 4. The play therapist will take care to understand the neurodivergent child's play preferences and interests. They will work with the child's play instead of trying to force the child to play in a certain way or teach the child to play in a way the therapist believes is the correct or most common way to play. It is the play therapist's duty to meet neurodivergent children where they are in their play preferences – not to judge, and not to devalue. The therapist may even see a type of play they cannot categorize, this should still be honored and validated.

Respect Diverse Neurotypes (Identity Freedom) – Neurodivergent children are not an indistinguishable construct. Neurodivergent children are not all going to look the same, talk the same, present the same, process the same, and have the same needs. Each child will have a distinct neurotype. Respecting diverse neurotypes means the child has the freedom to be themselves and all that comes with presenting who they are in the way they are designed. It is the therapist's role to create this open and accepting atmosphere, meeting each child where they are without judgment and working with them within their neurotype.

Advocate for Inclusion – Defined as the state of being included or being made a part of something, inclusion is about offering the same opportunities to everyone, while providing support and services to accommodate people's differences. Inclusion benefits all within a setting by minimizing stereotypes while encouraging learning to occur between neurotypical and neurodivergent children. Inclusion application is not likely to be a part of a typical play therapy session. More so, it will be part of the play therapist's advocacy work for and with the child. Most inclusion efforts seem to focus on educational settings and extracurricular social settings.

Support Self Advocacy Skills – At its basic, self-advocacy means learning to communicate for your needs. The Organization for Autism Research (2016) stated that self-advocacy is having the right to make and express your own life decisions and choices. Self-advocacy refers to an individual's ability to effectively communicate, convey, negotiate, or assert their own interests, desires, needs, and rights. It involves making informed decisions and taking responsibility for those decisions. Numerous studies demonstrate a clear link between teaching children self-advocacy skills and their ability to be happy, well-functioning adults. The Organization for Autism Research furthered that self-advocacy includes these components:

- Encouraging use of language that is inclusive, respectful, and person-first.
- Knowing what services, modifications, and accommodations you require and being able to request them.
- Knowing whom to ask and where to go to get assistance and support.
- Understanding and expressing one's strengths, talents, and interests.
- Being able to create personal goals and follow a path to achieve those goals.
- Having the ability to make choices.

Respect Body Autonomy – The idea that a person gets to make decisions about what happens with their body. They have control over their body and get to make choices about how their body is treated by others. This has two implications for autistic and neurodivergent children. First, that the therapist does not physically touch, move, or control the child' body (any body part) in any way without the child and parent's consent. Child therapists are highly encouraged to read the Association for Play Therapy (APT) *Paper on Touch*.

The document can be found on the APT website (a4pt.org). Second, that children have literal and figurative right and say to what happens to them and with them. Other adults should not be making decisions for them without the child having a voice and providing their wishes, wants, and giving consent. For example, an adult decides it is okay for a child to be lifted out of their wheelchair and carried into a building for a new tutoring session. This is decided by the adult without the child having a say in how they feel about this experience. Another example would be an 18-year-old learning that their parents are going to take guardianship of them without discussing it with the teen and letting them have a voice in the decision-making process.

Remember that Play is the Natural language of the Child – It is well understood that children learn, process, experience, communicate, and grow through play. The play therapist fundamentally understands the therapeutic powers of play and welcomes and encourages the child to engage in play. Landreth (1991) described the importance of understanding and valuing the child's natural language of play:

> Children's play can be more fully appreciated when recognized as their natural medium of communication. Children express themselves more fully and more directly through self-initiated spontaneous play than they do verbally because they are more comfortable with play. For children to play out their experiences and feelings is the most natural dynamic and self-healing process in which children can engage. Play is the medium of exchange and restricting children to verbal expression automatically places a barrier to the therapeutic relationship….The therapist's responsibility is to go to the child's level and communicate with children through the medium with which they are comfortable.
>
> (p. 10)

Case Example – Isaac

Isaac was brought into therapy by his parents. He lived with his biological father and mother and had two older sisters. Isaac was 10 years old when he began play therapy. He entered therapy with a diagnosis of autism spectrum disorder which he received from a psychological evaluation when he was 5 years old. Isaac had not participated in any specific therapies. He attended public school for kindergarten through 3rd grade. His parents described the school experience as terrible. They stated that Isaac had high anxiety about going to school and struggled with the environment.

The school had Isaac on an IEP, but the parents reported that the school did not help with Isaac's issues. After third grade, they removed Isaac from public school and began home schooling using an online program. After third grade Isaac seemed to improve with his anxiety and depression but prior to coming into therapy, they began noticing he was struggling with negative self-talk, communicating he was stupid and bad (because of his autism), and having some elevated anxiety levels. They wanted play therapy to help Isaac with his emotions and improve his self-esteem.

Isaac's parents were informed about neurodiversity and neurodiversity affirming processes. They appeared to be supportive of Isaac as an autistic child and at home, spoke about this freely and positively. They were concerned that he seemed to be taking on a negative self-image and unsure why this was happening. They reported that Isaac had always seemed to struggle with anxiety, but it had gotten worse over the last few months and now he would become very anxious and upset about many things such as going out in public, worry that one of his parents might get hurt or killed when they were not at home, tornados, and many other things.

I meet with Isaac following the AutPlay Therapy protocol. The first four to five sessions focused on building relationship with Isaac, getting to know him better, understanding his play preferences, and helping him feel familiar and safe with myself and the play therapy process. Isaac very much enjoyed board games; this was his primary play preference. Isaac was not interested in any of the playrooms, technology play or the sandtray room – he wanted to play board games. Isaac's therapy goals focused on understanding and decreasing his anxiety issues, learning regulation ability, addressing any identity issues, and improving his self-worth. Isaac's father and mother would alternate bringing him to therapy and each participated in the therapy sessions.

Sessions 6 through 10 focused on strength-based and emotion exploration play techniques. I would introduce an intervention that helped Isaac better understand his strengths and things he was good at. Isaac's parent, Isaac, and I would all participate in the interventions. I also introduced some expressive interventions designed to help Isaac recognize and talk about his emotions. The strength-based interventions set the foundation for referencing Isaacs's strengths and using his strengths to address his therapy goals. Emotion expression interventions set the foundation for Isaac becoming more comfortable talking about his anxiety feelings. At the end of each session, I would reserve the last 15 minutes to play any board game Isaac chose – his go to board game was Chess.

Sessions 11–25 focused on game selection and play to help address Isaac's therapy goals. Isaac agreed that each session he and I would each choose a board game to play. I would go first, and we would play the game I selected for about half the session. We would then play the game he selected for the remainder of the session. I purposely chose games that would help Isaac express his feelings, recognize his strengths and value, and that he would enjoy playing. Some of the games I chose included Feelings Fair (a therapeutic board game with a carnival design which has many concepts that engage the players in talking about their emotions), Feelings Jenga (each time a piece is removed the person identifies and shares about a feeling or acts out a feeling), Strengths Checkers (each time someone jumps another person they must share about something they do well or have accomplished) and Secret Square (a cooperative memory game that highlighted one of Isaac's strengths – his memorization ability). For Isaac's turn he would mostly choose Chess which he was very good at. It provided a natural opportunity to point out many of his strengths and help him feel good about himself. The parent attending and I would take turns playing with him. There were a few times Isaac choice a Pop It Dice Game (a sensory based popping game). This seemed to be something he would choose on days when he was needing a bit more regulation for his system. Isaac and the parent attending, participated in all the games and the process seemed successful and enjoyable for Isaac.

Sessions 26–30 focused on integrating bibliotherapy into our play therapy times. I selected two books to read with Isaac – *It's Okay to be Different* by Todd Parr and *Some Brains: A Book Celebrating Neurodiversity* by Nelly Thomas. We begin (session 26) with *It's Okay to be Different* and Isaac and I took turns reading each page. After we had finished the book, we each (myself, Isaac and the parent attending) shared what we thought the book meant and how we could apply it to our life. In session 27, we read the book *Some Brains*, implementing the same process as we did with the previous book. Both book readings and discussions provided meaningful opportunity for Isaac to share about his own thoughts and feelings and things he has struggling with in how he has felt about himself. Sessions 28–30 involved us creating our own board game based on helping kids feel good about being different. Isaac was the lead in developing the concept, design, format, and how the game would be played. We all worked together in creating the board game. For materials, we used a piece of cardboard and sharpies. Once the board game was complete, we all played the game together several times. Isaac took the board game home to keep and play with his family.

Session 31–37 focused on maintaining and reinforcing our self-worth gains and anxiety reduction. At this point, Isaac was doing much better with both needs. His anxiety had deceased, and he was talking about and expressing his feelings in healthy ways. He also reported that he did not feel as anxious about things any longer. Isaac's self-worth had improved significantly. He was no longer making negative self-comments. He was actively acknowledging his strengths and talking about things he could do well. He was also preparing to join a community chess club and had been playing online chess with others for the past four to six weeks. Our session times mostly consisted of myself, Isaac, and the parent attending each choosing a game to play and playing together. On session 37, we discussed Isaacs's improvements with his therapy goals and graduating him from his therapy time. Everyone agreed and Isaac's final session was session 38 which was a celebration of Isaac and his parents, and the therapy work they had done.

Case Example – Liam

Liam was brought to therapy by his biological parents who were going through a divorcee. Liam was a 14-year-old male who had a diagnosis of autism, ADHD, and OCD. His parents were concerned with behaviors Liam was displaying. They presented that he seemed depressed and anxious and would often engage in behaviors at school and home that were inappropriate and destructive. They had never told Liam that he had been diagnosed with autism and OCD. Liam did know he had an ADHD diagnosis. The parents seemed to communicate a great deal of stigmatization about autism and as therapy progressed, I discovered they had actively tried to do things with Liam and direct his life so he would not "look" autistic.

Beginning sessions focused on working with Liam individually to better get to know him, help him feel comfortable and safe in therapy, and to build relationship. Liam did present as a young teen with depression and anxiety. He could talk about this and express these emotions. By the end of our intake and assessment phase, a few things were clear about Liam –

1 He had very low self-worth. There were a lot of "failures" in Liam's life. Much of this had to do with Liam being placed in multiple environments (having no awareness or support for being autistic) that were not a good fit for him, and the results were negative. Although Liam did not know he was autistic, he had a great deal of initialized ableism. He did not know that different neurotypes existed, but he clearly knew he was different from the peers he was being exposed to. Common names Liam would often be called by peer groups included "retard," "dumb fuck," "idiot," and "moron." He was often degraded and not treated well or equally. Liam believed he was these things – he was the odd one out, so these things must be true. As a result, he was extremely depressed and experienced a great deal of anxiety.

2 He was not handling his parents' divorce well. He was being regularly shuffled back and forth between two homes and there had begun to be new people in his life – the parent's new boy- and girlfriends and in some cases their children. Liam was not managing the changes well and it was creating a great deal of dysregulation which in turn was creating some destructive behaviors.

Session 5–10 focused on establishing the therapy goals of improving self-worth, decreasing dysregulation, processing through his parent's divorce, and working on identity issues (telling Liam he was autistic). Many of these therapy goals were going to involve working with the parents. It was clear that there would have to be parent education and a shift in the parent's attitudes and beliefs if Liam was going to progress.

Sessions 11–45 were a combination of addressing the therapy goals – working with Liam in individual therapy, working with Liam's parents, and working with all of them in family therapy. The earlier sessions involved meeting with the parents to provide education and help them understand the importance of telling Liam he was autistic. The parents also needed an understanding of neurodiversity, ableism, and addressing their own issues. This was difficult at times. The parents had to do a lot of work at deconstructing their own ableist beliefs about autism and work on how to support Liam in an affirming manner before Liam could be told about his diagnosis. While I was meeting with the parents, I was also having weekly individual sessions with Liam and we were addressing recognizing strengths, learning regulation interventions, and working on Liam's perspective – helping him understand that many of his past experiences were not about him being wrong but about others not accepting him.

We eventually progressed to a point to tell Liam he was autistic and help explain neurodivergence to him and how this has shaped his life and experiences. His parents needed a lot of support but did make improvement and were able to shift their parenting and relationship with Liam to be more affirming. Liam was not surprised by the autism diagnosis. It seemed he had already done some research and had some suspicion. His anxiety and depression decreased, and he and his parents began finding peers and social outlets that were a better fit for Liam. The final therapy sessions, approximately 46–56 were focused on helping Liam process his parent's divorce and the changes/disruption it had made in his routine and familiarity.

Liam entered therapy with a lot of strengths; it was simply a matter of him recognizing and valuing them. Looking back in reflection, much of Liam's needs were a product of his environments, how people were responding to his autism, and his own lack of awareness. Had Liam (his life) navigated differently – known who he was, been sent affirming and valuing messages about who he was, and "found his people" socially, – it's likely he would have never come to my office.

References

American Music Therapy Association. (2021). What is music therapy? https://www.musictherapy.org/about/musictherapy/

American Occupational Therapy Association. (2021). About occupational therapy. https://www.aota.org/about/for-the-media/about-occupational-therapy

Association for Play Therapy. (2022). Why play therapy? https://www.a4pt.org/page/WhyPlayTherapy

Axline, V. (1947). *Play therapy*. Houghton Mifflin.

Bettelheim, B. (1972). *The empty fortress: Infantile autism and the birth of the self*. Free Press.

Friedman, L. (1999). *Identity's architect: A biography of Erik H. Erikson*. Scribner.

Grant, R. J. (2017). *Autplay therapy for children and adolescents on the autism spectrum a behavioral play-based approach*. Routledge.

Gravitz, L. (2018). At the intersection of autism and trauma. *Spectrum News*. https://www.spectrumnews.org/features/deep-dive/intersection-autism-trauma/

Grinker, R. R. (2020). Autism, "stigma," disability: A shifting historical terrain. *Current Anthropology*, 61(21). doi: 10.1086/705748

Hoover, D. W. (2015). The effects of psychological trauma on children with autism spectrum disorders: A research review. *Review Journal of Autism and Developmental Disorders*, 2, 287–299.

Iannelli, V. (2020). A history and timeline of autism. *Very Well Health*. https://www.verywellhealth.com/autism-timeline-2633213

Jaarsma, P., & Welin, S. (2012). Autism as a natural human variation: Reflections on the claims of the neurodiversity movement. *Health Care Anal*, 20(1), 20–30. doi: 10.1007/s10728-011-0169-9. PMID: 21311979.

Jorgensen, C. (2022). Five reasons why presuming competence is always a good idea. https://swiftschools.org/talk/five-reasons-why-presuming-competence-is-always-a-good-idea

Landreth, G. L. (1991). *Play therapy: The art of the relationship*. Accelerated Development Publishers.

Lobregt-van Buuren, E., Hoekert, M., & Sizoo, B. (2021). Autism, adverse events, and trauma. In A. M. Grabrucker (Ed.), *Autism spectrum disorders* (pp. 33–42). Exon Publications.

O'Reilly, M., Lester, J. N., & Kiyimba, N. (2020). Autism in the twentieth century: An evolution of a controversial condition. In S. Taylor, & A. Brumby

(Eds.), *Healthy minds in the twentieth century. Mental health in historical perspective* (pp. 137–166). Palgrave Macmillan.

Organization for Autism Research. (2016). Help children learn how to self advocate. https://researchautism.org/help-children-learn-how-to-self-advocate/

Prizant, B. M. (2015). *Uniquely human: A different way of seeing autism*. Simon and Schuster.

Rosa, R. (2022). The autism checklist of doom. *Thinking Person's Guide to Autism.* https://thinkingautismguide.com/2022/01/autism-checklist-of-doom.html

Siri, K., & Lyons, T. (2010). *Cutting edge therapies for autism*. Skyhorse Publishing.

Tricaso, K. (2021). What does it mean to be neurodivergent? *Modern Intimacy.* https://www.modernintimacy.com/what-does-it-mean-to-be-neurodivergent/

4
Neurodivergent Play

Playing is a fundamental part of childhood, and it supports children in their physical, cognitive, social, and emotional development. Human development and play are extremely diverse and, depending on socio-cultural norms, some forms of playing are seen as more beneficial or competent than others. When differences in play do not align to socially constructed understanding of normalcy, as often happens to autistic and neurodivergent children, they are generally pathologized and considered faults of the child to be fixed (Waltz, 2020).

Approximately 20 years ago I sat in a training that was focused on working with autistic children. This particular training had a mostly behavioral approach and was targeting professionals outside of mental health. I had hopes it would provide me with some additional information I could use in my play therapy work with autistic and neurodivergent children. About two hours into the one-day training, the presenter began talking about play. I don't remember all of what was covered but I clearly remember the presenter proclaiming that autistic children did not play, they did not know how to play, and thus play approaches would not work for them. The presenter furthered that you could not even teach an autistic child how to play. For me theses proclamations were absurd – I had already been working with several autistic children who played in multiple ways. My takeaway was the clear awareness that there were people (professionals) who really believed that autistic children did not play and were putting forth this view to many other professionals who would walk away believing this was true.

It would be nice to blame this uninformed training/presenter on some behavior-based protocol that was antiquated and out of touch. Unfortunately, the sentiment that autistic children do not play has been a predominant historically belief. I recall finding my way to a popular play therapy training with a highly sought-out play therapist. The training and the presenter lived

DOI: 10.4324/9781003207610-5

up to the hype and 95% of the training was very beneficial. This training was not focused on autistic children, it was focused on a particular play therapy approach and the case examples and application were primarily about neurotypical children. Toward the end of the training, the presenter began talking about who would not benefit from this play therapy approach and who it would not work for. I believe the exact presentation heading was *Exceptions for Using This Approach*. Listed right at the top of three exceptions was autistic children. "Autistic children do not understand play and cannot do this type of play and we would not work with them." Ugh! If the behavioral focused training was not bad enough, now my sacred play therapy space had been tainted.

In another example, that was approximately 15 years ago, I was facilitating a resource booth at a local resource fair that was focused on services related to autism and developmental disabilities. My booth was highlighting AutPlay Therapy with information that could be given to parents to explain AutPlay and how it might be helpful for an autistic or neurodivergent child. At some point in during the fair, a person who oversaw a local "Autism Center" approached me with a smile on their face and said "Hello." I said "Hello" back and then this person said to me "You know play therapy does not work for children with autism, they don't play." "Oh" I said, having been down this road before I knew my response, "Well, what is play therapy?" I think this question surprised them and they begin to fumble a bit and then tell me they had taken a one-hour training about ten years ago on Child Centered Play Therapy so they knew it didn't help autistic children. I nicely began to accurately define play therapy to them, listing off multiple play therapy theories and approaches, talking about the integration of approaches in AutPlay Therapy and sharing multiple examples of autistic children's play. Their response at the end of my free educational lesson was "I didn't know that, well I have heard you are doing good things, I'll talk to you later."

These excerpts from history are arguably not the thoughts and approaches by many today (especially in the play therapy world), but they highlight the widely held beliefs not too long ago, across disciplines, that was wrong about and harmful to autistic children. How many of these self-proclaimed experts who emphatically knew what, how, when, and everything about autistic children were daily implementing "treatments" that were harmful to autistic children? Autistic and neurodivergent children play, they have always played – all throughout history. Historically, it has been "well intended" adults who have stifled, devalued, and failed to recognize the play of autistic and neurodivergent children.

The troubled history begs the question "Are we better now?" The short answer is yes! Over the last ten years there has been a steady and significant increase in understanding autistic and neurodivergent play and how that play can be used to address mental health and other issues. Play therapy theories and approaches began to understand how the therapeutic powers of play were beneficial for autistic children. AutPlay Therapy and other play therapy trainings became more common and play therapists began learning about the mental health needs of neurodivergent children and how play therapy could help meet those needs. Over the last 10–15 years, play therapy research for working with autistic and neurodivergent children has significantly increased. Not only are play therapists understanding that neurodivergent children play, but they are also affirming the play preferences of neurodivergent children and utilizing the therapeutic powers of play for healing and growth.

Outside of the play therapy community, awareness and understanding has also increased. Other disciplines such as speech therapy and occupation therapy purposefully use play in their work with autistic and neurodivergent children. Many professionals seem to be speaking about play as the avenue for working with and helping autistic children. While the shift in thinking is promising, there is a caution. Some of the new ways of awareness and acceptance of play have been contorted into the same historic processes of controlling the child and not letting the child use their natural language of play. For a professional to say they are using play but are controlling the play (typically from their adult perspective) the child does and using play manipulativly to coax the child into another protocol is neither understanding nor affirming the play of autistic and neurodivergent children. Five main constructs separate play therapy theories and approaches from many who advertise "using" play or implementing a "play-based" approach with neurodivergent children. The five main constructs include:

- Play is the natural language of children. It is the way they understand best to communicate with themselves and others. To suppress their natural language is equivalent to placing tape over the mouth of an adult whose primary mode of communication is verbal.
- Play is the change agent, not a manipulative tool to lure the child to something else that is considered the change agent. Play is not to be used as a manipulative tool.
- Play preferences and interests are understood, valued, and if possible, utilized (focused on) to help address mental health needs and goals. The child is met where they are, with their way of playing (without

judgment). The neurodivergent child is not forced to conform their play to a societal neurotypical view of what play looks like.

• Play is never withheld to get compliance. Play is not held back as a reward to get the child to perform.

• The therapeutic powers of play (defined further in Chapter 5) are understood and utilized in play therapy.

How Do Neurodivergent Children Play?

Play is the natural language of all children regardless of diagnosis, disability, or developmental issue. It is the most organic process for children to express troubling thoughts and feelings that are both conscious and unconscious. Play makes learning an enjoyable and engaging experience and provides the best method to impart information needed by children to overcome struggles (Schaefer & Drewes, 2014). When working with neurodivergent children, it is important to discover what their language of play looks and sounds like. The AutPlay Assessment of Play (in the appendix of this book) is an inventory designed to help therapists gain more information about the neurodivergent child's play preferences and interests (their unique language of play).

The AutPlay Assessment of Play is typically completed by a parent/caregiver of the child or another adult who knows the child well. It is divided into two sections. Section one lists several types of play (with descriptions). There is a 1–10 scale where the parents can circle the number they believe their child is currently at in terms of showing or not showing the particular type of play – a 1 means does not show, and a 10 means shows very much. Section two provides several open-ended questions about play. The parent is instructed to answer the questions as best they can. This is a tool that therapists can use to help learn more about the child and their play preferences. It is important to note that the neurodivergent child may play in a way or exhibit a type of play that is not listed on this inventory. The neurodivergent child can play in any way their system desires and it can be an original type of play. The child's play is their play. It does not have to fit a preconceived category, and it can be uniquely their own style of play.

The therapist must begin with a healthy understanding of the individualization and uniqueness of neurodivergent play and value the play preferences of each child. With this understand in mind, there are some common play themes and expressions. Some of the more common manifestations of play include constructive play, functional play, sensory play, exploratory play, reenactment play, and solitary play, etc. The following highlights several types of play with a discussion of the play type regarding neurodivergent children.

Constructive play – A type of children's play that resembles the meaning of the word. It is any play that involves constructing, building, putting together, and/or creating something with their hands. This might include playing with LEGO bricks, building a train track or race car track, playing with blocks or any building type materials (Lincoln Logs, etc.), Mr. and Ms. Potato Head, large cardboard blocks, etc. Neurodivergent children may enjoy solitary play when doing constructive play – preferring to build, create, etc. on their own without participation from others. For some neurodivergent children, constructive play may provide the opportunity for therapists to engage and help with the construction (working together to create).

I recall working with twin autistic boys. They very much preferred doing everything together and rarely displayed solitary play. Both of their play preference was constructive play. They would enter the playroom and create elaborate train tracks and racetracks utilizing sandtray miniatures and anything they could find to adorn the environment. They would work in unison and often without saying one word to each other. Their joint constructive play was powerful in helping their parents and other adults in their life understand their creativity, intellect, and abilities, much of which was not being noticed or even considered prior to them entering play therapy.

Functional play – Means playing with something in the way (or function) it is intended to be played with or how it would typically be understood in functionality. This might include setting up a plastic bowling set in the playroom and then bowling. Another example would be taking a toy piece of bread and placing it in a toy toaster, then serving the toast on a toy plate. Functional play stays within the perceived accurate function of the toy. Many autistic and neurodivergent children will participate in functional play, especially if is it something they have seen, done, or are familiar with in their real life. Sometimes functional play provides an opportunity for mastery, accomplishment, practice, and curiosity with happenings they have experienced in their day-to-day lives. Some functional play provides a natural opportunity to be involved in the child's play either by the child's initiative (placing the therapist in a role) or by the therapist joining in an obvious participate role.

Sensory play – Many neurodivergent children engage in sensory play. This sometimes relates to having sensory differences or needs and sometimes it is simply the play preference of the child. Sensory play can be regulating, calming, and enjoyable for the child. The play can vary but typically addresses a sensory related system (area) such as playing in the sand tray for a tactile sensory experience or maneuvering on an exercise ball for a proprioceptive or vestibular sensory experience. Therapists should think about the different sensory areas and be mindful to include toys and materials in their playroom that address each area.

Exploratory play – This type of play is characterized by the child exploring and investigating in their play. This usually involves the ability to have free play and within the free play process, the child can explore toys, materials, the environment as they desire.

Reenactment play – This has sometimes been referred to as scripted play. The child will play with various toys and materials and reenact a scene from a favorite movie, TV show, or video game. Typically, the child will reenact the scene repeatedly – possibly multiple times a day. This might be the primary way the child plays. The child may include others in the play but usually the "script" must be adhered to and there is no changing or adjusting from the original scene.

Solitary play – A child may prefer to be solitary and exclusively or primarily play by themselves. Solitary play would not involve another person. The child might be in a room with other children but would typically not notice them. The child would be focused on something they are playing with and not seek to include or get involved with others. The solitary play could include any type of toy, material, or game that the child is playing with by themselves.

Pretend play – A type of symbolic play where children might use a variety of toys, objects, actions, or ideas to represent something else (people, animals, ideas, fantasy) using their imaginations to assign roles to inanimate objects or people. Any variety of toy or material may be used, and children may do pretend play with others or solitary. The concept of metaphor is often a component of pretend play. This type of play gives the child the opportunity to create, imagine, and "go" with their play wherever they want. Pretend play is a type of play often used and seen in many play therapy theories and approaches.

Dramatic Play – Can be part of or like pretend or symbolic play. Typically, a child pretends to take on a role of someone else, imitating someone real or a character. When another person becomes involved in the play, it is called sociodramatic play. The elements of reality and make-believe are involved as children imitate real-life people like a mother or father, a doctor, a schoolteacher, etc. and situations (going to the dentist, getting their haircut, a funeral) they have experienced. Pretend play often becomes a part of dramatic play as children may embellish or change the person, character, or situation.

Group play – Some children may struggle with groups (playing with more than one person) and the complexities that they may bring. Some children may desire group play but struggle with dynamics of multiple peers, fast changing processes, and sensory issues. Some may not like group play and simply prefer one-on-one or solitary play. In my personal experience, I preferred one-on-one and solitary play. I did understand group play; I was not waiting for some well-intended adult to come along and explain group play to me and then I would love it because I finally understood it. I understood how it worked and what the processes were, what people were supposed to do in group play – I simply didn't like it as much as one-on-one or solitary play.

Movement play – This type of play is mostly what is sounds like. It is play that involves movement of some type. The movement play can vary greatly from running and playing a game of catch, acting out charades, or rolling around on the floor. Movement play has been shown to be beneficial for a variety of developmental areas including physical, communication, cognitive, and social/emotional. It is also helpful for children with sensory differences and needs. For the play therapist, this involves consideration of how movement play can be supported in the playroom. This might mean opening space for larger movement play and/or adding items into the playroom that promote movement. This type of play can be done in solitary or with one or more people. Many neurodivergent children find movement play interventions helpful for regulation needs.

Art play – This type of play involves the use of art-related materials. This might include musical instruments, singing, dancing, drama, drawing, painting, molding clay, and writing – many forms of creation. Some children are more inclined to art-related play and prefer this type of play. Art play provides a vast opportunity for exploration, expression, and commutation. Many neurodivergent children may find art play regulating. Therapists should be mindful to include a variety of art related materials in their playroom.

Adult Led play – Adults often coordinate, facilitate, and lead children through play times. This is referred to as adult-led play. This can be a variety of types of play, it can include many different toys and materials. The adult may introduce and facilitate playing a board game, playing one-on-one basketball, leading a group of children through the game of *Simon Says*, or in some fashion be the lead out in how the play is done. This can be the type of play that most adults are comfortable playing with children. It may or may not be a type of play the child would like to engage with. Many children need the opportunity of showing their play preference and having the adult join it or follow them in their play preferences. Adult-led play interventions and play times can be beneficial but adult-led play should not monopolize the child's play and the therapist should always be seeking to discover the neurodivergent child's play preferences.

Educational play – Situations or "play" times that are typically created by an adult with the goal to provide some type of education or learning experience through the play. The play is often seen as an engaging element to gain greater participation from the child and provide an element of enjoyment for the child while they learn a specific concept or skill. Educational play is often adult-led.

The Integration and Complexities of Neurodivergent Play

Play presents a popular pastime for all humans, though not all humans play alike (Spiel & Gerling, 2020). It should be well understood and expected that neurodivergent children play. Neurodivergent children may share some commonalities, but they also represent a wide spectrum or presentation of identity. Thus, they will also display a wide range of plays. The complexities of neurodivergent play are not complex for the neurodivergent child – they understand their play preferences and interests and value (without judgment) their play. It is often the adult (usually a neurotypical adult) that finds the neurodivergent child's play complex. This is often coming from a pre-determined and conditioned view of play. When the adult encounters neurodivergent play that does not fit the preconceived notion of play, the adult has a difficult time recognizing and valuing the neurodivergent child's play.

Consider the following excerpt from an autistic teen's transcript notes and script for their video presentation and keynote address at Autistics Present Symposium: Essential Youth Voices on October 19, 2019 (Mydske, 2019).

> When I was young doctors and therapists told my mom I needed to play differently. When I'm told that I play in the wrong way it makes me feel kind of upset. I liked lining up toys for lots and lots of reasons, but no one had ever asked me why. The pros of lining up toys is some people like to have things in order, some people like to look at patterns and they've helped... they helped me see all the parts to rebuild them in different ways and that is creativity more or less. It also made me feel good to look at my collection and it never hurt anybody either.
>
> I interact with the world in autistic ways and there is nothing wrong with that.

There is no right way to play but the most important thing is that everyone has fun. Just because you don't understand the value of doing things
my way, that doesn't make it wrong. Telling people how they have to
play kind of defeats the purpose of playing in the first place.

Play is not work; it holds a natural, intrinsic value (Landreth, 1991). Play
performs an important preventative function in the lives of children and
serves as an intervention to assist children in coping with personal challenges. Research continues to demonstrate that play performs an important
role in the development of the brain – rehearsing behaviors, creating neural
connections, learning to problem-solve, and developing creativity (Taylor,
2019). Unfortunately, play is sometimes misunderstood by adults who work
with children. Play can be seen a silly, meaningless, a waste of time, and is
often taken away in place of something "more important" or withheld as a
reward for some type of compliance.

Regarding play, there seems to be two fundamental questions and possible
issues with adults working with neurodivergent children. (1) Does the adult
understand the therapeutic powers and importance of play, or do they view
it as frivolous? (2) If the adult does believe in the therapeutic powers and
importance of play, does the adult believe that autistic and neurodivergent
children play, or do they believe that play, and its therapeutic powers, are
somehow lost on neurodivergent children? In AutPlay Therapy the growth
and healing dynamics of play are well understood and are the forefront of
the therapy work being done. Further, AutPlay protocol unequivocally recognizes that neurodivergent children play and their play is no less beneficial
and is no less important than any child's play. Figure 4.1 illustrates some
of the possible play preferences that neurodivergent children may exhibit.
They are presented in equal importance – one type of play or preference of
play is not more important that another.

There is no optimal way to play, and children cannot fail at play. Yet time
and time again, play is boxed into neat and contained categories, often ex-
cluding neurodivergent children. Think of the times you've heard someone
say that autistic children cannot role-play or be imaginative. It immediately
frames autism as 'lacking' when it comes to playing. The therapeutic powers
of play rejects rigid descriptions of play and acknowledges that it has endless
and unknown possibilities. Essentially, play cannot be fully defined because
it is so vast. Our role as therapists is to become play protagonists. We need
to become curious, rather than dubious, when we see play that we might not
understand. And we need to introduce a play-rich environment for autistic
and neurodivergent children (Murphy, 2021).

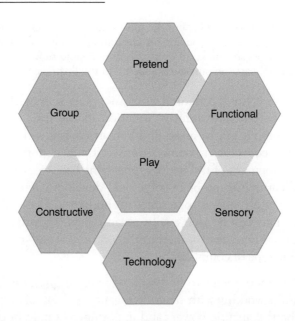

Figure 4.1 The Spectrum of Play. What Are the Neurodivergent Child's Play Preferences?

Murphy (2021) proposed several tips for working with and implementing play with autistic and neurodivergent children:

- Be open minded during play and challenge your conventional perceptions of what play "looks" like.
- Don't shut play down too early just because you don't immediately understand where it's going.
- Allow children control and ownership of their play.
- Use a "small dose" approach to learning, and don't be afraid to break tasks down further to support development.
- Focus on the unique child, what they need and assess how best to support them. Help them find out who they are and flourish in what they find, instead of 'fixing' them and looking at their behavior through a neurotypical lens.
- Always start with the characteristics of effective learning for an insight into who the child is as a learner.
- Don't separate the child from the process of play for the purpose of intervention.
- Make sure to read signs of engagement, involvement, and non-consent when interacting with a child.

Neurodivergent children will play if they are given the space to do so. They will play and they will access the value and benefits of play. For adults who wish to join children in their play and/or utilize the child's play for therapeutic work – it all starts with relationship! For the therapist, it is the interwoven nature of the natural language (play) of the child and the development of the therapeutic relationship that creates the atmosphere for growth and healing. The way the play therapist understands the integration of these two constructs and facilitates their existence in a naturalistic rhythm is the key to laying the foundation for neurodivergent children to address their mental health needs.

Consider the writing *How to Play with an Autistic Child* (Vance, 2020). It beautifully illustrates the importance of building relationship, attuning to the child, and respecting and entering their play.

> If your autistic child is playing by lining up toys or doing something repetitive, bring your own toys, assume a reasonable distance, and play happily and silently. Use sparkly toys, blocks, cars, spinning toys, pots and pans, kinetic sand, magnets, canned food, stickers, dry pasta, colorful dough, etc.
>
> Try something new if it doesn't work the first time. Make a craft. Spin something that sparkles. Meditate and quiet your mind. Find contentment in not worrying, fixing, controlling. Let it all go and stare into a shiny pinwheel. Watch the way the light bounces and bends, sending a spattering of dancing lights over your face and chest. Grab a handful of raw pasta and let it fall from your fingers and try to feel and visualize how many have fallen.
>
> Put an individual drop of water on the back of your hand. See if you can feel each fine, barely-visible hair bend as it slides off. Don't think of autism. Don't think of bills. Don't think. Experience. Breathe consciously. Conjure a beautiful or a fiery song in your head.
>
> See if you can make your mind play each note in memory. If you can't, listen harder next time. Don't hear. Listen. Once you have learned to be still, present, breathing, realize how connected you feel to your child, and to all things, in that moment.
>
> Your child might be curious to join you. They might give you the most profound gift of communicating without the baggage and bondage of words. You will learn nothing. You will unlearn. If your child doesn't join, just feel. Feel close. Don't feel disappointed. Feel love. Relax.
>
> Your child might be so sensitive to your tension, worry, and fear that they internalize it. Just be. Think like your child. Lie opposite your child

and color in a coloring book. Knit. Blow bubbles in the house. Color on the walls and laugh at how fun it is. Magic erasers work.

Eat your dinner while sitting on the floor. Use your fingers. Do this more often, and watch your relationship transform. Play like an autistic and watch your life improve. Laugh at yourself for playing, not in a performative way. Belly laugh at the rebellion.

If your child joins, great. If not, great. You have spent quality time together. You have communicated something profound. You have said: I enjoy being me while you're being you – together.

Respecting neurodivergent play means challenging assumptions about what play is and how to measure it. It means reminding ourselves that just because a child does not play with pink and blue plastic toys doesn't mean they are not playing. It means not asking a child to show you their play "skills" and devaluing their play preferences. It means understanding their play can look anyway they like, and our job is to join them in their play without judgment. Respecting neurodivergent play means the mental health community needs to apologize for decades of mistakenly insisting that autistic and other neurodivergent children do not play and play therapy approaches would not work for them. It means asking what I can do differently to honor the child's play instead of forcing the child to play the way I deem is play.

Case Examples of Play

The following case examples are vignettes that highlight the child's play preferences. In each example there were some additional processes and components that are not covered in the example. The purpose of the examples is to better illustrate the variety of play preferences of neurodivergent children.

Len

Len entered AutPlay Therapy as a 12-year-old male diagnosed with ADHD and sensory issues. His parents described Len as having a difficult time regulating and expressing his emotions and challenges socially with peers. Len presented as a quite pre-teen and was cooperative and seemingly interested in being in therapy. He concurred with his parent's description of himself and added that he also has challenges dealing with his younger sister. As part of the AutPlay intake and assessment phase, Len was given a tour of the whole clinic and shown all the playrooms, the sandtray room, and the outdoor play area. Len did not seem interested in much play (he did not like pretend play or technology play) and the beginning sessions he mostly wanted to stay in my office and talk, although his conversional talk was usually minimal. He had indicated on a play assessment that he liked sports, especially football, so we explored some outdoor play such as throwing the football back and forth, but it really didn't seem to engage Len.

Around session 6, Len asked if he could "Go to that room that had all the little things and sand." I said "yes," and we went to the sandtray room. Len had never participated in any type of sandtray work, but he was highly interested. I introduced the sandtray room to him giving him a basic description. I asked him if he wanted to create a sand tray and he did. I told him he could create whatever he wanted, or I could give him a theme. He requested a theme, so I asked him to create a sand tray describing himself and his life. Len created a tray and shared about himself and his life for about 10 minutes. This was the most expressive and communicative Len had been since beginning therapy. After he was finished, I asked him if he wanted to create a tray any way he wanted. He did, and he created another tray and again thoroughly shared about his tray.

We continued to do sandtray work with Len each session and occasionally implemented other forms of expressive techniques. Len responded most positively to these types of play and interventions. These approaches served the basis for our work toward his therapy goals. It is important to note a few things about Len's example:

- Len discovered a type of play that resonated with him (something he had not been doing in his life) and could be used to help Len work on his therapy goals. I was comfortable with and allowed this process to unfold for Len to find his play preferences.
- Initially, I tried some different things (outdoor football play) based on my understand of Len, but I did not force anything and if something was not a fit, we moved on.
- Len's play preferences were not just a discovery of play; they provided an avenue for him to express himself and address his therapy needs.

Brent

Brent entered AutPlay therapy as a nine-year-old male diagnosed with autism. His parents were concerned that Brent seemed depressed and had a great deal of anxiety – mostly associated with going to school and interacting with peers. Brent presented very interested in play therapy but was minimally active. He did not say much but seemed focused and attuned. His play assessment did not show any specific play preferences. His parents indicated that he did not do much play at home. Brent had received a tour of the clinic (including the playrooms) and he seemed most interested in being in one of the playrooms that had a specific type of toy – Goo Jit Zu figures. These are characters that are stretchy, squishy, and have different materials inside of them for different tactile experiences when you play with them. Brent really liked the Goo Jit Zu figures and wanted to play with them every session. He would set them up to battle each other and enjoyed simply stretching and squishing them in his hands.

I quickly noticed that Brent was drawn to sensory play. My office and all the playrooms are healthily stocked with sensory toys and materials. Brent would often play with tactile sensory toys manipulating them in his hands. He also enjoyed play that moved his body. He would balance on the wobble board and his favorite was hopping on an exercise ball in my office and then bouncing his body off the ball. He would do this play repeatedly. Through observation I discovered that Brent sought tactile and proprioceptive sensory input, and this was the type of play he was most drawn toward. I worked with Brent and his parents to establish a regulation/sensory playtime at home that the family could do together. This was successful and greatly helped reduce Brent's feeling of anxiety and depressions. Throughout therapy, he became more regulated and emotionally felt in a positive place. A few things to note about Brent's example:

- Brent was given the space and opportunity to discover and show his play preference. I was keenly aware of Brent and observing his play to better understand his play interests.
- The discovery of Brent's sensory play and further his sensory needs were new to Brent and his parents. This enabled a referral for Brent to access sensory based therapy at school which helped with some of Brent's school issues.
- Brent's anxiety and depression (his overall dysregulation) was greatly improved by utilizing Brent's play preferences and involving his parents in creating a regulation play time at home, which not only helped Brent, but he also enjoyed.
- There were additional issues addressed in this case. There were some school advocacy issues that needed work and some additional parent sessions, but the focus of the example is on highlighting the play of Brent.

Ella

Ella entered AutPlay Therapy as a ten-year-old female diagnosed with autism and sensory processing disorder. Ella's parents were concerned about her becoming dysregulated very easily and this would usually lead to physical aggression toward others. She was also struggling in school with peers, sensory issues, and becoming overwhelmed. Ella's play assessment indicated that Ella enjoyed expressive activities, and anything related to art and craft creation. She did not like or participate in pretend, movement, or technology play.

The majority of Ella's sessions focused on expressive art play. Ella would create many things and we explored a variety of feelings and thoughts about herself through the expressive play. Ella would share much of this with her parents which increased dialogue and understating between Ella and her parents. One key intervention was the creation of a sensory mandala. This is a technique I created for Ella. It combined the expressive play she enjoyed with a sensory regulation technique. The idea come from contemplating a way that Ella could regulate herself when she noticed she was feeling overwhelmed. She liked creating mandalas and found this process calming. I gathered several tactile items (cotton balls, ribbon, pipe cleaners, sandpaper, buttons, beads, etc.) and several olfactory items (scented stickers, scented markers, essential oil spray, etc.) and introduced the idea to Ella for creating a sensory mandala.

The basic instruction for a sensory mandala is to draw the mandala circle on a piece of card stock (this is heavier than regular paper and holds the material better). The child can then draw or write anything they want in the mandala, but they also add sensory (tactile and olfactory) items into the mandala. They typical glue or tape the items in the mandala. The child takes time to manipulate, feel, and smell each item to choose the ones they enjoy. The items along with whatever the child draws/colors forms the mandala. Figure 4.2 provides an example of a sensory mandala. Once they have finished, they can keep the mandala for refence.

Ella loved the sensory mandala. She began to create several of them in play sessions and at home. Her parents supported this play by stocking her room with sensory mandala materials. Over time, Ella began to notice when she was feeling dysregulated at home and would go into her room without any prompting from her parents and create a sensory mandala to help her regulate. This would take her around 30 minutes and then she would return to the rest of the family feeling regulated. The sensory mandala play became a

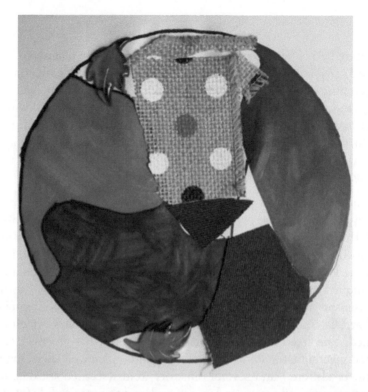

Figure 4.2 Sensory Mandala Example.

great tool for Ella in helping her address her therapy goals. A few notes about Ella's case example:

- Ella is a great example of her play preferences and interests being used to help address her needs. In the process, she leaned about herself and discovered sustainable things she could do to help her system regulate.
- I did not try to force her to play in any other way. We went with her play preferences. Not only was this helpful but it also facilitated health relationship development.
- I did address some additional things in this case. Similar to Brent's case, there were some school advocacy needs and some parent sessions but the focus of this example is highlighting the preference and effectiveness of expressive play with some neurodivergent children.

Danny

Danny entered AutPlay Therapy as an eight-year-old male diagnosed with autism (with a presentation similar to pathological demand avoidance). Danny's parents were concerned that he was experiencing a great deal of anxiety, often debilitating, resulting in him not being able to leave his home. Going to school was especially challenging. Danny's play assessment and observations clearly displayed that Danny liked pretend play. During his play observations, he was fully engaged with many toys in the playroom creating scenes, symbolism, and engaging in pretend play. His parents acknowledged this was typical of Danny, he spent most of his time in pretend play and preferred this activity over all others.

Danny's sessions were very similar to child centered play therapy sessions. Danny would enter the playroom and immediately begin to engage in pretend play. One of his favorite things was to use several of the puppets and create an elaborate story about them all competing in a contest. They each had names and personalities and ways they would interact with each other. Danny created a running story about the puppet characters competing in a contest where each week one of them would get limited. There was a great deal of fantasy play happening and Danny would always include me, putting me in the role of several of the puppet characters. As sessions went on, I began to see play themes emerging in Danny's puppet play. There were consistent themes of the unknown, unpredictable, how things could change and surprise you and you were not prepared. These were all played out in a negative context – the unpredictable was bad and scary for the puppets. He also began to play out themes that looked very similar to issues he was having at school. The characters would struggle (in their own way) with things he was struggling with at school. When Danny would have a victory at school, the puppets would have a victory in their journey.

Danny's fantasy/pretend puppet play provided many natural opportunities to address and express his emotions and concerns. There was depth, elaborateness, and healing elements in his pretend play. It was important that I recognize this and see the expression of his natural language as essential therapeutic process. A few notes about Danny's case example:

- It was easy to identify Danny's play presences as he went right to the playroom and began engaging in pretend play. It created an easy understanding for me (the therapist) to support Danny through a more nondirective (child centered play therapy) process.

- Danny expressed himself through his characters – his worries, his struggles, his victories. It provided a space of expression and exploration and well as resolution.
- Danny is a good example of not devaluing the play preference of pretend play. As sessions went on, Danny began to talk more about himself and his experiences/needs. Some solutions he came to on his own through his play, others we were able to talk about together. The valuing of his play preference instead of trying to force him into a more directive or "talk therapy" process gave him the space to feel safe, heard, and express himself.

References

Landreth, G. L. (1991). *Play therapy: The art of the relationship*. Accelerated Development Publishers.

Murphy, K. (2021). Neurodiverse play is the way. https://www.famly.co/blog/neurodiverse-play-is-the-way

Mydske, L. W. (2019). Respecting autistic ways of playing, interacting & making friends. https://neurodiversitylibrary.org/2019/10/20/respecting-autistic-ways-of-playing-interacting-making-friends/

Schaefer, C. E. & Drewes, A. A. (2014). *The therapeutic powers of play: 20 core change agents* (2nd ed.). John Wiley & Sons.

Spiel, K., & Gerling, K. (2020). The purpose of play: How HCI games research fails neurodivergent populations. *ACM Transactions on Computer Human Interact*, 28(2). https://doi.org/10.1145/3432245

Taylor, E. R. (2019). *Solution-focused therapy with children and adolescents: Creative and play based approaches*. Routledge.

Vance, T. (2020). How to play with your autistic child. https://neuroclastic.com/how-to-playwith-your-autistic-child/

Waltz, M. (2020). The production of the 'normal' child: Neurodiversity and the commodification of parenting. In H. Rosqvist, N. Chown, & A. Stenning (Eds.), *Neurodiversity studies* (pp. 15–26). Routledge.

5
Play Therapy and the Therapeutic Powers of Play

Play Therapy

Play is a child's form of improvisational dramatics. Playing is how the child tries out and learns about their world, and it is therefore essential to their healthy development. For the child, play is serious, purposeful business through which they develop mentally, emotionally, physically, and socially. Play is the child's form of self-therapy, through which confusions, anxieties, frustrations, pain, and conflicts are often processed. Play performs a vital function for the child. It is far more than just the frivolous, lighthearted, pleasurable activity that adults usually make of it. Play also serves as a language for the child – a symbolism that substitute words. The child uses play to formulate and assimilate what they experience (Oaklander, 2007).

Origins of play therapy can be traced back to the early 1900s. Anna Freud and Melanie, Klein, and David Levy are often credited with being pioneers in the field for introducing play in therapy and setting the foundation for further development. In the 1940s, Virginia Axline applied the philosophy and constructs of person-centered therapy in her work in counseling children. Ray (2011) stated that Axline was especially influential on play therapy's development as she was the first play therapist to undertake extensive investigation of her therapy methods through research. Second, she provided a structure to the theory and delivery of play therapy in her publication *Play Therapy* (Axline, 1947). Third, she published the book *Dibs: In Search of Self* (Axline, 1964) detailing the course of play therapy over a year with a child.

Play therapy as a field became more formalized and established by forward-thinking clinicians in 1982 with Charles Schaefer and Kevin O'Conner founding the Association for Play Therapy (APT) and Garry Landreth, Louise Guerney, and others envisioning a movement of individuals joined by a common interest in play as a therapeutic model. In 1983, a small group of

DOI: 10.4324/9781003207610-6

people gathered to have the first national play therapy conference in New York. The gathering included around 50 professionals (Gil, 2021).

The play therapy field has always been exciting in its evolution. The Association for Play Therapy (APT) (2022b) recently developed and published a list of the seminal theories of play therapy that are valid and reliable methods for guiding its practice. Those foundational theories include Psychoanalytic, Behavioral, Humanistic, Adlerian, Developmental, and Jungian, to name a few. These theories are well articulated and established, and ongoing research and practice efforts are underfoot to target key issues that might benefit from different forms of play therapy, such as ADHD, OCD, anxiety and depression, anger and dysregulation, gender identity concerns, suicidal tendencies, and other symptomatic behaviors or conditions. In addition, play therapists have documented methods for providing services to specific target groups: traumatized children, witnesses of interpersonal violence, children with sexual behavior problems, children with anxious attachment behaviors, developmental disabilities, etc. And still other play therapists have developed and shared expertise on working with infants and toddlers, elementary-aged, or teen clients, as well as couples and families. And thus, the plethora of approaches and interventions continue, likely falling into one of the seminal theories, and allowing therapists to customize their techniques to meet unique needs of the target groups mentioned, and those that will emerge (Gil, 2021).

"Play therapy" can best be thought of as an umbrella term, as there are currently several play therapy theories and approaches that exist. Play therapy approaches range from being nondirective to directive in terms of the therapist's involvement in the process with their clients. Some theories and approaches of play therapy rely heavily on the use of toys and props while other theories use toys minimally. Most play therapy approaches involve some use of toys, props, art, music, movement, or games as an avenue to help clients achieve their therapeutic goals. The Association for Play Therapy (2022a) defines play therapy as the systematic use of a theoretical model to establish an interpersonal process wherein trained play therapists use the therapeutic powers of play to help clients prevent or resolve psychosocial difficulties and achieve optimal growth and development.

Currently, the Association for Play Therapy recognizes ten seminal and/or historically significant play therapy theories and approaches. The list includes Adlerian, Child-Centered, Cognitive-Behavioral, Developmental (Viola Brody), Ecosystemic, Filial, Gestalt, Jungian, Object-Relations, and Theraplay. Beyond these ten recognized, there exist several established and emerging play therapy theories, approaches, and modalities such as Sandtray Therapy, Family Play Therapy, Experiential Play Therapy, Expressive Play Therapy, Relationship Play Therapy, First Play, AutPlay Therapy, Digital Play Therapy, TraumaPlay, Solution Focused Play Therapy, Synergetic Play Therapy, and Animal Assisted Play Therapy – to name a few.

Many play therapists self-identify as an integrative play therapist (combining different therapeutic methods, interventions, and approaches to best fit the needs of the individual client) or prescriptive play therapist (selecting and implementing a particular play therapy approach that research has indicated is likely to be the most effective for a specific problem or symptom). The possibilities of what "play therapy" might mean or look like in implementation are so varied that I often teach parents if someone tells you they do play therapy, the next question you should ask is "What type of play therapy do you do?" (Grant, 2021).

Play therapy is not the same as regular, everyday play. While spontaneous play is a natural and essential part of the developmental process, play therapy is a systematic and therapeutic approach. Play therapists have earned a graduate mental health degree and are licensed mental health professionals with extensive training, supervision, and education in Play Therapy (The Association for Play Therapy, 2022a). Play therapy incorporates a growing number of evidence-based practices and techniques and should only be utilized by specially trained mental health professionals. While some play therapists do not possess a specialized play therapy credential, a Registered Play Therapist (RPT), Registered Play Therapist-Supervisor (RPT-S), or School Based-Registered Play Therapist (SB-RPT) are those professionals who have met the stringent standards set by APT to become a credentialed Play Therapist.

Play therapy approaches have been successfully implemented for children, adolescents, adults, families, couples, and groups. Play therapy offers the ability to communicate inter-processes and emotions without using verbal communication and provides awareness properties to help put words to otherwise unidentified issues. The freedom from judgment and the ability to create and explore through play therapy offers safety for clients and facilitates an almost innate desire that exists in all people – the desire to play. Kottman and Meany-Walen (2018) highlighted the variance and complexities within play therapy:

> There are many things to consider when you examine the logistics of play therapy: stages of play therapy; skills, strategies, and techniques; toys and play therapy materials; explanation of play therapy for parent and clients; the first session; what to do in sessions; how to end a session;

course of therapy, and termination. The process of play therapy can unfold in multiple ways depending on the theoretical approach to play
therapy and a therapist's personal preferences.

(p. 13)

Kevin J. O' Conner (2000) contended that there is a biological, intraper-
sonal, interpersonal, and sociocultural function of play behavior in the lives
of children and furthered the definition of play therapy: play therapy consists of a cluster of treatment modalities that involve the systematic use of a
theoretical model to establish an interpersonal process wherein trained play
practitioners use the therapeutic powers of play to help clients prevent or resolve psychosocial difficulties and achieve optimal growth and development
and the re-establishment of the child's ability to engage in play behavior as
it is classically defined.

The benefits of children engaging in play include cognitive development
(learning, thinking, and planning, etc.), social needs (practicing social interaction, roles and routines), language (talking to others, turn taking, etc.),
problem-solving (negotiation, asking for help, solving difficulties, etc.), and
emotional development (managing feelings, understanding others, empathy,
etc.). Children with play skills are more likely to be included with their
peers and play is a key learning tool through which children develop social
navigation, flexibility, core learning skills, and language. Play also provides
opportunities for children to practice events, situations, and routines in a
safe place, with no pressure to "get it right" (Phillips & Beavan, 2010).

Play therapy is a theoretical modality that uses a wide variety of methodologies
to communicate with clients, including adventure therapy, storytelling and
therapeutic metaphors, movement/dance/music experiences, sandtray activities, art techniques, and structured play experiences in addition to free, un-
structured play. Interactions in play therapy should always allow for and even
encourage self-expression, creative representation, and imagination. Play therapy is a relationship in which a trained therapist creates a safe space for clients
to explore and express themselves (Kottman & Meany-Walen, 2018, p. 6).

Hudspeth (2021) stated that for play therapists, their play therapy is an-
chored in one or more of the seminal play therapy theories. A play therapist's theoretical orientation runs like a thread through everything from
conceptualization to assessment to diagnosis to treatment planning to delivery and through termination. It unifies what they see and do into a tightly
woven bundle. For a play therapist, play is the language and toys are the
words clients use; play is more than a tool and a means to an end (Landreth,
2012). It is the developmentally appropriate and naturalistic conduit that

incorporates the therapeutic process and the relationship provided to help clients evolve positively in their overall growth and development. Kottman and Meany-Walen (2018) expressed that play therapy responds to the developmental level of the person and the area of the brain impacted by distressing events. Play therapy is different from "just playing" because the presence of an empathic and attuned witness helps clients process their experiences, feelings, and thoughts.

Play therapy isn't just a nice idea. To date, there are four peer-reviewed published meta-analyses on outcome effect of play therapy interventions; one meta-analysis includes a systematic review. Lin and Bratton (2015) conducted meta-analysis with 24 child-centered play therapy studies and concluded that play therapy demonstrated a statistically significant effect. Ray et al. (2015) performed a meta-analysis and systematic review of 23 child-centered play therapy RCTs conducted in schools and concluded that play therapy demonstrated statistically significant outcomes for children with disruptive behavior, internalizing, self-efficacy, and academic problems. Bratton et al. (2005) employed meta-analysis with 67 play therapy studies and found statistically significant effects with medium effect size, concluding that play therapy was effective with both internalizing and externalizing problems. LeBlanc and Ritchie (2001) used meta-analysis to explore findings of 42 RCTs on play therapy, reporting statistically significant effects with moderate treatment effect size. Table 5.1 highlights the published metanalysis (Ray & McCullough, 2016).

Ray (2011) developed a list of functions served by play in play therapy resulting from a review of the history and theories of play:

1 Fun: The use of play in play therapy provides the opportunity for fun, either for the child or for the therapist and child. Although it is recognized that play is not always fun for the child, especially in therapy, it can often be fun. The allowance of fun in a therapeutic environment lowers a child's resistance to the therapeutic relationship and offers an experience that is often missing from the life of a child who is experiencing several environmental conflicts.

2 Symbolic expression: Play in play therapy allows for the symbolic expression of thoughts and feelings. As eloquently presented by both Piaget and Vygotsky, children use symbols for the acquisition of language and expression of emotion and cognition. The symbolic expression of play in therapy invites the play therapist into the child's world. The child is no longer confined by reality and can pretend, creating scenes for the expression of emotion or building of coping skills.

Table 5.1 Overview of Four Peer-Reviewed Published Meta-Analyses on Outcome
Effect of Play Therapy Interventions

Authors	Number of Studies	Mean Age	Effect Size	Favorable Outcomes
Lin and Bratton (2015)	24	6.7 years	33[a]	Externalizing and internalizing behavior problems; caregiver-child relationship stress; self-efficacy
Ray et al. (2015)	23	Range 4–13 years No Mean Reported	.21–.38[a]	Externalizing and internalizing behavior problems; self-efficacy; academic; other
Bratton et al. (2005)	67	7.0 years	.72[a]	Behavior problems; social adjustment; self-concept; anxiety; development; relationships; other
LeBlanc and Ritchie (2001)	42	7.8 years	.66[a]+	Emotional adjustment; social adjustment; reaction to traumatic event; academic; behavior problems; family adjustment

Source: Ray and McCullough (2015; revised 2016).

[a] ES is statistically significant + Studies included parent-involvement.

3 Catharsis: Play in play therapy allows a child to work through those issues of greatest consequence to the child. Nondirected play provides an
   environment in which the child chooses direction of effort.
4 Social development: Play not only allows for the expression of the child's
   world, but also promotes communication between child and therapist –
   or in the case of group play therapy, between peers. The building and
   maintaining a nurturing relationship facilitated through play strengthens a child's social motivation and skills.
5 Mastery: In play therapy, play is used by the child to control their world.
   They have the power to be anything and the capability to do anything.
   They are not limited by real-world restraints. The child uses play in

play therapy to develop a sense of control and competence over the environment.

6 Release of energy: Although the use of play to release energy may not seem like a therapeutic endeavor, children are likely to use play therapy as a place of free expression for unused or confining energy. Children who spend the day attempting to "keep it together" in structured environments often need a safe place for energy release, which, once expanded, allows for focused therapeutic work.

(pp. 14–15)

Play Therapy and Neurodivergent Children

Play therapy has not always been considered a viable approach for working with autistic and neurodivergent children. In fact, using any type of play-based approach to working with autistic children and/or children with developmental disabilities was considered ineffective and a waste of time. The leading, misinformed, and often harmful belief that autistic children and those with intellectual developmental disorder did not play, did not understand play, and play held no therapeutic value for them, permeated many autism-focused "treatments" for decades. Ableist thinking and processes guided many autism-related therapies as autistic children were often viewed as the equivalent of an animal that required training.

It was in the 2000s that play therapy began to emerge as a therapy approach that could be beneficial to autistic children and their families. Play therapists began to see more autistic children and recognized the antiquated ideas that autistic children did not play were not true. Further, they began having experiences of growth and success in helping autistic children address various mental health needs utilize play therapy. Around the same time, autistic adults began to speak and write about their experiences as children – noting that they did play and engaged in various types of play and the adults around them did not understand and often mislabeled their play. Autistic adults began to share about their experiences with rigid and "training" oriented therapies and "treatments" that felt abusive and created anxiety, depression, and low self-worth issues. They began to share about the need for and importance of more relational and humanistic infused therapy approaches and the play therapy community began to listen. Research using play therapy with autistic children can be dated back to 1970, but arguably the last 10–15 years has amassed the greatest amount of research support for implementing play therapy with autistic and neurodivergent children. The following highlights important points in the history of play therapy and autism (including significant research):

1970: This study is published using group play therapy with 6 children ages 8–13. They were hospitalized boys with diagnoses of childhood schizophrenia or infantile autism (Pratarotti, 1970).

2005: Robert Jason Grant presented the training titled *Using Play Therapy with Autism* which highlighted the beginning of what would become the AutPlay Therapy framework.

2011: Kevin Hull published *Play Therapy and Asperger's Syndrome: Helping Children and Adolescents Grow, Connect, and Heal through the Art of Play.*

2012: Loretta Gallo-Lopez and Lawrence Rubin published *Play-Based Interventions for Children and Adolescents with Autism Spectrum Disorders.*

2013: Robert Jason Grant published *AutPlay Therapy: A Play Therapy Approach for Autism, Neurodevelopmental Disorders, and Developmental Disabilities.*

2014: Therplay was recognized by the U.S. Substance Abuse and Mental Health Services Administration for inclusion on the National Registry for Evidence-based Programs and Practices as an effective approach for autism spectrum disorder.

2022: Robert Jason Grant Published *The AutPlay® Therapy Handbook*

Today, we fully understand that play therapy approaches can hold many benefits for autistic children and their families, especially in addressing mental health needs with which they may be struggling. Play therapy is uniquely designed for and responsive to the individual and developmental needs of each child and recently, there has been an increase in child therapy literature emphasizing play as the ideal way to address social and emotional difficulties in children (Bratton, Ray, Rhine, & Jones, 2005; Josefi & Ryan, 2004). Research has shown that autistic children participating in play therapy have gained improvement in attachment issues, social needs, self-regulation, coping with changes, emotional response, and autonomy (Josefi & Ryan, 2004).

Sherratt and Peter (2002) suggested that play interventions and experiences are extremely important to autistic and neurodivergent children. They stated that simultaneously activating the areas of the brain associated with emotions and generative thought while explicitly involving children in play will lead to success. Further, Thornton and Cox (2005) conducted individual play sessions with autistic children specifically to address behavior concerns. They incorporated techniques which included relationship development, gaining attention, turn taking, enjoyment, and structure. Their research found that play interventions did impact on the child's behavior with a reduction in dysregulated behavior following the structured play interventions.

On a theoretical level, the therapeutic foundations provided by play therapy approaches of unconditional positive regard, empathy and congruence (e.g. therapists' use of their own feelings therapeutically as they arise within social interactions) and the method's more recent emphasis on a developmental approach to therapy – all point to the possibility that this modality can enable autistic and neurodivergent children to benefit both emotionally and socially. The therapeutic condition of unconditional positive regard concentrates on accepting children's current self, along with assuming they possess an innate drive toward growth and healing. In theory, this allows autistic children to choose the pace and focus of change themselves, thus enabling interaction to be instigated by children rather than adults, as well as increasing the children's autonomy under the very favorable conditions of the playroom. In addition, play therapy's emphasis on children and adults' emotional responses, and therapists' skilled use of empathy to enter children's unique inner worlds essentially target areas of development in which autistic children can benefit (Josefi & Ryan, 2004).

Play Therapy can be an appropriate modality in working with neurodivergent children especially when working with children who have challenges in traditional communication methods (Parker & O'Brien, 2011). Play therapy approaches are gaining more and more valid research as effective therapy approaches for neurodivergent children and adolescents' mental health needs. Play therapy approaches provide the opportunity for the therapist to individualize therapy and engage the child in a playful and natural way that other therapies may not offer.

Arguably, some play therapy approaches have more research support for addressing the mental health needs of autistic and neurodivergent children than others (Child Centered Play Therapy), some are more specifically designed for autistic and neurodivergent children (AutPlay Therapy and Theraplay), and some incorporate more evidence-based practices than others (Cognitive Behavioral Play Therapy). The variety of therapeutic response in what is play therapy provides opportunity to individualize and uniquely address the mental health needs of neurodivergent children and their families.

Play therapy approaches, in general, are neurodiversity affirming – valuing the child, giving the child a voice, and affirming the identity of the child.

Several approaches have shown successful clinical outcomes; most notably Filial Therapy (VanFleet, 2014), Theraplay (Booth & Jernbeg, 2010), Child Centered Play Therapy (Hillman, 2018), and AutPlay Therapy (Grant, 2017). Research has also demonstrated the benefits of implementing play therapy to address a variety of mental health concerns that may be present with a neurodivergent child.

Play therapy has been shown to help autistic and neurodivergent children understand social navigation, improve emotional expression and regulation ability (Salter, Beamish, & Davies, 2016), improve expression, communication, and provide improvement in the parent/child relationship (Howard et al., 2018). Banerjee and Ray (2013) proposed that some core mental health issues can be addressed through play therapy such as relationship development, and recognition and expression of emotion. Further, they reported that play therapy can be effective for gains in sensorimotor play, reducing problem behaviors, and improving self-worth.

As a play therapy approach, AutPlay Therapy is an integration (synthesis) of various play therapy theories and approaches designed to specifically focus on neurodivergent children. Arguably, many play therapy theories and approaches have had some effect or influence on the creation of AutPlay Therapy, but the play therapy approaches that have been the most influential on AutPlay Therapy include Child Centered Play Therapy, Theraplay, Filial Therapy, Gestalt Play Therapy, Family Play Therapy, and Cognitive Behavioral Play Therapy. Although play therapy as a whole is the base for AutPlay Therapy, the above-mentioned approaches have specific elements and constructs that have more directly impacted the protocols of AutPlay Therapy. Chapter 6 further describes these play therapy influences as well as the integrative process in AutPlay Therapy.

It is essential to note that play therapy is an umbrella term and can refer to many different approaches. While the Association for Play Therapy (APT) (2022b) defines ten seminal and historically significant play therapy theories, there exists approximately ten additional play therapy theories and approaches. When parents are seeking out a play therapist for their autistic or neurodivergent child or a therapist is looking for a play therapist to make a referral, there are a few questions they might ask:

1 What type of play therapy do you offer and what are your credentials/-training for providing play therapy?
2 What is your experience working with autistic/neurodivergent children and their families?

3 Can you describe the types of issues you have worked on with neurodivergent children?

4 How might the play therapy you offer benefit my autistic/neurodivergent child?

5 What would a typical play therapy session look like and how would you involve the parent and/or family members?

6 What are some possible mental health needs and typical therapy goals when working with neurodivergent children?

7 How would you conceptualize neurodiversity and describe a neurodiversity affirming approach?

The Therapeutic Power of Play

One unifying feature throughout the myriad of play therapy approaches is Schaefer and Drews (2014), 20 core change agents of the therapeutic powers of play. These powers refer to the specific change agents in which play initiates, facilitates, or strengthens the therapeutic effect. Play powers act as mediators that positively influence the desired change in the client (Barron & Kenny, 1986) and provide the foundational framework for the clinical understanding and use of play therapy (VanFleet & Faa-Thompson, 2017).

Under the umbrella of play therapy, the therapeutic powers of play can be recognized throughout various theories and approaches. Some powers may be more evident or primary in some theories versus others but certainly the therapeutic powers of play serve as a unifying component in the vast world of play therapy. This book does not capture all the play therapy theories, approaches, and methods that currently exist, but it does provide a snapshot of the variety that integrate and influence AutPlay Therapy.

Historically, Schaefer (1993) identified 14 therapeutic powers of play based upon a review of the literature and play therapists' clinical experiences. Later the list was expanded and revised to include 20 core therapeutic powers of play (Schaefer & Drewes, 2014). Based on similarity of therapy goals, the 20 powers were classified into the following four categories: facilitates communication, fosters emotional wellness, enhances social relationships, and increases personal strengths (Schaefer & Drewes, 2014). He proposed that play helps in relationship enhancement, expressive communication, growth of competence, creative problem-solving, abreaction, role-play, learning through metaphor, positive emotion, and socialization. Children can learn social skills, develop relationships, learn how to communicate and express themselves through verbal and nonverbal means, and develop problem-solving abilities through therapeutic play.

Schaefer and Drewes' (2014) therapeutic factors refer to specific clinical strategies, and the therapeutic powers of play refer to the specific change agents in which play initiates, facilitates, or strengthens their therapeutic effect. The change agents include self-expression, access to the unconscious, direct teaching, indirect teaching, catharsis, abreaction, positive emotions, counterconditioning fears, stress inoculation, stress management, therapeutic relationship, attachment, social competence, empathy, creative problem-solving, resiliency, moral development, accelerated psychological development, self-regulation, and self-esteem.

Through specific consideration and selection of the core change agents, all children, including autistic and neurodivergent children, can learn regulation ability, develop healthy relationships, learn how to communicate and express themselves, improve emotional modulation, decrease stress and anxiety, address trauma issues, improve their awareness of self and positive self-esteem, increase advocacy ability, and develop problem-solving/coping strengths. Figure 5.1 displays the therapeutic powers of play.

The therapeutic powers of play are the mechanisms in play that actually produce the desired change in a client's dysfunctional thoughts, feelings, and/or behaviors (Peabody & Schaefer, 2016). Indeed, the prominence of these powers are evident in the definition of play therapy by the Association of Play Therapy. Just as an in-depth understanding of child development is foundational to play therapy, training in the therapeutic powers of play creates an understanding of why and how play creates therapeutic change.

These therapeutic powers of play have been referred to in the literature as the "heart and soul" of play therapy (Schaefer & Drewes, 2014, p. 4), exemplifying their essence in initial play therapy knowledge. With this foundational knowledge, therapists are better positioned during their comprehensive individualized assessment of each client to identify the core cognitive, affective, and interpersonal processes involved in the presenting clinical concern, and to apply specific powers of play designed to activate the desired change. Without this strong grounding, a clinician may operate with more of a "hope this works" mentality, rather than a purposeful understanding of how the therapist can initiate, facilitate, and strengthen play to impact change (Peabody & Schaefer, 2019).

The AutPlay Therapy protocol can potentially incorporate and address any of the 20 core agents of change of the therapeutic powers of play. AutPlay utilizes non-directed play and structured play therapy interventions that are specifically chosen and or created for the individual child. Therapeutic play

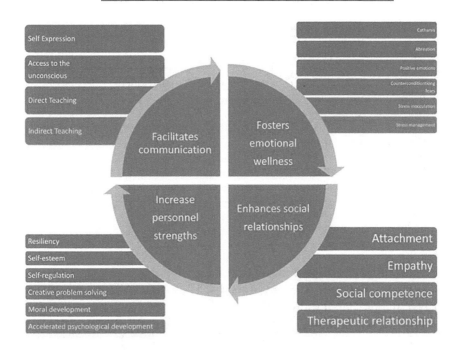

Adapted from Schaefer, C. E., & Drewes, A. A. (2013). *The therapeutic powers of play: 20 core agents of change*. Wiley and from Parson, J. (2017) Puppet Play Therapy – Integrating Theory, Evidence and Action (ITEA) presented at International Play Therapy Study Group. Champneys at Forest Mere, England. June 18, 2017.

JStone, Ph.D., 2020

Figure 5.1 The Therapeutic Powers of Play: 20 Agents of Change.

processes and play interventions are mindfully chosen with input from both the parent and the child. Each intervention embodies one or more of the 20 core agents of change depending on the child's assessed needs. Although any of the core change agents could be identified and addressed with a neurodivergent child, children typically benefit from a focus on specifically identified agents of change.

Ultimately, play is the natural language of all children and holds many benefits including therapeutic components. Play is also the agent of change that propels children forward in healing and growth. Within the therapeutic powers of play, neurodivergent children have a validating and naturalistic process to address needs and work on mental health growth and goals. AutPlay Therapy protocol is mindfully infused with play core agents of change that specifically align with the neurodivergence of autistic children and children with other neurotype needs. Table 5.2 shows the most common therapeutic powers of play in AutPlay Therapy protocol.

Table 5.2 Therapeutic Powers of Play in AutPlay Therapy

Common Core Agents of Change

Direct teaching	Positive emotions	Therapeutic relationships	Stress management	Social competence
Positive peer relationships	Stress inoculation	Empathy	Counterconditioning fears	Self-regulation
Moral development	Attachment	Self esteem	Creative problem solving	Resilience

The therapeutic powers of play are organized into four major categories: facilitate communication, foster emotional wellness, enhance social relationships, and increase personal strengths. These four categories are then described in more detail through the core agents of change as they are assigned to each category. A play therapist could recognize that a dynamic within the play interaction enhanced social relationships. To describe this dynamic further, the therapist could choose from the core agents under the therapeutic power of play As an example, the notes would then explain that the play therapy session met the goal of enhanced social relationships, and the appropriate core agents were enacted through play (Stone, 2022). The following provides some examples of common core agents in AutPlay Therapy when working with neurodivergent children. Each of the core agents could have multiple and varying examples. The following is simply providing a better understanding of the possibilities.

- Positive Peer Relationships – The therapist might select the AutPlay Intervention *Paper Friend*, which helps children identify what they would like in a friendship and who they would like to have as friends. The therapist would introduce the intervention and complete it with the child focusing on friendships. The therapist would continue to follow up with the child after the intervention had been completed to ensure the child was making gains toward their friendship goals.
- Therapeutic Relationship – The AutPlay process begins with a focus on building relationship. One of the primary goals of the Intake and Assessment Phase is to develop relationship with the child. Additionally, early in therapy, the therapist might play the intervention *Make My Moves*, designed to help develop trust, connection, and work on relationship development between the child and therapist or child and parent. The

therapist might also let the child choose an intervention to play or read the child a social story about being in play therapy.

- Direct Teaching – The therapist could choose any play intervention with a purposeful therapy goal focus to help the child progress toward their goals. For example, the therapist could choose the intervention *Backward Moves*, designed to help children regulate their system. The therapist would introduce the intervention, provide the instructions to the child for how to complete the intervention, and follow through with assessing to make sure the intervention is a good fit for the child and helping the child with their regulation needs.

- Positive Emotions – The therapist would be active in reflecting emotions presented by the child and co regulate emotions as needed. Further, the therapist could choose the intervention *Me and My Feelings*, which is designed to help the child identify positive emotions they experience. The therapist's ongoing relationship with the child also enhances the opportunity for the child to recognize and experience positive emotions.

- Self Esteem – The therapist is continually attuned to the child's self-worth and identity recognition and expression. The therapist can reflect acceptance and create and open and safe atmosphere in the playroom for exploring and expressing identity. The therapist could also implement the intervention *Look at My Strengths*, which is designed to help children identify one or more strengths they possess.

- Stress Management – The therapist would be active in co regulating with the child any stress-related feelings. The therapist could also implement the intervention *10 Cloud Relaxation* or some other guided deep breathing exercise to help the child relax and calm.

- Self-Regulation – The therapist can continually be modeling regulation and co-regulating with the child as needed. The therapist can introduce regulation play interventions that are a good fit for the child and help the child regulate. The therapist can work with the child to help them discover regulation ideas that do not involve another person for implementation.

- Social Competence – The AutPlay process begins with an assessment (the AutPlay Social Navigation Inventory) which helps identify any social-related needs the child might be experiencing. Through the therapeutic relationship and utilization of directive interventions, the therapist can help address any social- related therapy goals. For example, the therapist might implement the intervention *Safety Wheel*, which is designed to help children identify safe and unsafe places and people.

Kaduson, Cangelosi, and Schaefer (2020) stated that the heart and soul of play therapy is contained in the therapeutic powers of play. They are the specific, essential ingredients in play that produce therapeutic change. In application, the play therapist focuses on selecting the specific change agents(s) in play that will best resolve the client's presenting problem. For example, the "direct teaching" power of play would be indicated for a child who has difficulty making friends because of their anger management struggles. The "stress inoculation" power of play would be a good match for a child with medical-related fears or anxieties. Likewise, the "moral development" power of play would be a logical match for a child with conduct disorder. The idea is to individually match the power of play with the child who would most benefit from that particular power of play.

In AutPlay Therapy, the therapeutic powers of play 20 core agents of change can materialize in a number of different ways. They can also overlap and be integrated in their implementation with some children. Because of the variance in the spectrum of presentation with neurodivergent children, it is likely the AutPlay therapist will experience a variety of the therapeutic powers of play. Thus, it becomes important for the therapist to have a grounded knowledge in the therapeutic powers of play. The intersection between the therapeutic powers of play and the therapist's understanding of the neurodiversity paradigm creates the most beneficial, safe, and healthy environment for neurodivergent children to address their mental health needs through play therapy.

References

Association for Play Therapy. (2022a). Why play therapy? https://www.a4pt.org/page/WhyPlayTherapy

Association for Play Therapy. (2022b). *Credentialing standards for the registered play therapist* (pp. 11–12). https://cdn.ymaws.com/www.a4pt.org/resource/resmgr/credentials/rpt_standards.pdf

Axline, V. (1947). *Play therapy.* Houghton Mifflin.

Axline, V. (1964). *Dibs: In search of self.* Houghton Mifflin.

Banerjee, M., & Ray, S. G. (2013). Development of play therapy module for children with autism. *Journal of the Indian Academy of Applied Psychology, 39,* 245–253.

Barron, R., & Kenny, D. (1986). The moderator-mediator variable distinction in social psychological research: Conceptual, strategic, and statistical considerations. *Journal of Personality & Social Psychology, 5,* 1173–1182.

Booth, P. B., & Jernberg, A. M. (2010). *Theraplay.* Jossey-Bass.

Bratton, S. C., Ray, D., Rhine, T., & Jones, L. (2005). The efficacy of play therapy with children: A meta-analytic review of treatments outcomes. *Professional Psychology: Research and Practice, 36,* 376–390.

Gil, E. (2021). Foreword. In R. J. Grant, J. Stone, & C. Mellenthin (Eds.), *Play therapy theories and perspectives: A collection of thoughts in the field* (pp. xii–xiv). Routledge.

Grant, R. J. (2017). *Autplay therapy for children and adolescents on the autism spectrum a behavioral play-based approach.* Routledge.

Grant, R. J. (2021) *Understanding autism: A neurodiversity affirming guidebook for children and teens.* AutPlay Publishing.

Hillman, H. (2018). Child-centered play therapy as an intervention for children with autism: A literature review. *International Journal of Play Therapy, 27*(4), 198–204.

Howard, A. R. H., Lindaman, S., Copeland, R., & Cross, D. R. (2018). Theraplay impact on parents and children with autism spectrum disorder: Improvements in affect, joint attention, and social cooperation. *International Journal of Play Therapy, 27,* 56–68.

Hudspeth, E. F. (2021). Play therapy versus a play-based therapy. *Play Therapy, 16*(2), 14.

Josefi, O., & Ryan, Y. (2004). Non-directive play therapy for young children with autism: A case study. *Clinical Child Psychology and Psychiatry, 9,* 533–551.

Kaduson, H. G., Cangelosi, D., & Schaefer, C. E. (Eds.). (2020). *Prescriptive play therapy: Tailoring interventions for specific childhood problems.* The Guilford Press.

Kottman, T., & Meany-Walen, K. K. (2018). *Doing play therapy: From building the relationship to facilitating change.* Guildford Press.

Landreth, G. L. (2012). *Play therapy: The art of the relationship* (3rd ed.). Routledge.

LeBlanc, M., & Ritchie, M. (2001). A meta-analysis of play therapy outcomes. *Counseling Psychology Quarterly, 14,* 149–163.

Lin, D., & Bratton, S. (2015). A meta-analytic review of child-centered play therapy approaches. *Journal of Counseling & Development, 93,* 45–58.

Oaklander, V. (2007). *Windows to our children: A Gestalt therapy approach to children and adolescents.* The Gestalt Journal Press.

O'Conner, K. J. (2000). *The play therapy primer.* John Wiley and Sons.

Parker, N., & O'Brien, P. (2011). Play therapy reaching the child with autism, *International Journal of Special Education, 26,* 80–87.

Peabody, M. A., & Schaefer, C. E. (2016). Towards semantic clarity in play therapy. *International Journal of Play Therapy, 25,* 197–202.

Peadbody, M. A., & Schaefer, C. (2019). The therapeutic powers of play: The heart and soul of play therapy. *Play Therapy, 14*(3), 4–6.

Phillips, N., & Beavan, L. (2010). *Teaching play to children with autism.* Sage Publications.

Pratarotti, A. R. (1970). Group play therapy with autistic children. *Revista de Psicologia Normal e Patologica, 16*(3–4), 305–312.

Ray, D. C. (2011). *Advanced play therapy: Essential conditions, knowledge, and skills for child practice*. Routledge.

Ray, D., Armstrong, S., Balkin, R., & Jayne, K. (2015). Child centered play therapy in the schools: Review and meta-analysis. *Psychology in the Schools, 52,* 107–123.

Ray, D. C., & McCullough, R. (2016). Evidence-based practice statement: Play therapy (Research report). Retrieved from Association for Play Therapy website: http://www.a4pt.org/?page=EvidenceBased

Salter, K., Beamish, W., & Davies, M. (2016). The effects of child-centered play therapy (CCPT) on the social and emotional growth of young children with autism. *International Journal of Play Therapy, 25,* 78–90.

Schaefer, C. E. (1993) *The therapeutic powers of play*. Rowman & Littlefield Publishers.

Schaefer, C. E., & Drewes, A. A. (2014). *The therapeutic powers of play: 20 core change agents* (2nd ed.). John Wiley & Sons.

Sherratt, D., & Peter, M. (2002). *Developing play and drama in children with autistic spectrum disorders*. Fulton.

Stone, J. (2022). *Digital play therapy: A clinician's guide to comfort and competence*. Routledge.

Thornton, K., & Cox, E. (2005). Play and the reduction of challenging behavior in children with ASD's and learning disabilities. *Good Autism Practice, 6*(2), 75–80.

VanFleet, R. (2014). *Filial therapy: Strengthening the parent-child relationships through play* (3rd ed.). Professional Resource Press.

VanFleet, R., & Faa-Thompson, T. (2017). Animal assisted play therapy with reticent children. In C. Malchiodi & D. Crenshaw (Eds.), *What to do when children claim up in psychotherapy* (pp. 217–237). Guilford Press.

6

An Integrative Play Therapy Approach

What Is an Integrative Approach?

An integrative therapy approach can be traced back to the 1930s (Seymour, 2011). There are many different types of psychotherapy that are integrative, and the concept of integrative therapy has changed and developed since the 1930s. This chapter is not a complete overview of integrative therapy but a snapshot for the purposes of further explaining and supporting the AutPlay Therapy framework. Integrative therapy is defined as an approach to therapy that involves selecting the techniques from different therapeutic orientations best suited to a client's particular problem. By tailoring the therapy to the individual, integrative therapists hope to produce the most significant effects (Cherry, 2021).

Gilbert and Orlans (2011) furthered that the definition of integration involves the combination of two or more models of psychotherapy into a new and more effective model. The practice of an integrative therapy approach includes the considered and intentional use of an ethical relationship, grounded in a therapeutic alliance, in the service of the goals of the client. It is not a random eclectic "little bit of this and a little bit of that" approach. The following highlights an adaptation of Gilbert and Orlans' four components of integration definition with commentary on their application to the AutPlay integration process of working with neurodivergent children:

1 A holistic view of the person, a view that sees the person as an integrated whole: affectively, cognitively, behaviorally, physically, and spiritually. This includes a focus on the developing self as a central integrating principle. The therapist will view each neurodivergent child as a holistic child worthy of value and respect. Historically autistic and neurodivergent children have been devalued, viewed as less than neurotypical

DOI: 10.4324/9781003207610-7

children and not as a whole child. The therapist will strive to make sure the integration supports the neurodivergent self of the child.

2 The integration of theories and/or concepts and/or techniques from different approaches to psychotherapy. There is a purposeful integration at the level of theory and technique and involves drawing together a model of integration from different orientations. The therapist must understand that neurodivergence is a wide spectrum of presentation. While neurodivergent children share some common experiences, needs, and manifestations, there is still a great diversity in presentation, strengths, needs, and intersectionality. To fully meet the mental health needs of neurodivergent children, a carefully focused and assessed integrative and prescriptive approach is essential.

3 The integration of the person and professional. The integrative therapist is faced with personal and professional challenges that need to be worked through in order for the person to feel comfortable with who they are in the world. The therapist must be aware of their own self and careful not to project this onto the client. The therapist must take care to explore their own ableism and not project their ableist beliefs onto the client or into the play approaches they are implementing. Exploring one's own ableism is often an ongoing work, as many systems and processes to which the therapist has been exposed are conditioned with ableism. The therapist must understand the neurodiversity paradigm and movement and be prepared to implement a neurodiversity affirming approach with their neurodivergent clients.

4 The integration of research and practice. The therapist studies current research and integrates these findings into their framework. Also, the therapist observes their own practice and feeds these observations back into their model of practice and into their own research endeavors. Mental health therapists must take note of the historically ableist bias present in research focused on autistic and neurodivergent children. Only recently has neurodiversity affirming research been produced. As research related to neurodivergent children is viewed and conceptualized, the therapist must have a critical eye for ableist methods and practices. Many therapies boosting research support and findings do cite research which produced results, but at the same time, were harmful and abusive to neurodivergent children. Although the research showed a result, the abhorrent lack of consideration of the harm the research was causing has unfortunately been a terrible miss in the mental health community.

Integrative play therapy is a relatively new developing approach to working with children and adolescents. It offers promise in its flexible use of integrating play therapy theory and techniques in order to offer clients the best therapy for their presenting problems. Some examples of integrative play therapy include Ecosystemic Play Therapy (O'Connor, 2001), Flexibly Sequential Play Therapy (Goodyear-Brown, 2010), and AutPlay Therapy (Grant, 2017).

Arguably the most developed thought on integrative play therapy comes from the Play Therapy Dimensions Model (Yasenik & Gardner, 2012). The Play Therapy Dimensions model is an integrative approach that provides play therapists with a framework from which to conceptualize the play therapy process and evaluate their therapeutic interventions when working with children. Essentially, it is a process which aids the play therapist in decision-making about the best approach and/or integration of approaches to meet the child's therapy goals. Yasenik and Gardner further conceptualized the dimensions model process:

> The Play Therapy Dimensions Model conceptualizes the play therapy process according to two primary dimensions: Directiveness and Consciousness. These dimensions help define the therapeutic space in a manner that most practitioners will recognize as fundamental to the change process. The Consciousness dimension reflects the child's representation of consciousness in play, and is represented by the child's play activities and verbalizations. The second dimension, Directiveness, refers to the degree of immersion and level of interpretation of the play therapist. These two dimensions intersect, forming four quadrants. Depending on the case conceptualization, and the theoretical approach of the therapist, a therapist might choose to focus therapy activities primarily in one quadrant. Alternatively, there may be a number of indicators that suggest movement is required amongst the quadrants. Furthermore, movement may occur within a session, or across sessions, as the therapy process evolves. As will be discussed, this conceptualization assists therapists in navigating the complex client-by-therapist-by-therapy interactions in order to tailor therapy approaches and optimize effectiveness. This integrative approach also offers a process-oriented framework, providing guidance for tracking important change mechanisms.
>
> (p. 33)

AutPlay Therapy's integrative framework is specifically chosen based on the conceptualization of best practices in working with autistic and neurodivergent children in mental health care. Four themes describe the importance of integrative efforts in neurodivergent care. (1) Integration provides the avenue to access the best course of action – allowing for the perfect intersection between the options available and the unique neurodivergent need. (2) An integrative approach provides for a greater depth in exploration of the plethora of opportunities to uniquely speak to and serve the neurodivergent child. It avoids the common pitfall of a one size fits all approach. (3) Integration provides the range needed to address the many manifestations across the spectrum when working with neurodivergent children. The therapist must notice the individual child and join their world as opposed to demanding the child fit into a therapy model. (4) Integration requires the therapist to gain a depth of knowledge across theories, approaches, and techniques. This allows for greater opportunity to conceptualize individual therapy for each neurodivergent child. As VanFleet (2014) stated, "the heart and soul of any form of therapy depends on the theories and assumptions behind it" (p. 3). The following presents an overview of the play therapy integration found in AutPlay Therapy.

Primary AutPlay Play Therapy Theory Integration

Child Centered Play Therapy

What is considered modern day Child Centered Play Therapy (CCPT) was founded by Virginia Axline in the 1940s (Ray, 2011). It is an approach to person-centered counseling that effectively blends Rogerian tenets with the natural way children communicate through play. The three core elements of person-centered therapy are congruence, unconditional positive regard, and empathy (Moss & Hamlet, 2020). CCPT practice is particularly concerned with providing an environment of safety to facilitate the child's exploration of self and letting go of rigid behaviors resultant from a threatened self-concept. CCPT occurs in a playroom supplied with carefully selected toys and materials (Ray & Landreth, 2019).

Landreth (1991) described CCPT as an encompassing philosophy for living one's life in relationship with children. It is not a reference of techniques that are implemented in the playroom. It is a way of being based on a deep commitment to certain beliefs about children and their innate capacity for growth. It is a complete therapeutic process and not just the application of a few rapport-building techniques. It is based on the belief in the capacity and resiliency of children. Landreth furthered that the following tenets guide the CCPT process:

1 Children are not miniature adults, and the therapist does not respond to them as if they were.
2 Children are people. They are capable of experiencing deep emotional pain and joy.

3 Children are unique and worthy of respect. The therapist prizes the uniqueness of each child and respects the person they are.
4 Children are resilient. Children possess a tremendous capacity to overcome obstacles and circumstances in their lives.
5 Children have an inherent tendency toward growth and maturity. They possess an inner intuitive wisdom.
6 Children are capable of positive self-direction. They are capable of dealing with their world in creative ways.
7 Children's natural language is play and this is the medium of self-expression with which they are most comfortable.
8 Children have the right to remain silent. The therapist respects a child's decision not to talk.
9 Children will take the therapeutic experience to where they need to be. The therapist does not attempt to determine when or how a child should play.
10 Children's growth cannot be speeded up. The therapist recognizes this and is patient with the child's developmental process.

(p. 50)

Ray and Landreth (2019) noted that refences to traditional therapy goals or objectives is inconsistent with child-centered play therapy philosophy. Goals are evaluative and imply tracking specific, externally established achievements required of the client. Children should be related to as persons to be understood as opposed to goals to be checked off or persons to be fixed. Because a central hypothesis of CCPT philosophy is that the therapist has an unwavering belief in the child's capacity for growth and self-direction, establishment of therapy goals is somewhat contradictory. However, CCPT therapists seek to facilitate an environment in which the child can experience growth, leading toward healthier functioning.

CCPT holds many benefits for addressing mental health needs of neurodivergent children. Research has been consistently increasing in showing support for CCPT to address various mental health needs of autistic children (Hillman, 2018; Salter, Beamish, & Davies, 2016; War Balch & Ray, 2015). The tenets of CCPT and person-centered philosophy align well with the primary philosophy of the neurodiversity paradigm and neurodiversity affirming principles. The non-directive approach in CCPT provides opportunity for the autistic child to explore, express, and be themself. Unfortunately, in many of the therapies the autistic and neurodivergent child participates, child-led experiences are taken way and/or not allowed.

CCPT influence and integration in AutPlay Therapy can be seen in basic foundational constructs. (1) Accepting the child, allowing the self of the child to be seen and be valued. (2) Meeting the child where they are without judgment. (3) Not controlling the child's play. Allowing for the child's play preferences to be realized and not viewed as wrong or an incorrect way to play. (4) A foundational focus on relationship development. (5) Non-directive and CCPT protocols of attunement, child-led play, tracking, and reflecting in the AutPlay Follow Me Approach. (6) The overall respect for the child. The awareness that the child is not to be turned into a version of something the therapist wants to see but allowed to be themselves and become their best self.

Theraplay

Theraplay has been defined as a playful, engaging, short-term therapy method that is intimate, physical, personal, focused, and fun. It is modeled on the natural, healthy parent–infant relationship, and therapy actively involves parents. The focus of Theraplay is on the underlying disturbances in the relationship between the child and their caretakers. The goal of therapy is to enhance attachment, self-esteem, trust, and joyful engagement and to empower parents to continue on their own healthy interaction with their child (Jernberg & Booth, 2001).

Theraplay is modeled on the responsive, attuned, co-regulating, and playful patterns of interaction between parents and their babies that lead to secure attachment and life-long social-emotional health. The focus of therapy is the relationship itself; parents are an essential part of the process so that they can carry on the newly developed patterns of interaction at home. In sessions, the therapist initially guides the interaction. Progressively, parents take the leadership role. Regularly scheduled parent-only sessions allow for additional reflection and problem-solving. Theraplay may be combined or sequenced with other modalities for complex problems (Booth & Lindaman, 2019).

Booth and Jernberg (2010) reported that there are four dimensions that are used in therapy planning to meet the needs of the child and the parent in therapy. The four Theraplay dimensions are structure, engagement, nurture, and challenge. The following is a brief explanation of each dimension:

> Structure – Parents are trustworthy and predictable, and provide safety, organization, and regulation. As a consequence of the caregiver's structuring of the child's environment, the child not only enjoys physical and emotional security, but they are also able to understand and learn about their environment and they can develop the capacity to regulate themselves.

Engagement – Parents provide attuned, playful experiences that create a strong connection, an optimal level of arousal, and shared joy. Engaging activities are especially appropriate for children who are withdrawn, avoid contact, or are too constrained and rigidly structured. Learning to be more engaging with their child is essential for parents who are disengaged or preoccupied, who are out of sync with their child, who rely primarily on questions to engage their child, or who do not know how to enjoy being with their child.

Nurture – Parents respond empathically to the child's attachment and regulatory needs by being warm, tender, calming, and comforting. They provide a safe haven and create feelings of self-worth. Nurturing activities reassure the child that their parents are available when they need them. These activities are important in building the child's inner representation that they are lovable and accepted as they are.

Challenge – While providing a secure base, parents encourage the child to strive a bit, to take risks, to explore, to feel confident, and to enjoy mastery. Challenging activities are used to support and encourage the child's sense of competence. These activities are designed for success and are done in playful partnership with the adult.

(pp. 21–25)

A therapist trained in Theraplay protocol works with the child and parents in a family play therapy context to help work on improvement and success in each of the four dimensions. Therapists typically meet with the child and parent together to model and implement play interventions designed to meet therapy goals. The overall goal of therapy is to establish a trusting emotional relationship between the child and their parents. Booth and Lindamen (2019) proposed that the Theraplay process begins with an assessment, including a detailed intake interview with caregivers, observation of parent and child interactions via the Marschak Interaction Method (MIM), and a collaborative discussion of the MIM experience with parents (Booth, Christensen, & Lindaman, 2011). Next, the therapist creates a therapy plan, employing the dimensions, and has a reflective and practice session with the parent.

Theraplay represents a significant piece of the play therapy integration in AutPlay Therapy. Theraplay dimensions help form the relationship development (connection) which is achieved by parent and child in process together to create engagement and connection through natural, fun, play-based techniques and playtime in the AutPlay Therapy Follow Me Approach. It is important to note that Theraplay is an established therapy option that has had a great deal of research-supported success in working with autistic children. Jernberg and Booth (2001) proposed that Theraplay is particularly helpful in working with autistic children because it does not depend on their being able to respond to language or having any particular language presentation. Further, Theraplay concentrates on the precursors to cognition and to representational thinking, mutual attention, and engagement making it an ideal therapy approach for children with relationship and communication difficulties.

Bundy-Myrow (2012), stated that what differentiates Theraplay for autistic children from other play therapy approaches is twofold: As the primary playroom object, the Theraplay therapist uses sensorimotor-based play to engage the child and address needs. To empower parents as therapeutic partners, the Theraplay therapist demonstrates and guides parents to provide the unique relationship building blocks their child needs for development. These constructs are supported and more fully realized in the AutPlay Therapy framework for autistic and all neurodivergent children.

Booth and Jernberg (2010) stated that Theraplay is ideally suited for autistic children because Theraplay treatment engages children in a playful, positive social interaction that focuses on establishing the basis of the capacity to engage with others and participate in relationships. Simeone-Russell (2011) furthered that the use of group Theraplay has been found to be very effective in developing engagement, interaction, communication, language, and social navigation in autistic children. In working with autistic children, typical goals of Theraplay might include increasing relationship and connection, adjusting to transitions and changes, helping parents to discover methods to calm and soothe their child, and stimulating communication.

Theraplay's influence on AutPlay Therapy is evident through several constructs. (1) The purposeful inclusion of parents/caretakers in the therapy process. (2) The emphasis on the role of the parent as a partner or co-change agent along with the therapist. (3) The therapy protocol of teaching parents how to interact or work with their child through natural/nurturing and directive play based interventions. (4) The emphasis on relationship development or connection and addressing therapy needs simultaneously using parent/child play experiences as the main catalyst to reach therapy goals.

Filial Therapy

The term "filial therapy" comes from the Latin filios or filias, technically meaning sons or daughters. Loosely translated, it means parent–child. Filial

Therapy is a theoretically integrative psychoeducational model of therapy in which parents serve as the primary change agents for their children. In essence, it is a form of family therapy that uses play therapy methods to enhance parent–child relationships and to solve a wide range of child and family problems (VanFleet, 2014). In Filial Therapy, the therapist teaches the parent how to have child-centered play therapy sessions at home. The parent learns the principles and conducts the play times with their child in the home setting.

Guerney (1964) stated that the basic model or goals of Filial Therapy include: reducing problem behaviors in the child, enhancing the parent–child relationship, optimizing child adjustment, increasing child competence and self-confidence, providing parents with an understanding of their children's feelings, motivations, needs, and behavior and how to respond appropriately with empathy and limit setting, and enhancing parenting skills involving empathy, attentiveness, encouragement, and effective implementation of parental authority via the recommended approach to limit setting. These goals are attained by including parents in the process and empowering them to become change agents in working with their child. The overall goal of Filial Therapy is to focus on improvement in the parent–child relationship and subsequently produce improvement in other areas as well.

Scuka and Guerney (2019) explained that through Filial Therapy parents could be empowered to help their own children by teaching them CCPT skills, most importantly, the skills of following the child's lead, showing understanding through empathy, and limit setting. By teaching parents these skills in Filial Therapy, parents would become the primary agents to achieve therapeutic goals by helping their children work through emotional challenges and/or behavioral issues. In this way, Filial Therapy would simultaneously leverage the natural parent–child bond to further therapeutic goals while strengthening the attachment between parent and child.

Van Fleet (2014) stated that Filial Therapy is comprised of several core values and the therapist must embrace these values and always incorporate them into their work. These values include honesty, openness, respect, genuineness, empathy, relationship, empowerment, humility, collaboration, playfulness and humor, emotional expression, family strength, and balance. Van Fleet furthered that Filial Therapy comprises eight essential features that are central to its conduct. These features can be found individually or in smaller combinations in other interventions, but it is the presence of all eight that define Filial Therapy.

1 The importance of play in child development is highlighted, and play is seen as the primary avenue for gaining greater understanding of children.
2 Parents are empowered as the change agents for their own children.
3 The client is the relationship, not the individual.
4 Empathy is essential for growth and change.
5 The entire family is involved whenever possible.
6 A psychoeducational training model is used with parents.
7 Tangible support and continued learning are provided through live supervision of parent's early play sessions with their children.
8 The process is truly collaborative.

(pp. 10–15)

Van Fleet (1994) stated that the overall aim of Filial Therapy is to eliminate the presenting problems at their source, develop positive interactions between parents and their children, and increase families' communication, coping, and problem-solving skills so they are better able to handle future problems independently and successfully. Van Fleet (2014) furthered that Filial Therapy offers several potential benefits to families of autistic and neurodivergent children. The Filial process provides autistic children with safety and choices without pressure and there is not a need for verbal communication ability, as communication can be done through play. Perhaps the greatest value is the empowerment of parents, giving them tools with which to better understand and communicate with their children.

Filial Therapy provides a significant influence and integration on AutPlay Therapy. The primary focus of parents as change agents and play as the avenue to growth and healing is integrated throughout AutPlay Therapy protocols. The AutPlay Follow Me Approach in particular highlights several foundations of Filial Therapy including Filial play skills such as tracking, reflecting, letting the child lead, and limit setting. Several constructs highlight Filial Therapy integration (1) Methods that incorporate a parent training approach where the parents are taught play times to do at home with their child. (2) Parents are considered change agents for their child and partners in the process with the therapist. (3) Relationship connection and parent empowerment are both central features and considered agents of change. (4) At home play session training and implementation is focused on the core values of openness, respect, genuineness, empathy, relationship, empowerment, humility, collaboration, playfulness, emotional expression, family strength. (5) The entire family is involved whenever possible.

Family Play Therapy

Family play therapy involves the parents and child together in therapy sessions. Although there are many methods and approaches to involving children in family therapy, in family play therapy, play therapy techniques become a part of the therapeutic family process and are utilized to help engage all members of the family and to help address therapy goals. Gil (1994) stated that the therapist can teach parents to observe, decode, and participate in their child's play in such a way that their understanding of their child's experience is enhanced, and the possibility for deeper emotional contact with their child becomes available.

Gil (2015) explained that in family play therapy family members are seen together as a system to achieve systemic changes. The application of play therapy and verbal therapy approaches are used. The therapist implements a variety of play therapy tasks and invites participation in the tasks from all family members. Play therapy tasks are designed to assess and understand underlying issues and promote positive change within the family system. There is not one identified client; the whole family is the client. The family play therapist will likely have several directive play therapy interventions in their "tool box" to implement with a family to address specific issues happening within that family with the purpose of addressing and reaching established therapy goals. Koehler, Wilson, and Baggerly (2015) provided an example of a popular intervention used in family play therapy – the *Kinetic Family Drawing*.

> The *Kinetic Family Drawing* is a structed projective assessment in which family members are asked to draw each member of their family, including themselves, doing something. The counselor asks each family member to describe all the family members in the picture and say what they are doing. Subsequently, they can tell a story about the picture stating what happened immediately before and after as well as what they would like to change if they could. Extreme caution must be used by not overly interpreting the drawing. The drawing should not be used to determine abuse or predict behavior. It is only to be used for identifying individuals' perceptions of their family.
>
> (p. 98)

Family play therapy can help individual family members' shift rigid perceptions of each other. When a child who has experienced their parent as stressed and not engaging is now having a play time where the parent is in a role, interacting with their child in a puppet story, the relationship takes a positive shift. At this point, the adult is meeting the child in their world and the emotional connection that follows is rewarding to both (Gil, 2015). Family play therapy can involve multiple members, one or two parents, all siblings, even relevant extended family members. It provides the opportunity for systems healing a growth. Gil (2015) further described the family play therapy process.

> Family play fosters attachment and breathes new life into families as they discover novel ways to interact and explore alternative solutions to their problems. Family play therapists are in a unique position to experiment with innovative ways to engage and help more than on[e] generation simultaneously. Play benefits everyone in the room (including the therapist) and can address both intrapsychic and interpersonal problems throughout the family system. It allows families to recapture the joy they once had as they laugh and play together, experiencing mutual delight in pleasure activities. Family play opens windows of opportunity to observe family interactions on a deeper level than achieved in traditional talk therapy, due in part to the rich metaphors clinicians can use to assess each family member's perceptions of the family's problems, which often become more transparent when a family is playing together. The play itself may suggest solutions that might never have emerged though verbal discussion.
>
> (p. 29)

Grant (2015) put forth that parents and other family members play an important role in the emotional, psychological, and social development of autistic and neurodivergent children. The process of including family members in therapy with their autistic child provides an opportunity for parents to become empowered in relating to and working with their child beyond which the play therapist can provide by working with the child in isolation. Family members are typically present for the majority of the child's experiences and are the people in the child's life that remain constant, while mental health professionals are transient. This level of social and familial consistency provides opportunity for parents to become effective healing agents for their child.

Family play therapy's integrative elements and influence on AutPlay Therapy involves several constructs. (1) The understanding that a parent's interaction with their child through play methods can have a deep and purposeful impact on their child and on the entire family system. (2) Families can participate together in play therapy interventions and in special play times. (3) AutPlay Therapy at its foundation is a family play therapy approach. (4) The understanding that the family system is arguably the "front line" of support and most important system for neurodivergent children. (5) The family unit as a whole is often affected by and engaged with the various needs and components of autistic and neurodivergent children. (6) Equipping parents with education and tools to help their child is a critical and sustainable process.

(7) Most established therapies working with neurodivergent children recognize the importance of a focus on the whole family and actively incorporate the parents and/or other family members in the process.

Family-focused relationship development approaches, especially those grounded in play therapy methods, heavily influence the AutPlay Therapy component area of connection. They transcend throughout the AutPlay Therapy approach that emphasizes the importance of parent involvement and the important role that parents have in the AutPlay Therapy process. Ideally AutPlay Therapy is implemented as a family play therapy approach. Parents/caregivers and/or other family members are actively involved in the therapy approach, engaging in and learning play times, directive play therapy interventions, and protocols to improve relationship connection and address therapy needs.

Gestalt Play Therapy

In the 1970s, Violet Oaklander presented the Gestalt approach to therapy with children (Gestalt Play Therapy). The principles of Gestalt Play Therapy are rooted in neuroscience, philosophy, organismic functioning, field theory, the arts, and knowledge of human development (Carroll & Orozco, 2019). Gestalt Play Therapy can be considered a psychotherapeutic technique that uses the principles of Gestalt Therapy during play therapy with the child. By developing a therapeutic relationship and contact, and according to a specific process, children are given the opportunity to confirm their sense of self verbally and non-verbally, to express their thoughts and to nurture themselves. Various forms and techniques of play are used during the different stages. Creative, projective, expressive, and dramatized play can all be used in Gestalt Play Therapy such as clay play, fantasies, story-telling, puppet shows, sand play, music, body movement, and sensory contact making exercises (Blom, 2004).

Oaklander (2007) identified several important elements of the Gestalt therapy process. These are areas to explore, usually non-sequentially, to co-create experiences that support the child's ability to use their contact functions in order to strengthen their sense of self and support integration. Table 6.1 presents the elements of therapy and possible modalities.

Blom (2004) noted that Gestalt Play Therapy is a therapeutic process focused on building the therapeutic relationship. Important aspects include the establishment of an I–thou relationship, a focus on the here and now, the responsibilities of the child and therapist, a focus on experience and discovery, handling resistance and setting boundaries. Children are viewed holistically by

Table 6.1 Elements of Therapy and Possible Modalities in Gestalt Play Therapy

Elements of Therapy	Possible Modalities
Experiencing the contact functions and the child's process of making contact	Sensory/body activities
Strengthening self-support and the child's sense of self	Sand tray, drawings, games
Understanding emotions and emotional expression	Books, music, role play, clay
Developing the capacity for an accepting, nurturing relationship with one's self	Puppets, drawings
Experimenting with new ways to get needs/ wants addressed	Role-play, homework
Building appropriate support with parents, teachers, etc.	Parent consultations
Closing the therapeutic experience	Family involvement, acknowledgements

Source: Carroll, F., & Orozco, V. (2019). Gestalt play therapy. *Play Therapy*, 14(3), 36–38.

taking the various aspects of their holistic self into account. As part of assessing children's unique process during Gestalt Play Therapy, the therapist should give attention to every child's unique temperament as it contributes to certain inborn characteristics and ways in which children will satisfy their needs.

Oaklander (2007) noted that Gestalt Play Therapy processes hold benefits for working with autistic children. Autistic children often made their needs known but in ways that were often being overlooked by adults. The focus should be to tune into the child, what the child wanted to do, rather than trying to force the child to do what the adult had planned. Oaklander highlighted the following case example involving a teacher (Saliba) working with a young autistic boy (Sean):

> One boy, age 5, stood in front of the full-length wall mirror, ignoring her call to work on a puzzle with her. Instead of insisting that he come to her, she went to him, sat by the mirror without a word, and watched as he looked at himself and felt parts of his face. She realized that he was actually seeing himself. Suddenly he noticed that her reflection was in the mirror as well, and he was so delighted and excited that he settled right

down into her lap. Twenty minutes had gone by, and the teacher had said not one word, issued not one command. Saliba began naming the parts of the face, as he continued to point to them, looking in the mirror. But when he came to the mouth, she did not respond. He looked at her expectantly through the mirror and shouted, "mouth!" Saliba describes that up until the first day when Sean showed an interest in the mirror, she had panned what each student would do during her hours of contact with them. She knew exactly what puzzle would be done by which student at what time, and for how long. She believed that autistic children needed a lot of structure, and in essence, she was demanding them to perform what, when, how, where, and to what extent, what she thought the needed all day long. When she allowed Sean that time in front of the mirror, she was taking a cue from him, which was, "Hey, I want to study my reflection, and I like doing it." From that time on, she was able to open herself up enough to see that Sean could make other needs and desires known. As a matter of fact, she just needed to let herself see and respond to those cues instead of always imposing her own demands on him.

(pp. 274–275)

Gestalt Play Therapy provides several integrative and influential elements within AutPlay Therapy philosophy and protocols. (1) The relationship established with the child is the central focus in the therapeutic process. (2) The child is viewed from a holistic perspective – the holistic self of the child is assessed, valued, and seen. (3) The recognition that autistic children can express their needs and the therapist should meet the child where they are instead of trying to force the child to consider to the therapists demands. (4) The sensory experience is a vital and crucial piece of therapy for autistic and neurodivergent children. (5) Play therapy approaches and interventions are supported that focus on sensory integration/experiences which can include a wide variety of play – tactile movement, art, expressive, etc.

Cognitive Behavioral Play Therapy (CBPT)

Susan M. Knell (1993) conceptualized that Cognitive Behavioral Therapy (CBT) underlies Cognitive-Behavioral Play Therapy (CBPT) practice. CBPT is a therapy approach that incorporates cognitive and behavioral interventions within a play therapy paradigm. Play activities as well as verbal and nonverbal forms of communication are used in resolving problems. Knell defines six specific properties related to CBPT:

1 CBPT involves the child in treatment via play.
2 CBPT focuses on the child's thoughts, feelings, fantasies, and environment.

3 CBPT provides a strategy or strategies for developing more adaptive thoughts and behaviors.
4 CBPT is structured, directive, and goal-oriented, rather than open-ended.
5 CBPT incorporates empirically demonstrated techniques.
6 CBPT allows for an empirical examination of therapy.

CBPT is predominantly a structured, directive, and goal-oriented therapy modality that systematically incorporates empirically demonstrated techniques. It includes cognitive and behavioral interventions within a play paradigm allowing the child mastery and control over their environment while being an active participant in change (Knell, 2011). CBPT focuses on the child's thoughts, perceptions, feelings, and environment, while providing a strategy for the development of more adaptive thoughts and behaviors. Traditional play therapy materials are used, especially puppets for role playing and gradual exposure, and books using a bibliotherapy approach. Play is used to teach skills, alter cognitions, create alternative behaviors, generalize positive functioning across various environments, and reduce symptoms (Drewes & Cavett, 2019).

In CBPT, the practitioner can present developmentally appropriate interventions that help the child master CBT methodology. A wide array of cognitive and behavioral interventions can be incorporated into play therapy to address a wide array of issues (Drewes, 2009). CBPT interventions provide an opportunity for children to understand how their thoughts affect their behaviors and ways to change thoughts and behaviors. CBPT's emphasis on doing, rather than talking, allows children to practice all the new skills they have learned and to generalize them to their lives outside of the play therapy session. Drewes and Cavett (2019) stated that coping skills, such as relaxation, mindfulness meditations, guided imagery, and sensory experiences are taught to reduce physiological arousal and affect dysregulation. CBPT utilizes exposure therapy through systematic desensitization for excessive fear combined with coping skills to decrease anxiety. Homework is given at each stage of therapy, so the child will practice skills in multiple settings, aiming for generalization of behaviors.

Drewes (2009) proposed that CBPT provides a wonderful opportunity to help children decrease anxiety (a common struggle emotion for autistic and neurodivergent children) and by incorporating play activities as a vehicle to involvement and exposure it may help a child manage and reduce anxiety and experience therapy in a more positive and fun atmosphere. Further, CBPT can be beneficial in helping children who experience emotional dysregulation. Children who experience emotional dysregulation (as many autistic and neurodivergent children experience), can have sudden explosions of out-of-control behavior, high levels of anxiety, and difficulties with concentration and focus. Through various cognitive methods paired with play activities, children with these issues gain a greater mastery of their emotions and thus experience less of the issues created by dysregulation.

The use of play to address needs or alternative behaviors is a common aspect of CBPT. Educating the child takes place in the CBPT model, such as, a puppet behaves in such a way that teaches the child to express emotions or gain a new skill. Through CBPT, children can address their feelings and issues and learn more adaptive ways of dealing with their feelings. Initially this could involve nonverbal expression and verbal labeling which is modeled for the child by the therapist. Later, if the child begins to talk to the therapist, more direct verbal labeling of feelings or addressing of issues can be explored (Knell, 1993).

Drewes and Cavett (2019) pretended a case example that highlights some basic ways in which CBPT can be implemented and how it might look in working with a child client:

> Jasmine (pseudonym), age 5, witnessed domestic violence and developed symptoms of defiance, mild aggression, anxiety, and depression. During the initial stage, affective psychoeducation, using dolls with feeling faces and a three-headed dragon in role play, along with a doll house, allowed Jasmine to play out scenarios from her family life while identifying and expressing feelings through her doll characters. Jasmine's mother assisted in identifying thoughts and feelings that preceded her negative behaviors, and helped her use relaxation techniques (i.e., otter breathing: breathing in and out with the waves as the "baby" otter puppet rode the waves on its mother's tummy). As therapy evolved, Jasmine used play therapy materials to reenact scenarios and verbalize witnessing domestic violence. She explored affect and beliefs that she will become like her parents, either the "hurter" or "hurted" in relationships. During the working phase of therapy, play-based techniques helped Jasmine learn non-hurtful ways to express her affect, along with systematic desensitization and exposure techniques to address separation difficulties.
>
> (para, 12)

CBPT provides integration and influence on AutPlay Therapy in a few ways. (1) The approach of having a specific agenda for each session where specific play therapy techniques are implementing with the child (and often the parent) is a component of AutPlay Therapy for some children who respond positively to directive play. (2) The goal of helping clients understand a connection between their thinking, feeling, and reactions is sometimes a therapy goal in AutPlay Therapy. (3) Incorporating "homework assignments" and practice for repetition to address therapy goals is a highlighted component of AutPlay Therapy. Parents and child may be taught several play therapy interventions to continue to play at home between sessions. Also, they may be taught special play times to have at home between sessions. For many parents, a therapist-led psychoeducation time to further understand advocacy, neurodiversity, and implementing neurodiversity affirming principles is needed and may be implemented.

This chapter highlights the primary play therapy integration that produces the AutPlay Therapy framework for using play therapy with autistic and neurodivergent children. Although the play therapy theories highlighted do indeed influence AutPlay Therapy to a great extent. It would be a miss to not acknowledge other play therapy theories and approaches. In some regards, Adlerian Play Therapy, Developmental Play Therapy, Exosystemic Play Therapy, and a variety of play therapy methods and interventions have influenced the framework of AutPlay. Table 6.2 highlights some the constructs in AutPlay Therapy and the play therapy theory integration/influences.

In the 1940s, Virginia Axline presented several tenets for Child Centered Play Therapy. Since that time, play therapy as a modality has grown and expanded with currently there being approximately 10–15 recognized play

Table 6.2 AutPlay Therapy Theoretical Constructs and Play Therapy Theories
          Integration

Theoretical Construct	*Play Therapy Theory Integration*
Parent/family involvement	Filial, Theraplay, Family PT
Family play therapy approach (systems)	Filial, Theraplay, Family PT
Emphasis on relationship development	CCPT, Gestalt PT
Connection and engagement through play	CCPT, Theraplay, Family PT
Parents considered co-change agents	Filial
Limit setting model	CCPT, Filial
Structured interventions to address specific needs	CBPT, Gestalt PT, Family PT
Interventions and processes to address sensory needs	Gestalt PT
Toys and materials utilized to encourage expression and address needs	CCPT, CBPT, Gestalt PT
Acceptance of the child a holistic and respected person	CCPT, Gestalt PT

therapy theories and approaches. Research support for many play therapy theories has grown significantly and continues to grow. Many play therapy approaches hold methodology that is helpful and affirming for autistic and neurodivergent children, yet no one theory or approach fully meets the needs across the spectrum of neurodivergence. This void created the need for AutPlay Therapy – an affirming framework for addressing needs across the spectrum using an integration of existing play therapy theories, approaches, and techniques. Essentially becoming a fusion of the best, most helpful, impactful, and affirming components of play therapy into one framework. AutPlay represents a celebration of play therapy for a population that has historically been forgotten and denied access to the therapeutic powers of play.

References

Blom, R. (2004). *The handbook of gestalt play therapy: Practical guidelines for child therapists*. Jessica Kingsley Publishers.

Booth, P. B., Christensen, G., & Lindaman, S. (2011). *Marschak interaction method (MIM) manual and cards (Revised)*. The Theraplay Institute.

Booth, P. B., & Jernberg, A. M. (2010). *Theraplay*. Jossey-Bass.

Booth, P. B., & Lindaman, S. (2019). Attachment theory and theraplay. *Play Therapy, 14*(3), 14–16.

Bundy-Myrow, S. (2012). Family theraplay: Connecting with children on the autism spectrum. In L. Gallo-Lopez, & L. C. Rubin (Eds.), *Play based interventions for children and adolescents with autism spectrum disorders* (pp. 73–96). Routledge.

Carroll, F., & Orozco, V. (2019). Gestalt play therapy. *Play Therapy, 14*(3), 36–38.

Cherry, K. (2021). What is integrative therapy. *Very Well Mind.* https://www.verywell mind.com/integrative-therapy-definition-types-techniques-and-efficacy-5201904

Drewes, A. A. (Ed.). (2009). *Blending play therapy with cognitive behavioral therapy: Evidence based and other effective treatments and techniques*. John Wiley & Sons.

Drewes, A., & Cavett, A. (2019). Cognitive behavioral play therapy. *Play Therapy, 14*(3), 24–26.

Gil, E. (1994). *Play in family therapy*. Guilford Press.

Gil, E. (2015). *Play in family therapy* (2nd ed.). Guilford Press.

Gilbert, M., & Orlans, V. (2011). *Integrative therapy: 100 key points and techniques*. Routledge.

Goodyear-Brown, P. (2010). *Play therapy with traumatized children: A prescriptive approach*. Wiley and Sons.

Grant, R. J. (2015). Family play counseling with children affected by autism. In E. J. Green, J. N. Baggerly, & A. C. Myrick (Eds.), *Counseling families* (pp. 91–105). Rowman & Littlefield.

Grant, R. J. (2017). *Autplay therapy for children and adolescents on the autism spectrum a behavioral play-based approach*. Routledge.

Guerney, B. G., Jr. (1964). Filial therapy: Description and rationale. *Journal of Consulting Psychology, 28*, 303–310.

Hillman, H. (2018). Child-centered play therapy as an intervention for children with autism: A literature review. *International Journal of Play Therapy, 27*(4), 198–204.

Jernberg, A. M., & Booth, P. B. (2001). *Theraplay: Helping parents and children build better relationships through attachment-based play.* Jossey Bass.

Knell, S. M. (1993). *Cognitive-behavioral play-therapy.* Jason Aronson.

Knell, S. M. (2011). Cognitive-behavioral play therapy. In C. E. Schaefer (Ed.), *Foundations of play therapy* (2nd ed., pp. 313–328). John Wiley & Sons.

Koehler, C. M., Wilson, B., & Baggerly, J. (2015). Play-based family assessment and treatment planning. In E. J. Green, J. N. Baggerly, & A. C. Myrick (Eds.), *Counseling families* (pp. 91–105). Rowman & Littlefield.

Landreth, G. L. (1991). *Play therapy: The art of the relationship.* Accelerated Development Publishers.

Moss, L., & Hamlet, H. (2020). *An introduction to child-centered play therapy. The Person-Centered Journal, 25*(2), 91–103.

Oaklander, V. (2007). *Windows to our children: A Gestalt therapy approach to children and adolescents.* The Gestalt Journal Press.

O'Connor, K. J. (2001). Ecosystemic play therapy. *International Journal of Play Therapy, 10*(2), 33–44.

Ray, D. C. (2011). *Advanced play therapy: Essential conditions, knowledge, and skills for child practice.* Routledge.

Ray, D. C., & Landreth, G. L. (2019). Child centered play therapy. *Play Therapy, 14*(3), 18–19.

Salter, K., Beamish, W., & Davies, M. (2016). The effects of child-centered play therapy (CCPT) on the social and emotional growth of young children with autism. *International Journal of Play Therapy, 25*, 78–90.

Scuka, R. F., & Guerney, L. (2019). Filial therapy. *Play Therapy, 14*(3), 20–22.

Seymour, J. W. (2011). History of psychotherapy integration and related research. In A. A. Drewes, S. C. Bratton, & C. E. Schaefer (Eds.), *Integrative play therapy* (pp. 3–18). John Wiley & Sons

Simeone-Russell, R. (2011). A practical approach to implementing theraplay for children with autism spectrum disorder. *International Journal of Play Therapy, 20*(4), 224–235.

VanFleet, R. (1994). *Filial therapy: Strengthening the parent-child relationships through play.* Professional Resource Press.

VanFleet, R. (2014). *Filial therapy: Strengthening the parent-child relationships through play* (3rd ed.). Professional Resource Press.

Ware Balch, J., & Ray, D. (2015). Emotional assets of children with autism spectrum disorder: A single-case therapeutic outcome experiment. *Journal of Counseling and Development, 93*, 429–439.

Yasenik, L., & Gardner, K. (2012). *Play therapy dimensions model: A decision making guide for integrative play therapists.* Jessica Kingsley Publishers.

7
The AutPlay® Therapy Process

Quickly out of graduate school and into a rural private practice group clinic, I began my mental health work with children. It did not take long (one session I believe) to realize I had not received what I needed from my graduate program to adequately work with children. I begin exploring play therapy and working toward receiving the play therapy credential of Registered Play Therapist (RPT). I found in play therapy the healing and growth-producing processes that spoke to children and gave them a voice and a therapeutic process. I discovered how their natural language of play could speak throughout the array of the therapeutic powers of play.

Shortly into my play therapy career I began to receive referrals for children with ADHD and sensory differences and then my first referral for an autistic child who was also diagnosed with intellectual developmental disorder, a chromosome disorder, and various medical conditions. I was initially drawn to neurodivergent children (although I did not understand the term neurodivergent at the time). I connected with them and much of what they were experiencing due to my own neurodivergence. Having sensory processing disorder, social anxiety disorder, and trauma issues in my childhood gave me an affinity for working with similar populations. I often reflected on my own childhood and what it would have meant if I could have found my way to a play therapist. I do believe the therapeutic powers of play would have been a great gift to me and changed the trajectory of my childhood.

After I began working with my first autistic child, I began to feel that there was something missing in the play therapy training I had received. I felt I needed something more to help address the myriad of needs and presentations I was seeing across neurodivergent children. I began to investigate additional trainings and therapy approaches. In the play therapy and greater mental health fields there was little available. Most of these children were not being seeing by mental health professionals and were being referred to

DOI: 10.4324/9781003207610-8

behavioral programs. I began to explore trainings outside of the mental health community – popular advertised trainings for working with autistic children. I attended many, and most had a strong behavioral focus and/or rigid child training protocol and none viewed play in the way I had learned and valued as a play therapist. Many of these "therapies" were adamant that autistic children and children with developmental disabilities did not understand play, did not play, and play-related therapies would not help them. I disagreed.

These training did provide me with a greater knowledge enhancement and there were some elements I could take and apply that increased my toolbox, but in general they were not a fit for me and the work I was trying to do as a play therapist. I began to conceptualize how the greater field of play therapy (the various seminal play therapy theories) collectively held a great deal of value for autistic and neurodivergent children. It was at this point I began to think integrative – how different methods and approaches in various play therapy theories could be integrated to form a framework or guide for working with autistic and neurodivergent children. This was the beginning of what would become AutPlay Therapy.

AutPlay Therapy Overview

This chapter is designed to present an overview of AutPlay Therapy. Specific protocols and processes in AutPlay are further explored in other chapters. AutPlay Therapy has been defined as an integrative family play therapy approach designed to address the mental health needs of neurodivergent children (autistic, ADHD, learning differences, sensory differences, Tourette Syndrome, giftedness/twice exceptional, intellectual developmental disability, developmental disabilities, etc.). The foundation of AutPlay Therapy consists of seminal play therapy theories and approaches integrated into a neurodiversity affirming framework. As a comprehensive model, AutPlay Therapy is designed to assist children and adolescents (across a spectrum of presentation) and their families with mental health needs.

AutPlay Therapy is a synthesis or true integration of various psychological and counseling theory including humanistic, developmental, and family systems methodology. AutPlay Therapy protocol involves assessing and addressing the developmental issues for children and adolescents, and provides continuous awareness of developmental levels, needs, strengths, and progress. Four overarching constructs guide the framework and implementation of AutPlay Therapy:

- Play Therapy – Consists of multiple theories and approaches that recognize the therapeutic powers of play. It is a form of psychotherapy and can be effective in helping children through emotional and mental issues and has a large research (evidence-based) support. Play Therapy can involve nondirective or directive play, various types of play preferences, and can be implemented with individual children and/or families.
- The Neurodiversity Paradigm and Movement – Neurodiversity defines the variance of neurotypes that exist across the human race. The neurodiversity paradigm illustrates the awareness and acceptance of this truth and a commitment to view children through this paradigm lens. The movement is action-oriented – attending to processes, approaches, and techniques to make sure they are neurodiversity affirming and children receive an affirming approach during their play therapy experience.
- The Social Model of Disability – Proposes that an individual is not disabled by their diagnosis, condition, or state of being, they are disabled by the attitudes and structures in society and the environments in which they navigate. There is often an ableist process which prevents or makes it very challenging for neurodivergent children to achieve and excel.
- Family Systems – Often defined as an approach to understand human functioning that focuses on interactions between people in a family and between the family and the context(s) in which that family is embedded. Family (parent/child) is a critical, foundational relationship and often presenting issues or needs involve the whole family in healing and growth.

AutPlay Therapy incorporates a combination of non-directive processes and directive play therapy interventions and approaches designed to meet children where they are and provide mental health support. Nondirective play therapists are trained to trust that children can direct their own process rather than the therapist directing their own ideas of what needs to happen in therapy to address therapy goals and needs. A nondirective approach requires the therapist to enter the emotional world of the child rather than expecting the child to understand the therapist's world, which is beyond their capabilities. Nondirective play therapy is based on respect for the child and confidence in their ability to direct their own process. It requires that the therapist maintain unconditional acceptance and positive regard for the child (Petruk, 2009).

Directive play therapy is an integrative approach that combines different theoretical models in a manner that responds to and addresses the needs of children. Other terms that have been used for this approach include structured, prescriptive, focused, and non-humanistic. Therapists use directive play therapy to focus attention, stimulate further activity, gain information, interpret, specifically address therapy goals, or set limits. Purposeful activities, such as games or play techniques, are structured by the therapist to elicit process and responses from the client. The therapist assumes the responsibility for the guidance and interpretation of the play interactions (Leggett & Boswell, 2017).

AutPlay Therapy process can be utilized to address a variety of concerns, and the need areas that neurodivergent children may present with include but are not limited to trauma issues, parent/child relationship struggles, emotional regulation, social navigation, sensory processing, anxiety reduction, and life adjustment issues. As needs are conceptualized and addressed in AutPlay, it is important to remember that when children can learn to understand and regulate their system, possess awareness of and receive support for the environments in which they are asked to function, and have meaningful relationship connection, they are far less likely to have any type of "behavioral issues" and more likely to successfully maneuver in their day-to-day environment.

Neurodivergent children and adolescents may have overlapping or intertwined needs. Often the internal processing ability, the child's environments, and supports (or lack of supports) are co-creating mental health needs for the child. There tends to be a relationship among need areas in regard to the child feeling or being "stuck" and needing help with forward movement (if a child has a need such as regulation struggles, they will likely have needs in the other areas, such as school challenges or anxiety issues. If a child addresses one need area, they will likely see resolve in the other need areas). For example, as a child makes gains in understanding their internal system and regulation, it will have a positive effect on their social navigation needs. As a child's social needs improve, it will have a positive effect on their self-awareness, identity, and self-worth.

AutPlay Therapy is often refenced as a play therapy approach. AutPlay protocol and processes are more like a framework for using play therapy with neurodivergent children. For conceptualization, the analogy of building a house is illustrated. The framework guides the larger and foundational purposes. It serves as a guide for implementing play therapy principles through an understanding of neurodivergence and neurodiversity affirming application (the basic framework and foundation of the house). In AutPlay we always start with a healthy understanding of the foundation (neurodivergence) and framework (play therapy). This is what creates the AutPlay therapist.

We then move to individualizing the therapeutic approach based on each unique neurodivergent child's strengths and needs (each individually designed room in the house). Each individual child is understood as unique on the spectrum of presentation and the play therapy process will be molded to the specific child. Considerations should include the child's play preferences and what seems to be a best fit for the child and their needs. Based upon the child, some processes may be more nondirective and some more directive, some may integrate multiple play therapy methods while some function in primarily one approach. The level of therapist involvement, the type(s) of play, the utilization of the playroom, will have an individualized look. Regardless of the design of each individual "room in the house," the totality of each child's play process, will always be governed by the neurodivergence and play therapy foundation and framework.

Partners

A partnership or "partnering" is often defined as relating to an agreement between people to work together. The purpose of this relationship is to work toward shared goals through a division that all parties agree on. The primary characteristics of partnership include commitment, coordination, trust, communication, participation; and a conflict resolution (disagreement) technique for joint problem-solving. Partnering with the parent, child, and whole family (when possible) is an important feature of the AutPlay Therapy framework. Both parent and child offer much to the therapeutic process. They are the experts on themselves and their families. On a pragmatic level, the "partnership" can take many forms (this is further discussed in a later chapter) but would manifest in some fashion.

Kottman (2003) explained the partnership or collaboration process in *Adlerian Play Therapy* when working with children and parents:

> I am extremely reluctant to see a child in play therapy without conjoint parent consultations because of my belief that the child is socially embedded. I believe that I must understand the child's lifestyle from the perspective of the child and from the perspective of other family members before I can help the family. To effect long-lasting change, it is essential for (a) the child to make shifts in the way he or she sees himself, others, and the world, and (b) the members of the family to be willing to make adjustments in the way they view and respond to the child.
>
> (p. 21)

AutPlay Therapy incorporates a parent partnering (training) component where parents are trained by the therapist in using various play therapy approaches and techniques at home with their child. Parents are viewed as partners with the therapist and are empowered to become co-change agents with the therapist in helping their child address and advance in therapy goals. AutPlay Therapy's parent training component teaches parents how to facilitate AutPlay Follow Me Approach play times and specific play therapy technique play times at home with their child between therapy sessions. Parents learn about play, procedures, and techniques and are shown how to implement play times at home to improve the parent–child relationship and work toward addressing therapy goals.

Children are also viewed as partners in the process with the therapist and the parent. As much as possible, the child's thoughts, feelings, and voice are included into the therapy process, goals, and plan. Children should have a say in what they want to achieve and the process to achieve it. Children should be clearly informed that they can freely share what they think, like, and don't like. In AutPlay, children are often asked if they liked a play intervention and if they felt the intervention was helpful to them. The level of "partnership" that a child participates in will vary from child to child. Much of this will depend on the child's age and their need level or ability to communicate and interact. It would be expected that an older child and/or a child with communication and interaction ability would participate more fully. Regardless of the child's age or level, the therapist should make every possible effort to include the child as a partner (even in small ways or increments). Any empowerment possible for the child should be extended.

AutPlay Therapy functions ideally as a family play therapy approach involving both the child and the parent in the therapeutic process. Using a play therapy base that is a natural language for the child enables the parent to be involved with their child in a way that builds healthy relationship and addresses therapy goals within a fun and connecting process. Further, when possible and appropriate, AutPlay Therapy involves other relevant family members including siblings and extended family members in the therapy process. For consistency purposes the term parent is used, but involvement of the "parent" means whoever is in the caregiver role with the child.

Play

Play is rooted in processes that lie deep within the brain (Kestly, 2014). Play provides an opportunity for children to see their world for what it is and what has come their way, and to resolve a new way to survive. It provides a way of understanding and healing each day. Play has a special place in the lives of children throughout the world. Playing provides an experience and purpose for joining. Children can connect, share, understand their reason for connecting, growing, and attachment (Bowers & Bowers, 2013). Models of play therapy highlight the power of play as an avenue for children to express, explore, and address a variety of mental health needs.

Given that play is a significant focus of models of play therapy and AutPlay Therapy specifically, it is important to examine what can be expected of play in the therapeutic process with neurodivergent children. What are the similarities and differences from a neurotypical child? What can a therapist expect a client's play to look like when beginning the AutPlay Therapy process?

Historically, autistic children, those with high needs, and children with developmental disabilities were described as lacking spontaneous, flexible, imaginative, and social qualities that are common with play. Playing with toys spontaneously, engaging in pretend and imaginative play, understanding metaphor in play, and successfully engaging in group play was not likely. At best, it was stated that autistic children would manipulate objects in a detached fashion rather than play either functionally or symbolically. Research and writings often described common play challenges that limited an autistic child or adolescent's play potential such as Cross's (2010) five problems with autistic play:

1 Repetitious play
2 Continual roaming around the playroom
3 Continual anxiousness about or during play
4 Continual detachment or unfriendliness during play
5 Continual rejection by playmates during play

These ideas are contrary to the view of neurodivergent play in AutPlay Therapy. The play of neurodivergent children is recognized, valued, and understood for its therapeutic merit. The historical views of neurodivergent play were incorrect and laden in ableist views of what play *must* look like and *must* be to be recognized as play.

When an autistic or neurodivergent child enters a play therapy room, it is possible that they will not engage in play in a tradition or socially deemed "correct" way to play. A neurodivergent child might be very hesitant when first entering play therapy. They may be feeling anxiety or dysregulation and may take some time to get comfortable or familiar with what is around them and then eventually begin to in play. Some children may prefer to isolate themselves and play with toys or materials paying no attention to the therapist or things around them. Some children may find an object not traditionally considered a toy and desire to play with the object and ignore what would be considered the popular toys.

When neurodivergent children are given the opportunity to play freely, they are likely to pursue preferences, interests, and activities that mean something to them. Some children may produce and participate in elaborate play scenarios in symbolic or pretend play. Some children might enjoy scripted play – playing out a favorite scene from a move or TV show. Some may prefer to play repetitively with the child coming back to the same scenarios over and over again for long periods of time. Often autistic children will enter a play therapy scenario and begin playing in a way that speaks to them and in a way they understand. If the therapist is patient and allows the child time to feel safe and familiar with the therapist and the surroundings, the child will begin to display their play preferences and interests. The therapist should avoid jumping to a conclusion that the child does not play. The therapist may see a hesitancy or what appears to be not understanding what to do, but this typical anxiousness and/or discomfort is associated with being around a new person, a new place, and not understanding the expectations.

Autistic and neurodivergent children may have struggles and needs related to social play with peers. Unfortunately, many neurodivergent children can become isolated in their play and withdraw from peer play groups. There is often a great deal of rejection and lack of acceptance from peers. The social model of disability and ableist ideas can often be present in children just as they are in adults and systems. After several attempts met with rejection and sometimes ridicule, many neurodivergent children stop trying to engage in peer and group play. This can present to others and has been misinterpreted to mean that autistic and neurodivergent children do not know how and/or do not want to play with peers. There is significant evidence to indicate that autistic children do desire peer relationships and to participate in peer play but are often met with blocks to success. Besides peer rejection, many neurodivergent children may have anxiety, sensory differences, or other issues that make it difficult to initiate and maintain such play. There is plenty of evidence to indicate that autistic and neurodivergent children do indeed play in a variety of ways and desire play. A neurodivergent child may play in non-traditional ways, may play with things that are not socially accepted as toys, and their play may not look the way an adult is used to seeing – but that does not mean it is not play.

Michael (an eight-year-old autistic child) is a proper example of the variability of play in autistic and neurodivergent children. He entered AutPlay

Therapy with a diagnosis of autism spectrum disorder, intellectual developmental disorder, a genetic disorder, and several compounding medical issues. Michael's verbal output consisted of very little speaking, when he did, approximately 80% of what he said was difficult for other people to understand. Michael mostly kept to himself and did not interact much with others. Due to some medical conditions, he had difficulty with large and fine motor skills and also had a feeding tube. I began working with Michael using the AutPlay Follow Me Approach (discussed more fully later in this book), with a more concentrated focus on nondirective play. Michael wanted to be in the playroom and spent the first couple of sessions roaming around the playroom not really participating with any toys or activities in the playroom and very little engagement with me.

The playroom that Michael had his sessions in also had a storage closet that was used to store various office supplies. Michael discovered the storage closet during session three. Inside the storage closet was a variety of cleaning supplies including a vacuum cleaner. Michael quickly took notice of the vacuum cleaner and wanted to vacuum the playroom floor and anything else he could find to vacuum. This often included vacuuming the puppets, plush chairs, and various toys. The vacuum cleaner quickly became his toy and type of play for the next several sessions. Michael would enter the playroom and go directly to the storage closet and retrieve the vacuum. He was very excited for the vacuum to be plugged in and begin his vacuum play. Michael expressed positive emotions while he was vacuum playing, he would smile, laugh, and generally seem happy. I would track Michael's play and reflect any feelings presented. I began to try and get involved in Michael's vacuum play. I introduced items to see if he would vacuum them, I asked him if I could have a turn vacuuming and he handed me the vacuum. We began taking turns giving each other specific items to vacuum. I introduced some vacuum sharing games between Michael and myself and his mother. I also introduced some problem-solving and coping skill games. Michael's overall interaction and connection with myself and his parents began to significantly increase.

Michael's interest in playing with the office vacuum carried over to his home setting. I was able to teach Michael's parents how to use the vacuum to have relational focused play times at home. This became a positive experience for Michael and his parents. They expressed this was the first time they had been able to have play times with Michael. Through Michael's "vacuum play" with myself and his parents at home, Michael began to make significant strides in his therapy goals. In line with AutPlay protocol, Michael showed me his play preferences and interests and I followed his lead and used his play preferences to help address this therapy goals. I did not discredit his play preferences because it was a vacuum cleaner and not a traditional toy from the playroom. This acceptance of him and his play was instrumental in developing therapeutic relationship with Michael. Eventually, he began to branch into other types of play which opened more opportunities for addressing additional therapy goals.

Each autistic and neurodivergent child will have a different assessment in terms of their play preferences, strengths, and interests. The therapist may not know the child's play preferences until they spend time with the child and observe their play. It is essential that proper assessment is done to learn the child's play preferences, strengths, and interests. It is not fair to assume that every neurodivergent child will play in the same way. Some children will play but in ways and with objects that may not seem like or look like traditional play. Some children will display multiple types of play preferences. It is the therapist's job to accept and value play preferences with judgment. The following present points to remember regarding the neurodivergent child's' play in therapy:

- Play is the natural language for all children.
- Play can look different from a neurotypical presentation – different is not wrong.
- Engage with the neurodivergent child in the way they prefer to play – explore their interests.
- Help parents understand the play preferences of their child and how to relationally play with their child.
- Play is the agent of change not a manipulative to get the child to do something.

Play Techniques

AutPlay Therapy does utilize a variety of structured and directive play therapy interventions and techniques to help address therapy goals. Although this directive and more therapist-driven element exists, it does not replace the foundational importance of therapeutic relationship. Relationship development is central to the successful implementation of any directive play intervention. It is the relationship that gives the interventions power and effectiveness.

The purpose of a therapeutic relationship is to assist the child and family in therapy to change their life for the better. Such a relationship is essential, as it is oftentimes the first setting in which the person receiving therapy explores intimate thoughts, beliefs, and emotions regarding the issue(s) in question. As such, it is very important that therapists provide a safe, open, and non-judgmental atmosphere where the child can be at ease. Trust, acceptance, and congruence are major components of a good therapeutic relationship. Therapists are encouraged to show empathy and genuineness. As with any other social relationship, the therapeutic relationship has boundaries which help to define acceptable and unacceptable behaviors (GoodTherapy.org, 2015).

Landreth (1991) emphasized the central importance on relationship development in the play therapy process. He conceptualized the following personal reflections about the play therapy relationship with children:

- I am not all knowing. Therefore, I shall not even attempt to be.
- I need to be loved. Therefore, I will be open to loving children.
- I want to be more accepting of the child in me. Therefore, I will with wonder and awe allow children to illuminate my world.
- I know so little about the complex intricacies of childhood. Therefore, I will allow children to teach me.
- I learn best from and am impacted most by my personal struggles. Therefore, I will join children in their struggles.
- I sometimes need a refuge. Therefore, I will provide a refuge for children.
- I like it too when I am fully accepted as the person I am. Therefore, I will strive to experience and appreciate the person of the child.
- I make mistakes. They are a declaration of the way I am – human and fallible. Therefore, I will be tolerant of the humanness of children.
- I react with emotional internalization and expression to my world of reality. Therefore, I will relinquish the grasp I have on reality and will try to enter the world as experienced by the child.
- It feels good to be an authority, to provide answers. Therefore, I shall need to work hard to protect children from me.
- I am more fully me when I feel safe. Therefore, I will be consistent in my interactions with children.
- I am the only person who can live my life. Therefore, I will not attempt to rule a child's life.
- I have learned most of what I know from experiencing. Therefore, I will allow children to experience.
- The hope I experience and the will to live come from within me. Therefore, I will recognize and affirm the child's will and selfhood.
- I cannot make children's hurts and fears and frustrations and disappointments go away. Therefore, I will soften the blow.

- I experience fear when I am vulnerable. Therefore, I will with kindness, gentleness, and tenderness touch the inner world of the vulnerable child.

(pp. 5–6)

Therapeutic relationship development is a core change agent within the therapeutic powers of play. In AutPlay Therapy there is a mindfulness of relationship development practices at the beginning of therapy and throughout the duration. Even when implementing directive play interventions, the therapist's focus should be on developing relationship which includes the following:

- Accept the child and the child's behavior where they are at.
- Do not place judgment on the child and/or parent.
- Provide unconditional positive regard to the child and family.
- Recognize the child is a fully functioning person and is more than their diagnosis or issue.
- Provide empathic responding, reflective responding, and active listing skills.
- Relationship development is an active process throughout the duration of therapy.

Autistic and neurodivergent children and children with developmental disabilities often do not track to the established developmental age charts. When deciding on directive play therapy techniques to help address therapy goals, it is important to remember that some of a child's developmental levels may be different from their chronological age. If a child or adolescent is having difficulty understanding a technique or has anxiety that is preventing them from fully engaging, it is important to adapt the technique so that anxiety is alleviated, engagement is increased, and the child can enjoy the intervention (Delaney, 2010).

AutPlay Therapy directive play therapy techniques are specifically designed to meet a child where they are at in terms of their development and play preferences. AutPlay Therapy directive play therapy techniques help increase relationship development and address therapy needs and goals. AutPlay Therapy takes into account the various issues that may be present with a child and is sensitive to introducing directive play interventions in a specific manner so that neurodivergent children can feel comfortable, participate, and gain from directive play techniques. Children and adolescents are thoroughly assessed at the beginning of therapy to identify their needs and play preferences. This assists the therapist in creating therapy goals and choosing directive play interventions to specifically address each child's needs.

It is important to remember that when working with any child, and using any play technique, the therapist will find they participate at various levels with a child. This is determined by the therapist when working with a child. If a child has higher needs and is having trouble with a concept, then the therapist will likely become more involved and may lead much of the play technique, taking on more of an instructional and psychoeducational role. If a child has less needs and easily understands the technique components, then the therapist will do less directing/instructing and will let the child create and develop in the play intervention on their own. The therapist should remember that they will, at times, be more instruction/participator oriented, but the therapist should always be looking for advancement in a child and allowing them to do as much as they can on their own.

Therapists should take note that there exist multiple play therapy books that highlight techniques and interventions. Although many of these books are not autism- or neurodivergence-specific, some of the interventions can still be used with neurodivergent children and adolescents, especially with some specific modifications. Some important points to remember about directive play therapy techniques with autistic and neurodivergent children and adolescents include:

1 It is the relationship with the child and family that makes the play technique work best. This book could be filled with examples of children who challenged and struggled with other professionals who lacked a relationship focus and those same children freely participated in working on all kinds of goals with therapists who promoted relationship development with an essential focus throughout therapy.
2 Techniques that are directive or structured, meaning the therapist will be introducing the technique to implement, should be an active and fluid process in which the therapist can shift focus and redirect as needed.
3 Fun is more important than form. Children should feel safe, comfortable, and have fun during play therapy interventions. Keep in mind that some neurodivergent children may experience a level of anxiety or dysregulation when participating in a play technique. Unfamiliar people, places, and things can create anxiety. Be mindful of this, stay attuned with the child and provide co-regulation during play interventions.
4 A difficult to measure and often undervalued skill is the therapist's playful instinct and attitude. Because some techniques involve structure and

may initially lack a great deal of enticement, the therapist's playful attitude is essential for making the child's experience more engaging and enjoyable.

5 The therapist should involve the child in decisions about directive techniques, ask the child's opinion, provide choices, and allow for the child's voice.

6 Techniques should have a purposeful focus and direct connection to therapy needs and goals.

7 The therapist should be comfortable with and flexible in their involvement in directive techniques. They may take on a minimal role or a more instructional role. The level of role will vary from child to child depending on how much assistance is needed by the therapist.

8 The therapist should be prepared to participate in the play technique with the child and/or family. Often the therapist will be actively participating with the child, playing with the child, taking on a role, or creating and sharing their own representation of the intervention.

9 The therapist should be an attuned observer during the session/technique to assess if the technique seems to fit the child well and is appropriate for helping the child or adolescent address therapy goals. Notice if the child is struggling and try to assess and reflect how to help the child with what they may be feeling or struggling with.

10 Techniques should align with and respect the child's play preferences and interests. The therapist should not implement a directive technique based in a type of play in which the child is not interested and does not respond.

11 Techniques can be implemented in which the therapist is unsure of the play preferences of the child or when introducing a type of play the child may have never been exposed to. In these situations, care should be taken to monitor the child's response. Ideally the child will respond favorably and seem to connect with the play and/or intervention. If the child does not respond favorably and seems disinterested or does not like the play/intervention, the therapist should discontinue the intervention.

12 Techniques should have the ability to be easily simplified or made more complex. This way, techniques can be adapted for any child or adolescent across ages and regardless of need level.

13 Directive play therapy technique should be introduced and explained by breaking down instructions to the technique into simple understandable steps. If the child or adolescent is struggling to understand or complete an intervention, the therapist may want to try completing one step at a time before giving the next instruction.

14 The therapist may model for the child or adolescent what they want
    them to do or create. Some children may have receptive language issues
    and/or prefer a visual representation of what is being asked of them. In
    these situations, auditory instructions would not be the primary method
    of instruction. The therapist would include visuals or demonstrations.

15 Techniques should be created that can easily be taught to parents and
    implemented by parents in the home setting. Parents should not be re-
    quired to purchase several toys, props, or materials to implement home
    play times and interventions.

16 Techniques will not always flow smoothly when being implemented. The
    technique may highlight additional issues that need to be addressed. The
    therapist may interject helpful statements, reflections, or questions dur-
    ing a technique. Additionally, the therapist may need to help some chil-
    dren understand the constructs involved with a particular intervention.

17 Therapists should be flexible when implementing a play technique.
    Therapists should be prepared to let go of the structure of the session if
    necessary and understand that some children may produce an approxi-
    mate of the completed technique, and this is okay.

18 Therapists can use prizes and incentives to help engage a child in partic-
    ipating and/or to create another playful element to the technique. Prizes
    and incentives should not be viewed or used as rewards for compliant
    behavior. Implementing a prize or incentive should always be discussed
    with the child's parents and the child prior to using them with a play
    technique.

19 Provide feedback for the child and family during and after techniques to
    encourage them in how they did and what they accomplished, especially
    when the child and/or family member is hesitant.

20 Ask the child questions about the play technique. Ask the child or ado-
    lescent if they enjoyed the technique or if they felt it helped them with
    their needs or goals. Try to process the technique with the child and
    apply the technique to the child's real life. Remember the child is a part-
    ner in the process and their voice should be heard. Take time after the
    session to evaluate how the session went and if the technique seems to
    have been successful for the child or adolescent.

21 Technique options are many but should always be selected and imple-
    mented with the individual child in mind. Inspiration can be found in
    many places for play therapy techniques. Therapists should try to im-
    plement techniques that will be most beneficial for the individual child
    or adolescent and the family. Play therapy techniques should follow the
    following equation, understanding the individual child + understanding

the child's play preferences + knowing the child's therapy needs and good + understanding the family = ready for play therapy technique selection.

Once a play therapy technique is introduced, the technique is made a part of the child's awareness from that point forward. The therapist, parents, and child may practice the same play technique for several sessions in a row. A technique may be completed in one session and revisited several sessions later and completed again if it would be relevant and helpful for therapy goals or evaluation purposes. Many techniques could serve as coping and accommodation aids that the child could use throughout their lifetime. It is preferred that a child and parent use and reference play techniques as often as appropriate. Parent and child can begin to accumulate a "toolbox" of ideas and interventions that they can implement any time they feel it would be beneficial.

Pragmatics

AutPlay Therapy is most appropriate for children aged 3–18 across the neurodivergent spectrum.

Session Protocols

Starting a session – Sessions should begin with a structing statement such as "This is the playroom or space and you can play with anything you want, and I will be in here with you."

Ending a session – The therapist should let the child know when five minutes are left of the session and then again when one minute is left of the session. The therapist should position themselves where the child can see them and give them the minutes left. It is also helpful for the therapist to use a visual such as holding up their hand with five fingers then one finger. Often in AutPlay Therapy a transition item (small toy, sticker, balloon) is provided at the end of the session for the child to take home. This is not a prize or a reward for participating in the session or exhibiting some type of behavior. If a transition item is established, it is part of the routine to provide consistency and is always given regardless of the session components.

Playroom cleanup – This depends on the developmental level of the child. Typically, children help (partner) with cleanup if it relates to a therapy goal (such as working together to complete a task). This can be turned into a playful game. In AutPlay, the process of cleanup is at the discretion of the therapist based on the induvial child they are working with.

Toys, Games, and Materials

AutPlay Therapy sessions consist of both nondirective play and directive play therapy techniques which usually involves toys, games, and expressive materials that have been selected by the therapist and placed in a play therapy room and/or as part of a directive technique. Purposeful toy selection is essential as it pertains to toys or materials that will be most representative of the variance in play preferences of neurodivergent children and used in completing directive play therapy techniques. Therapists should also consider that some neurodivergent children will want to engage in free play in the playroom setting, may want space for movement play, may have a play preference in technology play, and these opportunities should be made available to the child. Many therapists have successfully combined session times to include both implementing directive techniques and allowing the child time to have nondirective play time. Much of this is decided by the therapist and child/parent in establishing the therapy needs and goals and the play preferences of the child.

Toys, art, games, movement, sensory, and expressive materials are often used in AutPlay Therapy (a list of suggested toys and materials for AutPlay is provided in the appendix section). When using toys in AutPlay Therapy, there are some issues for consideration regarding the autistic and neurodivergent child. First, many typical or popular toys for children or adolescents may not be interesting to the neurodivergent child. Do not assume that traditional toys and mainstream marketed toys will appeal to neurodivergent children. Second, having too many toys in the playroom or toys displayed in a disorganized manner may feel dysregulating to the child. Playrooms should not be cluttered, and toys should be easily seen and accessed. Third, it is likely that a child or adolescent will choose to focus on one or two particular toys and want to play with them repeatedly from session to session. Fourth, more reality-based toys such as a doctor's kit, play phone, and kitchen toys, or sensory based toys such as sensory balls, sand, or fidget toys will likely be more popular or appealing for many neurodivergent children. Finally, therapists will want to select toys and materials that align with therapy goals and directive interventions they will be implementing.

Many autistic and neurodivergent children and adolescents will enjoy and may find more appealing – board games, card games, movement based games, technology games, or prop based games. Several AutPlay Therapy interventions do involve a game-based format. Therapists should pay careful attention to games that involve certain skill levels or physical ability and make sure the game matches the child's level. Expressive materials cover a wide range of materials from art related such as painting and drawing to sand and other sensory trays to electronic apps. The main consideration regarding expressive materials involves being sensitive to the child's sensory differences. Many neurodivergent children have sensory differences and may have an aversion to the feel of sand or clay or may have a strong negative reaction to the smell of paint or markers. Other neurodivergent children will not have any problems with these materials and may find them comforting and relaxing. Therapists should pay special attention to the sensory needs of each child and adolescent when selecting toys and materials and implementing play interventions.

Play Therapy Rooms

AutPlay Therapy sessions can be facilitated in a play therapy room, practitioner's office, school counselor's office, special education classroom, or almost any environment. Since sessions may involve pre-selected play therapy techniques, the therapist can collect the materials and toys needed and have them ready in any office space. The exception to this would be implementing the AutPlay Therapy Follow Me Approach (discussed in a later chapter). This approach does utilize a traditional child-centered playroom. Typically play therapy rooms include several toys and materials, so if the therapist needs to change or adjust an intervention during a session, it will be more likely that the therapist will have the needed materials or toys close by for an easy transition.

Some children or adolescents may have a preference in regard to going into a play therapy room or to staying in the therapist's office or another space. If a child or adolescent has a distinct preference, then that preference should be given priority. If the child does not have a preference, then sessions might be better facilitated in a play therapy room as the play therapy room does provide a good environment and opportunity to continually evaluate and assess a child's play preference and space for the child to utilize play for growth and advancement. Therapists should note that some autistic and neurodivergent children may find a playroom too distracting, overwhelming, or anxiety producing. If this is the case, the therapist should facilitate sessions in their office or a more benign, less stimulating setting.

In AutPlay, play therapy rooms are typically used during the intake and assessment phase (discussed more fully later in this book) of therapy when the therapist conducts a child observation and a parent and child observation in a play therapy room. Also, during the intake and assessment phase, children should be given a tour of the building, office, playroom(s) that may be accessed. The tour helps the child become familiar with the space and gives the child the awareness that they can choose a playroom or some other space depending on their preference. After the intake and assessment phase is complete, therapy sessions can occur in any office setting as long as the needed toys and materials are present to implement interventions and allow for play preference expression.

The following are some considerations and guidelines for setting up a playroom or office space when working with neurodivergent clients:

- Develop a normal routine that the child or adolescent follows as they enter the office and/or playroom to begin a session. Try to keep things the same from session to session – keep toys and materials in the same place in the playroom and make sure playrooms are back to their organized state before bringing the child into the playroom. Most neurodivergent children will respond more positively to things being predictable.
- Some children and adolescent may have strong sensory integration issues. Therapists should assess for these needs and adjust their office and/or playroom accordingly. This might include being able to adjust the lighting, attending to noise levels, being flexible in where the child wants to sit and having a variety of options (soft chair, hard chair, rug, exercise ball, etc., and avoiding certain odors like a scented candle or air fresheners.
- Make sure toys and materials include a healthy variety of sensory and regulation products. This might include play doh, clay, sand trays, various sensory trays, sensory balls, fidget toys, various tactile experiences, a mini trampoline, a balance board, stepping stones, hula hoops, an exercise ball, etc.
- It is best to begin with a traditional child-centered play therapy playroom setup and modify as needed from there. Some considerations for modification include placing some of the toys and materials out of view in a cabinet or behind a curtain to help with children becoming overwhelmed, establish space for full body movement play and interventions, try to represent the various play preferences a neurodivergent child may have including technology play. Make sure the space is accommodating for children with differing abilities such as a wheel chair, certain walking

aids, augmentative and alternative communication supports, and fine and large motor issues.

Limit Setting with the AutPlay Follow Me Approach

There may be times when the therapist needs to set a limit on something that is happening in the session. When this occurs a limit setting model should be implemented. Limit setting should be kept to a minimum, so the child and therapist do not get distracted and disrupted by continually setting limits. When a limit needs to be set either by the therapist in the playroom or by parents in the home setting, they should be consistent, follow the limit setting model, and moved on from. Limits should consist of situations that would be dangerous for the child, for others, or situations where the child might be destroying property. If one of these situations arises, then the therapist could implement the three R's AutPlay Therapy limit setting model. The three R's limit setting model stands for redirect, replacement, and removal.

Redirect – If the child begins to or is breaking a limit. The therapist could begin with redirection which means redirecting the child's focus and energy away from a problematic situation to something that is allowed. For example, away from throwing sand all over the playroom to shooting baskets in the basketball hoop. The therapist would simply try to redirect the child to another activity, toy, or object to transition their attention off the limit violation. There does not need to be any dialogue about a limit being broken or that the child needs to stop. In this situation, the therapist realizes the limit is being broken and moves to see if redirecting will suffice.

Replacement – If the child begins or is in process of breaking a limit, the therapist could begin with implementing a replacement activity. Redirecting and replacing are two processes that can be used interchangeably. Replacement means literally replacing what is happening (something that is likely meeting a need for the child) with something new or different that is acceptable (continues to meet the need for the child). For example, the child is smashing a toy truck into the floor which is breaking the truck. The therapist or parent would quickly select another object such as a rubber hammer and play doh and put it in the child's free hand showing them how to smash the play doh while taking the truck away from the child. Replacement can also be replacing a game that is being played with the child with a different game. Where redirection is the act of transitioning the child's attention or trying to distract the child away, replacement is giving the child a tangible, acceptable alternative that continues to meet their need. As with redirecting, there does not need to be any dialogue about the limit being broken when using the replacement strategy.

Removal – If a child is beginning to or in the process of breaking a limit, redirecting and replacement should be implemented first. If these processes do not work, then removal is the final option. The first step in removal is verbally explaining to the child that they need to discontinue a limit setting behavior, or a toy/material may be removed from the playroom or the play session may end. In situations where a toy or material can be removed, the therapist might say "Michael in here you cannot cut the dolls' hair, if you keep trying to cut the hair, I will take the doll and scissors out of the playroom." If the verbal prompt does not stop the behavior, then removal is implemented. The therapist would remove the doll and scissors from the playroom and continue with the session. If removal involves the child needing to leave the playroom (usually due to unsafe behavior), the therapist could try guiding the child into another location, possibly where the child can be alone or minimally supervised while the child calms. In an extreme case, removal might involve ending the session and physically taking the child out of the clinic. If physical removal is necessary, then a parent should be the one to physically remove the child. This is done in extreme cases where the child or others are in danger due to the child's behavior, and action is needed to keep everyone safe.

When limits need to be set, the therapist could also try the Child Centered Play Therapy Limit Setting Model. Landreth (2001) outlined the ACT limit setting model. (A) Acknowledge the child's wants/needs (C) Communicate the limit in a non-punitive way (T) Target acceptable alternatives. For example, (A) "Sarah, I know you want to paint on the wall." (C) "but in here we cannot do that." (T) "You can paint on the easel or on this paper." The therapist decides what is a limit to set and limits should be set as little as possible. If the child did not respond to the limit, the ultimate action the therapist would take is ending the session time.

Additionally, the therapist could try implementing the Filial Therapy Limit Setting Model. VanFleet (2014) described a simple three step approach to limit setting. (1) Reflect the child's desire and state the limit – "You want to paint on the wall, but in here we can't do that, you can do almost anything else." If the child continues to break the limit, the therapist would restate the child's desire and state the limit and add a warning – "You want to paint on the wall, but in here we can't do that, you can do almost anything else." "If you continue to choose to paint on the wall, you choose to lose the paints." If the child continues to break the limit, the therapist would follow through on taking the paints away and making the statement "You chose to lose the paints."

Some children will be challenging a limit, maybe on purpose, maybe because they are dysregulated or uncomfortable, or possibly because they don't know that something is a limit. Regardless of the limit setting model chosen, the therapist should be nonjudgmental when setting limits. Many autistic and neurodivergent children may not understand that a behavior is inappropriate, or they are experiencing dysregulation and anxiety, and this is creating the behavior. Some autistic and neurodivergent children may produce a behavior that is a limit multiple times because they are still learning about regulating their system, social understandings, and communication. The limit setting model implemented should be based on an awareness of the child and what the therapist believes will work best with the particular child. This may involve trying different limit setting approaches until a good fit is discovered.

Basics of the AutPlay Therapy Process

AutPlay Therapy is an integrative family play therapy framework (approach) where children and parents/caregivers participate as co-change agents/ partners in the therapeutic play therapy process. It is designed primarily for mental health professionals, play therapists, and child therapists. It addresses children and adolescents aged 3–18 who are autistic, neurodivergent, and/or have developmental or physical disabilities. This includes ADHD, learning disorders, sensory differences, and social anxiety.

AutPlay is designed to help address the mental health needs of autistic and neurodivergent children and their families through a neurodiversity affirming therapeutic play process. It serves as a guide for therapists in using an integration of play therapy theories and approaches and the therapeutic powers of play to address a variety of possible mental health needs for optimal growth and healing.

AutPlay is a neurodiversity informed approach which strives to value neurodivergence and support non-ableist processes – respecting, valuing, and appreciating the identity and voice of the child client. AutPlay framework highlights affirming evidence based and research informed practices to address identified needs and therapy goals. It is a guide for establishing therapeutic relationship, assessing for individualized therapy needs, and implementation of play therapy approaches and interventions.

AutPlay is focused on an understanding of needs related to mental health/ life issues such as trauma, bullying, depression, anxiety, sensory challenges, education challenges, parent/child relationship issues, etc. Also important are needs such as understanding autism, advocacy needs, social navigation, regulation goals, family awareness, and mental health needs related to co-occurring issues such as developmental disabilities, physical disabilities, and chronic medical conditions.

Research

According to Parker and O'Brien (2011), the literature over many years abounds with case studies where changes are noted as a result of an intervention using play therapy. Various issues addressed with play therapy approaches include regulation struggles, depression, anxiety issues, child abuse, trauma issues, family issues, and general life adjustments concerns.

Multiple single case study designs have shown that autistic and neurodivergent children who participate in AutPlayTherapy once a week for six months show gains in original therapy goals such as emotional regulation ability, social navigation needs, anxiety reduction, and connection (relationship development). Parent rating scales also support an increase in targeted therapy goals for those who have participated in AutPlay Therapy once a week for six months. Parents also report gains in feeling more knowledgeable and empowered in their parenting abilities and less stress/strain regarding their relationship with their child.

Although single case study designs continue to be done and continue to show positive results for autistic and neurodivergent children, it is challenging to produce controlled studies as AutPlay is conceptually a framework and not a theory with specific tenets. It is an integration of play therapy theories and guide for how to use play therapy with neurodivergent children. Thus, therapy sessions do not always look uniform from client to client. It is important to note that the AutPlay Therapy integration/framework consists of theories/approaches rich in research that have shown positive outcomes in working with the autistic and neurodivergent population.

A great deal of caution should be taken when discussing research, evidence-based practices and "treatments" concerning autism and neurodivergence. The history of research with these populations is laden with ableist practices that have often been harmful. Bottema-Beutel et al. (2021) stated that autism research can easily reflect and perpetuate ableist ideologies (i.e., beliefs and practices that discriminate against people with disabilities), whether or not researchers intended to have such effects. In the past, autism research has mostly been conducted by non-autistic and non-neurodivergent people. Researchers have described autism as something bad that should be fixed. Describing autism in this way has negative effects on how society views and treats autistic people and may even negatively affect how autistic people view themselves. Some interpretations of research findings have tacitly or explicitly questioned the humanity of autistic and neurodivergent people.

Even sources such as The National Professional Development Center (NPDC) on autism spectrum disorder and the National Standards Project (NSP) must be highly scrutinized. There review of literate is predominately literature that implemented ableist ideas and practices and viewed autism as a problem that needed to be treated and cured. Evidence-based practices that focus on strict behavioral training and "correcting deficits" which are basically labeled as anything the does not look neurotypical, should be discounted. These practices have been shown to be harmful and degrading to autistic and neurodivergent children and even create trauma responses.

Bottema-Beutel et al. (2021) explained that participatory models of autism research have been developed. A hallmark of these approaches is that autistic people are included in the research process conducted by non-autistic investigators, and editorial decisions made by non-autistic publishers elevate autistic voices into roles with greater power. This can help break down conventional barriers and lead to research that better matches the preferences and priorities of the autistic community. Below are seven questions created by Bottema-Beutel et al. (2021) that may help researchers determine if they have adequately considered the impacts of their language process choices on autistic communities. If the answer to question one is "no" or the answers to questions two through seven are "yes," researchers should consider alternative ways of speaking, writing, and conducting research.

1 Would I use this language if I were in a conversation with an autistic person?
2 Does my language suggest that autistic people are inherently inferior to non-autistic people, or assert that they lack something fundamental to being human?
3 Does my language suggest that autism is something to be fixed, cured, controlled, or avoided?
4 Does my language unnecessarily medicalize autism when describing educational supports?

5 Does my language suggest to lay people that the goal of my research is behavioral control and normalization, rather than granting as much autonomy and agency to autistic people as reasonably possible?

6 Am I using particular words or phrases solely because it is a tradition in my field, even though autistic people have expressed that such language can be stigmatizing?

7 Does my language unnecessarily "other" autistic people, by suggesting that characteristics of autism bear no relationships to characteristics of non-autistic people?

AutPlay Therapy empowers the therapist by providing a comprehensive therapy framework that addresses mental health needs autistic children and adolescents and other neurodivergent children may be experiencing. Through AutPlay Therapy training, the therapist can feel knowledgeable in the realm of neurodiversity and neurodivergence and be prepared and equipped to establish and assist in meeting therapy goals for autistic children and adolescents and their families. Further, AutPlay Therapy empowers therapists to assist parents/caregivers in feeling confident and knowledgeable in helping their child.

AutPlay Therapy is a flexible and prescriptive therapy process that focuses exclusively on the neurodivergent child and adolescent population. AutPlay Therapy can be done in conjunction with other therapies and may be part of a collaborative approach to helping children and adolescents address a variety of therapy needs. AutPlay Therapy consists of three phases of therapy: intake and assessment, directive play intervention, and termination. It also includes the AutPlay Follow Me Approach, a nondirective infused family play therapy approach for working with younger children and children with higher needs. The phases of therapy and Follow Me Approach are further presented and explained in later chapters.

Case Example "Leah" by Sarah Moran

Leah began AutPlay Therapy at age 6. She engaged in therapy via telehealth, due to Covid-19 restrictions. Leah's parents sought therapy for her due to concerns about her inattention, impulsivity, behavioral problems at school, and difficulties with emotional regulation. Leah lived with her mother and father and had one younger brother. Leah had no previous encounters with mental health therapy. Leah possessed strong cognitive ability and thrived in learning skills for a variety of interests. Leah demonstrated a precocious vocabulary and was excelling above grade level academically. Leah demonstrated an ease in entering new social situations and making friends but demonstrated difficulty maintaining close friendships. Typically, Leah would do most of the talking and often interrupted her friends and friends would respond negatively.

Leah attended online school while at a daycare facility. This school environment was challenging for Leah. Leah and other school-aged peers would be directed to a specific area of the room to engage in their individual online classes, each child wearing headphones. Leah often struggled to focus on her zoom-class, because she was surrounded by toys and people to socialize with. Leah would often get distracted or share an idea with a neighboring peer while she was supposed to be focused on class. If a daycare teacher redirected her, Leah would quickly become frustrated and verbally defend herself, often talking louder and becoming more of a distraction to her peers. Other times, the redirection would cause Leah to shut down and instead she would communicate by pretending to be a kitten, meowing at her teachers and feigning understanding. Leah's daycare would often call home with reports of her misbehavior and outbursts. Leah's parents expressed feeling helpless in supporting Leah at school.

Leah began AutPlay Therapy by participating via telehealth from her home. The therapist facilitated a modified version of the Intake and Assessment Phase through telehealth. A play observation was conducted with Leah and the therapist observed a play time between Leah and her mother. The parents also completed AutPlay inventories and returned them to the therapist – including the AutPlay Assessment of Play and AutPlay Emotional Regulation Inventory (child version). Leah presented as excited and talkative. She was eager to share her toys, thoughts, and ideas. Leah basked in the one-on-one attention she received from the therapist during their sessions.

Therapy goals were established to work on increasing Leah's ability to name and express her feelings, increasing her emotional regulation ability and impulse control. The Structured Play Intervention Phase began around session four. Structured play therapy interventions and bibliotherapy were implemented by the therapist to address these therapy goals. Leah participated in these interventions, and engagement differed depending on Leah's buy-in to the specific play activity. One intervention, *What Are They Feeling?* was a favorite of Leah's. This intervention requires participants to recognize and identify different emotions, and process why a person might be feeling that way. This intervention suggests the use of pictures cut from magazines; however, this was modified on telehealth by using a collection of images the therapist had found and shared with Leah through screen-share. Leah demonstrated the ability to recognize a person's emotions and was eager to use her imagination to create a backstory about each person and how they came to be feeling that way. Over time, *What Are They Feeling?* was repeated to increase variety in Leah's emotion vocabulary.

Another intervention called *Action Identification* was also implemented with Leah. In this play intervention the child is asked to recognize expected versus unexpected behavior to do in certain situations. The therapist prepared this intervention by writing various behaviors/actions on index cards. The therapist included some general actions, as well as some specific to Leah, such as "meowing like a kitty" and "interrupting someone." The therapist acted out an action, and engaged Leah to guess what it was, then name expected and unexpected environments or situations to do the behavior. Leah enjoyed this activity and often requested it, engaging the therapist in taking turns to act out the behavior. Once Leah understood, for example, that "meowing like a kitty" was expected to do at home or while playing with friends, she was able to better control her impulse to do so at school. This play intervention worked on improving Leah's emotion regulation and impulsivity in a non-shaming, affirming way.

Leah progressed quickly with her therapy goals participating in telehealth. Her parents reported improvement in her emotional regulation ability, improvement in problem-solving strategies when frustrated, and a decrease in major meltdowns. Leah's understanding of why she behaved in certain ways allowed her to have buy-in to change her actions in certain situations. Leah's frequency of therapy quickly reduced, and her therapy goals shifted to focus on increasing positive self-concept and coordination of care with an occupational therapist for ongoing body regulation and sensory processing challenges. Around session 41, the therapist, Leah, and her mother discussed graduating therapy and began the Termination Phase. Leah participated in AutPlay Therapy through telehealth for approximately 11 months, and then graduated from therapy having completed her therapy goals.

References

Bottema-Beutel, K., Kapp, S. K., Lester, J. N., Sasson, N. J., & Hand, B. N. (2021). Avoiding ableist language: Suggestions for autism researchers. *Autism in Adulthood*, 3(1), 18–29. http://doi.org/10.1089/aut.2020.0014

Bowers, N. R., & Bowers, A. (2013). Play as a voice for our children. In N. R. Bowers (Ed.), *Play therapy with families: A collaborative approach to healing* (pp. 1–6). Jason Aronson.

Cross, A. (2010). *Come and play: Sensory integration strategies for children with play challenges*. Redleaf Press.

Delaney, T. (2010). *101 games and activities for children with autism, aspergers, and sensory processing disorders*. McGraw Hill.

GoodTherapy.org (2015). Therapeutic relationship. https://www.goodtherapy.org/blog/psychpedia/definition-of-therapeutic-relationship

Kestly, T. A. (2014). *The interpersonal neurobiology of play: Brain building interventions for emotional well-being*. W. W. Norton & Company.

Kottman, T. (2003). *Partners in play: An Adlerian approach to play therapy*. American Counseling Association.

Landreth, G. L. (1991). *Play therapy: The art of the relationship*. Accelerated Development Publishers.

Landreth, G. L. (2001). *Innovations in play therapy: Issues, process, and special populations*. Routledge.

Leggett, E. S., & Boswell, J. N. (2017). Directive play therapy. In E. S. Leggett & J. N. Boswell (Eds.), *Directive play therapy: Theories and techniques* (pp. 1–15). Springer Publishing Company.

Parker, N., & O'Brien, P. (2011). Play therapy reaching the child with autism. *International Journal of Special Education, 26*, 80–87.

Petruk, L. H. (2009). An overview of nondirective play therapy. *Good Therapy*. https://www.goodtherapy.org/blog/non-directive-play-therapy/

VanFleet, R. (2014). *Filial therapy: Strengthening the parent-child relationships through play* (3rd ed.). Professional Resource Press.

8
The AutPlay® Therapist

The Play Therapist

The AutPlay therapist begins with a fundamental understanding of what it me means to be a play therapist. Across the planet, organizations like the Association for Play Therapy and the British Association for Play Therapy have established characteristics and standards for becoming a play therapist. Kottman and Meany-Walen (2018) stated that there are specific personal qualities that are important in becoming a play therapist and there are professional trainings and experiences that are essential in preparing people to become play therapists. Kottman and Meany-Walen (2018), Kottman (2011) furthered:

> Effective play therapists should like children and treat them with respect and kindness, have a sense of humor, and be willing to laugh at themselves and with others, be fun loving and playful, be sufficiently self-confident and not to depend on positive regard from other people to bolster their self-worth, be open and honest, be flexible and be able to deal with ambiguity and uncertainty, be accepting of others perspectives without feeling vulnerable or judgmental, and be willing to think of play and metaphor as vehicles for communication with others. They should also be relaxed and comfortable being with children and have experience building relationship with them, be capable of firmly and kindly setting limits and maintaining personal boundaries, be self-[a]ware and able to take interpersonal risks, and be open to considering their own personal issues and the impact of those issues on what transpires in play therapy sessions and relationships with clients and their families.

In general, it is important for those who practice play therapy or want to become play therapists to be creative, cognitively flexible, fun, passionate, caring, trustworthy, and responsible. This isn't a whole lot different from counselors and or therapists who do other types of therapy. We think an important consideration for professionals who do play therapy is a willingness to enter into the creative world of the client and to

DOI: 10.4324/9781003207610-9

think symbolically. These qualities are important because your primary "tool" in play therapy is you – the person who loves to play – the person who loves to listen to stories and have adventures and dance and tell stories and make up songs and mess around in the sand and do art…It is essential that you are open to thinking about the play (or what the client does), rather than words (what the client says), as the healing channel – the path for communication and facilitation of movement and growth.

(p. 8)

The British Association for Play Therapy (2014a) created the essential personal qualities for a play therapist which demonstrate identified personal qualities of a play therapy practitioner to promote public protection and ethical practice. This includes *Empathy* – to empathize with the emotional and psychological expressions, experiences and needs of clients and significant others. *Sincerity* – commitment to being sincere and genuine to self and others. *Honesty* – to act truthfully and with integrity toward self and others. *Respect* – to acknowledge and show acceptance toward other people's understanding, experiences, and abilities. *Ethical* – to be committed to ethical practice and able to comply with the ethical code and values defined by the British Association of Play Therapists. *Knowledgeable* – to be able to apply knowledge, evidence and experience critically. *Self-awareness* – to assess, review and consider own competencies, strengths, and weaknesses as a play therapist. *Self-responsibility* – to operate and practice efficiently within own level of competencies. *Congruence* – to be authentic and genuine in conduct with clients and significant others. *Compassion* – to be emotionally warm, caring, and concerned toward others. *Critical reflection* – to critically reflect upon the emotional, social, and psychological world of clients, significant others, and the self and to integrate reflection into practice. *Commitment to professional development* – to continue professional development as a play therapist in a responsible and effective manner. *Commitment to personal development* – to be reflexive, to integrate personal insights into future practice, to continue personal development in a responsible and effective manner.

The British Association for Play Therapy (2014b) furthered that ethical principles are essential for the play therapist and created the following intended to guide and inspire play therapists toward achieving the highest ideals of the profession.

• Play therapists need to be motivated, concerned, and directed toward good ethical practice.

- Play therapists strive to benefit those with whom they work, acting in their best interests and always working within their limits of competence, training, experience, and supervision.
- Play therapists are committed to not harming those with whom they work.
- Play therapists establish relationships of trust with those with whom they work.
- Play therapists recognize that fairness and justice is an entitlement for all persons.
- Play therapists respect the dignity and worth of all people and the rights to privacy, confidentiality, and autonomy.
- Play therapists respect the needs of individuals, including emotional, psychological, social, financial, educational, health, and familial needs.
- Play therapists apply all of these principles to themselves. This involves a respect for the play therapist's own knowledge, needs, and development.

O'Conner (2000) stated that the play therapist seeks to maximize the child's ability to engage in behavior that is fun, intrinsically complete, person-oriented, variable/flexible, non-instrumental, and characterized by a natural flow. High-quality play therapy as practiced by a given play therapist represents an integration of the therapist's specific theoretical orientation, personality, and background with the child's needs in working toward therapy goals. Play therapists universally recognize that therapy has been successfully completed when the child demonstrates an ability to play with joyous abandon – this is what makes play therapy unique. The Association for Play Therapy (2022) identified the following areas of competencies (knowledge and understanding of play therapy, clinical play therapy skills, and professional engagement in play therapy) as essential to the competent practice of play therapy, irrespective of theoretical orientation.

The play therapist will:

- Demonstrate knowledge of the history of play therapy.
- Demonstrate understanding of the therapeutic powers of play.
- Demonstrate knowledge of the therapeutic relationship in play therapy.
- Demonstrate knowledge of seminal/historically significant play therapy theories and models.
- Apply theories and stages of childhood development in play therapy.
- Identify and apply ethical practices in play therapy.
- Demonstrate an understanding of the play therapy treatment process (e.g., treatment goals and plans, documentation, intake/termination, and tracking of treatment progress).

- Demonstrate knowledge of family and systemic theories in play therapy.
- Demonstrate knowledge of childhood-related problems and mental health diagnosis/disorders.
- Demonstrate an understanding of the diverse impacts of childhood trauma (e.g., neurobiological, systemic, social) and the implications in play therapy.
- Demonstrate knowledge of assessment in play therapy.
- Apply and articulate the therapeutic powers of play.
- Demonstrate relationship and rapport-building skills (e.g., empathy, safety, unconditional positive regard) by utilizing 'self' in relationships with children, caregivers, stakeholders in play therapy.
- Apply assessments that highlight various aspects of the child and/or system and the play therapy process (e.g., conceptualization, diagnosis, family dynamics, treatment suitability and effectiveness, termination).
- Articulate and explain the play therapy process.
- Demonstrate basic play therapy skills (e.g., tracking, reflection of feeling, limit setting, pacing with the client).
- Identify play dynamics (e.g., types of play, themes, stages) and incorporate clinical considerations in treatment.
- Develop play therapy treatment goals and plans congruent with theoretical orientation.
- Demonstrate understanding of own cultural and social identity and its influence in the play therapy process.
- Exhibit multicultural orientation to diversity, equity, and inclusion through a culturally and socially diverse playroom and play therapy process.
- Demonstrate play therapy treatment skills congruent with theoretical orientation (e.g., conceptualization, interventions).
- Maintain play therapy credentials and involvement in professional play therapy organizations.
- Consistently evaluate and adjust play therapy practices to meet state and discipline ethical guidelines and codes.
- Apply ongoing integration of APT's guidelines within the Best Practices and Paper on Touch.
- Recognize and adhere to the limits of professional scope of competence in play therapy.
- Seek and integrate play therapy-specific continued education, research, and literature.
- Seek and integrate play therapy-specific supervision and consultation.
- Practice self-care to maintain quality play therapy services.

- Seek and integrate ongoing knowledge regarding cultural and social diversity in play therapy.

(pp. 11–12)

Landreth (1991) described play therapy to be a dynamic approach to counseling with children which allows the play therapist to fully experience the child's world as the therapist ventures forth in the process of presenting the person they are and opening their selves to receive the delicate and subtle messages communicated by the child. Landreth furthered the following descriptors for defining the play therapist.

- The play therapist is a unique adult in children's lives, unique because the therapist responds out of their own humanness to the person of the child.
- The characteristics of acceptance of the child, respect for the child's uniqueness, and sensitivity to the child's feelings identify the play therapist as a unique kind of adult.
- The play therapist is intentional about creating an atmosphere. Therapists must be aware of what they do and why they do it. This makes therapists unique because they are not stumbling through a relationship with a child, but rather are being careful about their own words and actions.
- The therapist is working hard at treating an atmosphere conducive to building a relationship with the child.
- The play therapist is an adult who intently observes, empathically listens, and encouragingly recognizes not only the child's play but also the child's wants, needs, and feelings.
- The uniqueness of the play therapist is heightened by listening actively not only to what the child verbalizes but also to the messages conveyed through the child's activity.
- The therapist should be open-minded rather than close-minded. Openness and sensitivity to the child's world are basic prerequisites for play therapists. Children are considered and related to primarily on the basis of their own merit, who they are rather than who they have been described to be.
- Play therapists have a high tolerance for ambiguity which enables them to enter into the child's world of experiencing as a follower, allowing the child to initiate activity, topic, direction, and content with encouragement from the therapist.
- The play therapist acts and/or responds out of personal courage by admitting mistakes, by being vulnerable at times, and admitting inaccuracies in personal perceptions. The play therapist is personally secure and thus

recognizes and accepts personal limitations without any sense of threat to their feelings of adequacy.

(pp. 87–93)

Deconstructing Ableist Ideas

When I began (around 22 years ago) compiling the protocol/integration for AutPlay Therapy, I had an understanding of neurodiversity. I had read about the term and concept from Judy Singer and had my own lived experience as a neurodivergent person. I also had an awareness and understating of ableism, most specifically as it pertained to individuals with physical disabilities. As the tenets of AutPlay were being realized, I believed I was celebrating neurodiversity, not being ableist, and providing a new way of viewing and working with children. To some degree I was doing all this and while I had learned much, there was still more to learn. I had deconstructed a great deal of the ableist education I received. I fully believed that autistic and neurodivergent children were not receiving the therapeutic benefits of play therapy approaches and was committed to advocating for this change, but unbeknown to me, my work was not finished, there was still much to unpack, unlearn, and understand.

The beginnings of AutPlay certainly contained affirming ideas and a distinct difference from the behavioral focused "therapies" that permeated at the time, but it was not a fully realized affirming approach that it is today. In the beginning, there were still elements of the medical model, deficit thinking, person first language, and uneven views of "skill" development. Even as a neurodivergent person, I was not immune to the societal and systems conditioning of ableist thought that still found its way into the AutPlay protocol.

My understanding of the neurodiversity paradigm, movement, and anti-ableist processes has grown exponentially since the beginning of AutPlay. Luckily, I have been able to grow AutPlay as I have grown, fine-tune the framework to comprehensively highlight a neurodiversity affirming approach and continually eradicate ableist pieces. The process has been challenging and rewarding and some of the most important work I have done. Along my own growth journey, I have discovered a few truths that I try to share with therapists to help them in their own journey of deconstructing ableism and non-affirming beliefs and rebuilding a neurodiversity informed and affirming awareness and practice.

1 Ableism is a powerful conditioning process. To deny its power historically and in our current society is to set ourselves up to produce ableist

(and harmful) processes, likely without realizing it. There is always a benefit to question your own thoughts, especially through an ableist filter. Why do I think this? Why am I doing this? Where did I get this idea? Is this really important? Who is this important for? Why do I think it is important? It's never wrong to stop, reflect, and question.

2 Neurodivergent individuals can be ableist. No one is immune from conditioning and ableist thoughts and beliefs. As a matter of fact, until recently most individuals in the US would have grown up in a society where every system was laden in ableist ideas and processes. This is beginning to change but it is far from a healthy place.

3 Ableism exists in levels and/or degrees of ableist thought. Just because you are not like "that professional" who believes that autistic children need to be cured from their autism, doesn't mean you don't have your own ableist beliefs. Many professionals who work with neurodivergent children seem to have good intentions with a sincere desire to help children. Often these professionals are furthering ableist ideas and lacking affirming practices and they do not realize what they are doing. This is why it is so critical to ask, "Could this be me?" No one should assume they do not need to work on being better at affirming practices.

4 We must continually commit to listening to, hearing, learning from, and contemplating the words, insights, and experiences of neurodivergent individuals. There may currently be nothing better in terms of learning about ableism and affirming practices than spending time listening to neurodivergent adults. Commit to reading published works by neurodivergent adults who are affirming – watch their YouTube channels, read their blogs, take their trainings, and follow them on social media.

5 To become non-ableist and affirming is a mindful, consistent, lifelong pursuit to deconstruct societies' conditioning and create new self-awareness. This simply must be understood. Growth is progressive. Maintaining an attitude of life-long learner will help ensure that therapists stay the course and avoid pitfalls.

6 Ideal change happens on a systemic level but starts with one person making changes within themselves. I have often contemplated how basically every system seems to be embedded in ableist and non-affirming processes. How will anything every improve until these systems change and how can something that seems so massive ever change? Often these questions can feel overwhelming for us and our clients. The realization of what is and the work that needs to be done requires the therapist to engage in meaningful self-care. Change often does and can start with one person. One therapist shifting, being better, can have an impact.

Am I ableist? It is not always easy to tell if you are biased or implementing an ableist belief. Many people have biases, and many are very well conditioned in ableist practices and thoughts and don't realize it. It can be because of the way they grew up or what they learned from their education, media, and/or society. Vormer (2020) developed a set of questions to ask yourself to help identify your ableist biases:

- Do you feel that people with differences need to be cured?
- Do you think that all disabled and neurodivergent people have intellectual challenges?
- Do you think that people with disabilities can't be full members of society?
- Do you feel pity for people with disabilities and/or differences?
- Do you think that all disabilities are visible?
- Do you think that all neurodivergent people and those with a disability rely on other people their whole lives?
- Do you believe that a person's disability is the most important thing about them?

(p. 32)

The AutPlay therapist should be mindful of ableist influences. They should be active in exploring and recognizing ableist and non-affirming ideas within the mental health culture, approaches, techniques, etc. and within themselves. They will make a commitment to keep learning about the neurodiversity paradigm and movement. They will take care to view all play therapy techniques and interventions through a neurodiversity affirming filtering process.

Issues of Diversity and Intersectionality

Intersectionality is widely described as the acknowledgement that everyone has their own unique experiences of discrimination and oppression, and we must consider everything and anything that can marginalize people – gender, race, class, sexual orientation, physical ability, etc. Mallipeddi and VanDaalen (2021) stated that intersectionality means that many different social influences make up a person's experiences. Examples of these social influences are gender and sexism, ethnicity and racism, and disability and ableism. This topic is important because different autistic and neurodivergent people may have different experiences depending on these other social factors. The theory of intersectionality calls for an understanding of issues in terms of multiple intersecting power structures and social positionalities. In other words, when seeking to understand the experiences of persons with disabilities, it is important to also seek to understand how they may differentially experience, benefit from, or enact racism, sexism, or heterosexism, among other forms of power and privilege.

Intersectionality can encompass many different scenarios. Considering neurodivergence, this identity could overlap with one or multiple other minorities and/or oppressed identities. Mette (2020) provides a snapshot of one possible example of intersectionality:

> As a mixed-race woman with autism, I have three identities that give me unique lived experience that a white man with autism would not have. I experience disadvantage on account of my gender, race, and neurodiversity. What is meant by this is that I go through something different by having a three-part identity. For many marginalized people who have multiple difficulties, intersectionality is a really useful way to describe how different parts of you can be discriminated against at one time.
>
> (para. 1)

O'Conner (2000) proposed that there are two key issues with diversity in play therapy. One is the therapist themselves and the other is the role of culture in modern society and the mental health field in particular.

> The persona of the therapist plays an incredibly important but often neglected role in the way they practice psychotherapy. The therapist's philosophy, values, experiences, cultural background, family background, and so forth influence every nuance of the therapy. These variables in turn affect the style and pattern of the therapist's speech and the way the therapist dresses and moves in the session, the way they react to different clients, and the way clients react to them. Even the theoretical orientation that the therapist adopts and the techniques they choose to implement are not without their determinants in the persona of the therapist. It is critical that therapists recognize themselves in their work and not hide behind rationalizations that hold that what they do in a given case is the one best intervention. Otherwise, the therapist risks becoming blind to the client's needs. And therapy may not only cease to be effective, but it may also even become iatrogenic.
>
> (p. 59)

O'Conner (2000) explained that the play therapist must understand that in many cases the child's difficulties are best characterized as conflicts between the child and any one of a number of other systems in which the child is embedded (the social model of disability). The play therapist's role is to work with the child and family to develop strategies for meeting as many of the child's needs as possible within the different environments in which the child is embedded. This places the therapist in much more of an advocacy role (a component of AutPlay Therapy) than is typical of some play therapy theories and approaches. The play therapist must consider their own and their client's similarities and differences in neurodiversity (neurotype), ethnic and culture background, race, class, language, gender identity, religion, sexual orientation, family experience, age, and nationality. O'Conner (2000), furthered that there are specific guidelines for practicing therapy in general and play therapy in particular in a culturally competent manner:

1 Awareness/Sensitivity/Empathy – Practicing culturally competent play therapy requires developing awareness of one's own and other's cultures to facilitate the ability of the therapist to empathize with the client. The therapist should respect historical, psychological, sociological, and political dimensions of a particular diversity group, culture, race, and/or ethnic group and be certain the child and family feel the therapist accepts their belief system and diversity experience. The therapist should display an appreciation for strengths of different cultures. The therapist should be forthcoming and acknowledge to the client an awareness of differences between themselves and the client and ask the client in a supportive way if they have any concerns.
2 Dynamic sizing – The ability to understand and evaluate the meaning of culture for a specific client and the ability to assess the impact that a history of discrimination may have on the therapy process. The therapist should not generalize about all clients that belong to a particular group and focus on understanding the particular individual with whom the therapist is working. The therapist should be aware that many factors contribute to a person's orientation and values and recognize that social, economic, and political discrimination and prejudice are real problems for minority and diversity groups.
3 Knowledge – Two types of knowledge make it more likely that the therapist will be successful with clients from diverse backgrounds. One is the knowledge about how to modify the therapeutic process to suit a given cultural group. The other is knowledge of the culture itself and the way it is manifested in the system(s) in which the client is embedded.

(pp. 80–82)

AutPlay Therapists must be prepared for diversity and intersectionality in play therapy. A neurodivergent child may be of a different race, gender, sexual orientation, etc., from the therapist. It will not be only a neurodivergent child that will come into the playroom. Consider a white American neurotypical male therapist. A new referral the therapist receives is a BIPOC, female, autistic child or a LGBTQIA+ Chinese child with a developmental disability. The combinations (intersectionality) can consist of many experiences. AutPlay Therapy training (framework protocols) and/or neurodiversity affirming training will likely not be sufficient to address all the diversity needs that can present in the playroom. The AutPlay therapist will need to take care to be trained, informed, aware, and ready to be a healing, helpful support to their clients regardless of diversity.

Understandings of the AutPlay Therapist

Understandings are fundamental. They are not "nice ideas." The AutPlay therapist realizes that each understanding presented is an active and happening component of therapy, and it is the therapist's responsibility to ensure they encompass and reflect each understanding. The understandings are presented as follows:

- The development of the therapeutic relationship is the grounding focus throughout therapy. This process begins with first contact with the child and family and continues until termination of therapy services. The AutPlay therapist makes a distinct effort to understand relationship development principles and to apply those principles. They also take care to evaluate that effective relationship development is occurring in the therapist/client experience.
- The foundation and framework of AutPlay Therapy consists of an integration of seminal play therapy theories and approaches. Without play therapy there is no AutPlay Therapy. The AutPlay therapist values, supports, and understands the therapeutic powers of play, that play is the change agent, and play is the natural language of neurodivergent children. The AutPlay therapist supports play therapy as a viable option for addressing the mental health needs of autistic and neurodivergent children.
- The foundation and framework of AutPlay Therapy also consists of neurodiversity affirming and informed constructs and practices. The AutPlay therapist will have a working knowledge and understanding of the neurodiversity paradigm and movement as well as how to implement neurodiversity affirming constructs in play therapy work. The therapist will be able to conceptualize how play therapy theories and approaches can be implemented in an affirming way. The therapist will also ensure

that play therapy techniques have been evaluated to ensure non-ableist messages and protocols before implementing with children and families.

- The children deserve the right to have their play preferences and interests recognized and valued. The AutPlay therapist will strive to ensure that the child's play preferences and interests are realized and utilized in play therapy approaches and techniques. Therapy goals will, if at all possible, be addressed through the child's play preferences and interests. The therapist should implement AutPlay processes that observe and assess for play preferences and assist parents in understanding and valuing their child's play preferences.

- The parent and child are considered partners (co-change agents) in the play therapy process. The AutPlay Therapist will make every effort to include the parents and child in therapy goals and planning. The therapist will value and listen to the parents and understand that parents possess a knowledgeable input about their child and family and parents and family are a critical and foundational relationship for the child. The therapist will also listen to and value the child as a partner in the play therapy process. The therapist will provide space and opportunity to empower the child to express themselves – their wants and needs related to therapy. The therapist will realize that the child is an expert on themselves, and their voice is critical in accomplishing the best therapy outcomes.

- Each child is an individual and developmentally will have unique strengths, presentations, and needs. Therapy goals and planning should reflect the individual child and not be a standard protocol based on a diagnosis. The AutPlay therapist will implement processes to gain an understanding of the individual child, how they navigate, think, process, play, and experience their world. Significant time will be spent (as much as necessary) to conceptualize the individual self and identity of the child. This individual awareness will shape the direction of therapy and therapy goals.

- A systems approach, including family members and other individuals actively in the child's life, is important. Family systems theory looks at the mutual influences of family members on each other. It moves away from an identified patient (usually the child) model to a way of understanding the problem or issue in the context of the whole family. The therapist will understand that the family unit is the foundation for children – it has the greatest impact on the child's development. The family is the main environment for a child – little else has the same influence as the family environment. What the parents do greatly affects the child and what children do greatly affects parents. As the AutPlay therapist works with each family, they will consider and assess: What is the definition of this family, how does the family play, does the family not play, how does play contribute to the family's relationships, and how does/can the family heal through play?

- Children and families should be engaged and accepted where they are at, and diligence is ensured to provide empathy and support. The AutPlay therapist will provide unconditional positive regard, defined as showing complete support and acceptance of a person no matter what that person says or does. The AutPlay therapist accepts and supports the client, no matter what they say or do, placing no conditions on this acceptance. The application for providing unconditional positive regard includes having respect for the parent and child, being non-judgmental and impartial, valuing the parents and child and accepting them as a unique individuals and families, being accepting of the parent and child, and their views, opinions, and beliefs, providing a nurturing and caring support for the parent and child, and being conscious of their needs and being compassionate about, and understanding the parent's and child's struggles and needs.
- The therapy should have an assessed and identified purpose ensuring that therapy goals maintain healthy expectations and are clearly identified and explained – the reasons for participation in play therapy. As much as possible, the parent and child will participate in creating and adjusting therapy goals and in implementing the process toward achieving therapy goals.
- The therapy should involve formal and/or informal periodic evaluation to monitor for progress toward therapy goals. The evaluation process should include the therapist, parent, and child. Each should have an active voice in assessing how therapy is progressing. This can be done through a consultation/meeting discussing the therapy process or can be done through providing formal inventories that assess for progress and or growth.
- The therapist will stay current with research regarding neurodiversity, neurodivergent individuals (autistic, ADHD, sensory differences, learning differences, Tourette's syndrome, developmental disabilities, etc.), and play therapy. The AutPlay therapist will take care to recognize and avoid research that includes ableist processes. The therapist will also clearly understand their role and scope of practice when working with neurodivergent children. The therapist will not falsely advertise or claim to address needs in which they are not qualified to do. The therapist will not attempt to establish therapy goals that are outside their scope of practice and will ensure to make referrals as needed.
- The therapist brings their unique culture, values, and beliefs to their play therapy work. Therapists may have also been impacted by racism,

classism, sexism, ableism, homophobia, xenophobia, or other systems of oppression. Each child and family client may also bring these experiences into therapy. AutPlay therapists intend to practice ethically and from a diversity-informed space. Diversity-informed is defined as a dynamic system of beliefs and values that strives for the highest levels of diversity, inclusion, and equity. Diversity-informed practices recognize the historic and contemporary systems of oppression that shape interactions between individuals, organizations, and systems of care. Diversity-informed practices also seek the highest possible standard of equity, inclusivity, and justice in all spheres of practice: therapy, teaching and training, research and writing, advocacy, and direct service (Irving Harris Foundation, 2018).

Fundamentally, the AutPlay therapist will strive to follow the legal, ethical, and best practices of their given license and profession. Beyond the basics of professionalism, the AutPlay therapist will understand the therapeutic powers of play, play therapy theories, and work within the construct of play as the change agent in mental health care. Specially, the AutPlay therapist will be neurodiversity informed and affirming – committed to non-ableist practices and doing no harm to neurodivergent children. Realistically, the AutPlay therapist has no distinction from what should be expected from any play therapist working with autistic and neurodivergent children and their families. The commitment to providing best practices and the most valuing and affirming therapy should be something all professionals are continually striving toward.

References

Association for Play Therapy. (2022). *Credentialing standards for the registered play therapist* (pp. 11–12). https://cdn.ymaws.com/www.a4pt.org/resource/resmgr/credentials/rpt_standards.pdf

British Association for Play Therapy. (2014a). Play therapy core competencies. https://www.bapt.info/play-therapy/play-therapy-core-competences/

British Association for Play Therapy. (2014b). Ethical basis for good practices in play therapy. https://www.bapt.info/play-therapy/ethical-basis-good-practice-play-therapy/

Irving Harris Foundation. (2018). *Diversity-informed tenets for work with infants, children and families.* https://diversityinformedtenets.org/

Kottman, T. (2011). *Play therapy: Basics and beyond* (2nd ed.). American Counseling Association.

Kottman, T., & Meany-Walen, K. K. (2018). *Doing play therapy: From building the relationship to facilitating change.* Guildford Press.

Landreth, G. L. (1991). *Play therapy: The art of the relationship.* Accelerated Development Publishers.

Mallipeddi, N. V., & VanDaalen, R. A. (2021). Intersectionality within critical autism studies: A narrative review. *Autism in Adulthood.* http://doi.org/10.1089/aut.2021.0014

Mette. (2020). I'm an autistic, mixed race woman – let's discuss intersectionality. *Learning Disability Today.* https://www.learningdisabilitytoday.co.uk/im-an-autistic-mixed-race-woman-lets-discuss-intersectionality

O'Conner, K. J. (2000). *The play therapy primer.* John Wiley and Sons.

Vormer, C. R. (2020). *Connecting with the autism spectrum: How to talk, how to listen, and why you shouldn't call it high functioning.* Rockridge Press.

9
Phases of AutPlay® Therapy and Therapy Goals

Therapy Phases in AutPlay Therapy

Ultimately AutPlay Therapy is a framework or guide for the therapist to implement play therapy with neurodivergent children. The phases of therapy exist to help provide a level of structure for the therapist to follow. The phases can be considered as flexible phases where the therapist has room to adjust and navigate as needed to best address the mental health concerns of the child and their family. The phases of therapy begin with the Intake and Assessment Phase which typically lasts four sessions. The second phase is the Structured Play Intervention Phase, which continues until therapy goals have been completed. The third and final phase is the termination phase which typically last two to three sessions. Table 9.1 displays the typical progression through the phases of therapy.

Intake and Assessment Phase

The intake and assessment phase of AutPlay Therapy is all about the beginning of meeting, being with, learning about, and building relationship with the child and family. This phase of therapy typically lasts three to five sessions, with the most common being four sessions. The Intake and Assessment Phase begins with first contact. Once the therapist has established

Table 9.1 The Three Phases of AutPlay Therapy

Phases of Therapy		
Intake and assessment phase	Structured intervention phase	Termination phase

DOI: 10.4324/9781003207610-10

an initial session, the therapist should send the family a social story about going to see a play therapist. The parents are instructed to read the social story to the child a few times a day the week before the first appointment. The social story should include information about what the child can expect and pictures of the therapist and the office and playroom. If a social story is not appropriate, the therapist could send an email that welcomed the child and family and included pictures of the therapist and the clinic. The parents could share the email with the child. The following presents an example social story:

> A play therapist is someone who plays with kids and tries to help
>
> them with their problems.
>
> My mom or dad or both may take me to see a play therapist.
>
> The play therapist usually has an office.
>
> Sometimes my parents may see the play therapist with me.
>
> Sometimes I may see the play therapist by myself.
>
> There are toys to play with and other things to do at the
>
> play therapist's office.
>
> I can play with the toys, games, and art materials.
>
> The play therapist may talk to me.
>
> I can talk to the play therapist and that's okay.
>
> I don't have to talk to the play therapist and that's okay.
>
> I can go to the play therapist's office and not feel nervous.
>
> I can go to the play therapist's office and have fun.
>
> I can go to the play therapist's office and feel better.

The first session is a general intake session with the parents. Typically, children are not involved in this session. The therapist meets with the parents to complete all necessary paperwork and to acquire information on presenting issues and child/family background. The therapist should begin establishing relationship with the parents. As parents share their concerns and presenting issues, the therapist should listen and provide empathic response. The therapist will answer any parent questions and explain the therapy process, including how AutPlay Therapy works. The therapist provides the parents with the AutPlay Emotional Regulation Inventory (child or adolescent), the AutPlay Social Navigation Inventory, the AutPlay Connection Inventory (child or adolescent), and the AutPlay Assessment of Play Inventory (all inventories are in the appendix section) to take home, complete, and bring back in the second session. The therapist may give parents additional inventories to complete if it is deemed necessary. A helpful additional inventory might include a sensory inventory or checklist such as Biel's (2014) Home Screening Tool and School Screening Tool.

Session two involves both the child and parent(s) with the therapist conducting a family play observation. The observation can include both parents with the child or one parent with the child. The therapist will observe the child and parent together in a play therapy room. If possible, the therapist will observe via monitor or two-way mirror. If this type of process is not available, then the therapist should stay in one corner of the play therapy room and try just to observe. The parent should be told in session one that they will be participating in a play observation with their child in session two. The therapist should be sensitive to any anxiety this might create for the parent. The general instruction to the parents is "I'm going to observe you and your child playing together for about 25–30 minutes. There are really no guidelines or rules, just keeping everyone safe. Try to play just as you normally would at home." Koehler, Wilson, and Baggerly (2015) stated that family play therapy approaches typically begin with some type of family play assessment or observation. They identified three reasons why this type of process is beneficial:

1 Observations of family play interactions enhance and enrich the information gathered throughout the traditional data collection process of clinical interviews and self-report measures.
2 Family play-based assessment is developmentally appropriate for children.
3 Play-based family assessment facilitates rapport between a family and the therapist, which increases the family's trust, comfort, and motivation to participate.

The child/parent observation should last approximately 30 minutes. The remaining time should be used for the therapist to join in with the child and parent in their play. During the child/parent observation, the therapist should use and complete the AutPlay Child/Parent Observation Form (in the appendix section). This form is designed to help the therapist note anything of interest during the child/parent observation. The observation is conducted to help the therapist better understand and build relationship with the child and parent. Observing the family playing together can provide valuable insight for conceptualizing therapy goals. Some areas to consider when conducting the observation include general child and parent interaction, how the child and parent play together, parent initiations toward the child, the child's initiations toward the parent, communication styles, and how limits are addressed. The therapist should make notes that will be shared with the parent and child in session four. Typically, session two will end with the therapist taking the child on a tour of the clinic or facility including any playrooms or office spaces they may use during therapy sessions.

Session three involves the therapist working with the child. The therapist will meet with the child to continue to develop therapeutic relationship and help the child feel familiar and comfortable with therapy. The therapist will informally observe the child in a play session. Typically, this is done in a play therapy room or some type of play space setup. A play therapy room provides a wonderful opportunity to allow the child to express and display their play preferences and interests, their communication style, and to facilitate relationship development between the therapist and child. The therapist will use and complete the AutPlay Child Observation Form (in the appendix) to better understand and conceptualize the child. The therapist and child will typically participate in the observation play time for the entire session, approximately 45 minutes. The therapist should focus on relationship and rapport- building as well as completing the areas on the Child Observation Form. Observation areas include communication style, play preferences, relational interaction, executive functioning, sensory issues, and frustration tolerance.

The therapist should introduce the play session (observation) like any other session with a structuring statement – "This is the playroom, and you can play with anything you want in here and I will be in here with you." The therapist should begin the observation in nondirective play therapy mode. The child should lead the play and the therapist should follow, staying attuned to the child. The therapist can periodically make tracking and reflective emotion statements and set a limit if needed. Some example tracking statements include "You filled the whole bucket up with sand," "You colored the picture just the way you wanted," and "You were finished with the dollhouse and now you are playing with the puppets." Some example reflective statements (done when the child displays or communicates emotion) include "That's frustrating you that the lid won't come off," "Bouncing that ball makes you feel happy," "You don't like that," "That makes you mad," "That feels good to you."

If the child invites the therapist into their play (gives the therapist a role), the therapist should join the child but stay in the role the child gives the therapist. The therapist should not change the play or try to direct. Approximatively halfway through the session, the therapist should naturally introduce some directive elements into the observation. This might include occasionally asking the child a question (something simple and play related). It could also include seeing if the child would respond to playing a game or activity the therapist introduced. The totality of the observation play time is designed to help the therapist build relationship and better know and understand the child.

Parents should have completed and returned all inventories given to them from the therapist by session three. Between sessions three and four, the therapist should review the parent completed inventories and the observation forms. The therapist should note any questions they may have for the parent to ask in session four. The therapist should also begin to formulate possible therapy goals and a therapy plan to share with the parents and child.

Session four begins with the therapist meeting with the parent(s) and child (if appropriate) to review the inventories, observations, and ask any additional questions. Often, parents like to hear some feedback from the therapist about the observations and the inventories. There may be some natural comments or questions the therapist wants to give the parents. If there is not, the therapist should still try to provide some feedback to the parents, ideally something positive or encouraging that the therapist noted during the observations. This is a time of discussion with the parents. Session four is designed to establish therapy goals and a therapy plan. The therapist should talk with the parents and child about possible therapy goals to address. The therapist will want feedback from the parents and child if they feel the goals are in line with the child and family's needs. There may be multiple identified therapy needs and goals. In this case, there will need to be a prioritization process. Typically, around two therapy goals can be chosen to address. The other therapy needs and goals can be addressed systematically as goals are accomplished. The therapist, parent, and child can work together to decide what therapy needs are the priority to begin with.

Involving the child in session four should be done if at all possible and appropriate. The child's voice is important, and the therapist wants to hear from the child as much as possible. The child is considered a partner in the therapy process from the beginning to the end of therapy. In some cases, the child may be too young or in a developmental state where they may not participate in session four or they may have a limited amount to contribute. The therapist needs to be mindful of the partnering/participation level of the child and if the child will attend session four or not. Even if the child is in a developmental position or age which decreases their participation in partnering, the therapist should look for every option throughout the therapy for the child to express decisions and contribute to their thoughts and feelings.

Once the therapy goals have been established, the therapist should explain the AutPlay Therapy process. The therapist will explain what happens next as therapy enters the Structured Intervention Phase. Ideally the child and parent will participate in sessions together during the Structured Intervention Phase. It should be established with the parents how the child and parent sessions will be facilitated. This can happen in several ways and is usually decided by what works best logistically for the therapist and family. The most common way is for the child and parent to attend weekly sessions and participate together. Another option would be one week meeting with the parents and the next week meeting with the child. If it is possible to meet twice in one week, then one time can be with the child and the other with the parent. Another possible combination is meeting each week with both parent and child by dividing the session time. The first half of the session is the therapist and child together and then the parent is brought in for the second half of the session. If the parent cannot be present with the child in person during their session time, the parent could join the session via a video conferencing platform. The level of parent involvement and the application of involvement will depend somewhat on the therapist's discretion. Considering the child, family, needs, and therapy goals, the therapist should determine what would work best for addressing therapy needs. This might mean more or less parent involvement or parent involvement that looks a specific way.

Step Guide for the Intake and Assessment Phase:

Session One

1 Therapist meets with the parents only to conduct a general intake process which includes completing intake paperwork and any legal documents.
2 Therapist gives parents AutPlay inventories to compete and return in session two.

3 Therapist collects background information on the child and family and all relevant documents including any previous psychological evaluations, sensory evaluations, and IEP documents.
4 Parents provide presenting issues and reasons for seeking therapy.
5 Therapist explains AutPlay Therapy and provides information on neurodiversity affirming practices.
6 Therapist explains that session two will be a child/parent observation play time.

Session Two

1 Therapist collects the AutPlay inventories from the parents.
2 Therapist facilitates a child/parent play observation in a playroom setting. Therapist should observe through monitor equipment or station themselves in one corner of the playroom. Therapist should utilize the AutPlay Child/Parent Observation form when conducting the observation. This observation should last approximately 25–30 minutes.
3 Therapist joins the child and parent in their play time after the observation time is over.
4 Therapist takes the child on a tour of the facility including all playroom(s) and office spaces that may be used.

Session Three

1 Therapist focuses on relationship development and helping the child become familiar and comfortable with the facility and the therapist.
2 Therapist facilitates a child/parent play observation in a playroom setting. The parents should observe via monitor or in a corner of the playroom. The therapist should utilize the AutPlay Child Observation form when conducting the observation. This observation should last approximately 45 minutes.
3 Therapist should explain that session four will be a meeting with the child and parent to discuss therapy needs and goals and answer any questions.

Session Four

1 Therapist meets with the child and parents. The therapist should discuss the observations and AutPlay inventories with the family and answer

any questions they may have. The therapist works with the child and parent to establish priority therapy goals and discuss moving forward with the therapy process.

2 Therapist uses any reaming session time to meet with the child in a play-room and continues to develop relationship and rapport.

3 Therapist prepares therapy goals and a therapy plan which may include selecting structured play therapy interventions to complete with the child and parent before session five.

Structured Play Intervention Phase

The Intake and Assessment Phase is an important time to begin developing therapeutic relationship with the child and parent. It is also an important time to get to know the neurodivergent child and their parent and begin to individualize the play therapy process for the child. The Intake and Assessment phase sets the stage and helps establish what will happen during the Structured Play Intervention Phase. Once the Intake and Assessment phase has been completed, the next session begins the Structured Play Intervention phase. This phase typically begins around session five, continues until the therapy goals have been completed, and includes both the child and parent.

The Structed Play Intervention Phase is where play therapy approaches and/or interventions began to be implemented to address the established therapy goals. Much of the direction in this phase is determined by information gathered in the Intake and Assessment Phase. The therapist may move forward with a more nondirective approach, may begin implementing structured play interventions to address specific needs, or may do some type of combination. This will depend heavily on the individual child – their needs, their play preferences, the totality of their self, and how much or little parent participation is happening. The therapist will want to conceptualize this plan and be open to adjustments, changes, and feedback from the child and parent. Typically, the Structured Play Therapy Phase will involve a level of structure from the therapist. This may include what types of play therapy approaches or methods to implement, the facilitation play therapy interventions, or an individualized integration designed for the child. The following should be considered when creating the structure of the Structed Play Therapy Phase:

• Who is this child? What do I understand about them? What do I understand about their neurodivergence? Based on what I understand would a less structed, or more structured play therapy process be appropriate?

- What are the child's therapy needs? What seems to be the best level of structure to address their therapy needs?
- Will I have parent participation? What level of parent participation will I have? What type of play approach or level of structure would be best based on the level of parent involvement?
- If I am going to implement structured play therapy interventions, what interventions would best address the therapy needs and goals? Have I filtered the play therapy interventions to make sure they are affirming and non-ableist?
- Will the structure involve an integration of nondirective and directive approaches? If so, what will this look like in each session?
- Will there be a focus on home play times or interventions? If so, how will I teach, support, help implement home play times? What seems like the best fit for the family and to address therapy needs?
- How does the child and parent feel about the plan for the Structured Intervention Phase? Have I shared it with them and gotten their feedback and opinion?

The structured Play Intervention Phase can have different "looks." Ideally there is a level of parent involvement and a participation where parents become co-change agents, working with their children at home to implement what they are learning in therapy sessions. As much as possible, parents should be taught how to implement play therapy techniques and/or play times at home that mimic what the therapist is doing with the child in sessions. There could be some directive play therapy techniques or approaches that the therapist does with the child in session that may not, by nature of the design of the activity, transfer to the home setting. This is fine but should be the minority of experiences. The majority of the play therapy techniques and/or approaches implemented should be able to be taught to the parents and transferred to the home environment. The following presents a few examples of the different ways the Structured Play Intervention Phase can manifest. Each conceptualization would be based on an understanding of the individual child, their therapy needs, their neurodivergence, and the level of parent involvement:

- It is evaluated, discussed, and decided that the Structed Play Intervention Phase will consist of directive play therapy interventions to be introduced each session by the therapist. The child and parent will participate in the session together and in the play interventions. The child and parent will continue to play the interventions together at home between sessions. The therapist will choose play interventions that align with the child's play preferences and interests and ensure that the interventions can be easily taught to parents and implemented at home.

- It is evaluated, discussed, and decided that the Structed Play Intervention Phase will involve the therapist primarily working individually with the child to address therapy needs. The therapist will meet every 4–6 sessions with the parent for a parent consultation. The therapist will implement an integration of nondirective play and directive play interventions that involve the child's play preferences and address identified therapy needs. This will involve the therapist structuring sessions at the beginning (the first half of the session) with a directive play intervention designed to address therapy goals. The second half of the session involves a nondirective play session time designed to continue to address therapy goals.

- It is evaluated, discussed, and decided that the Structed Play Intervention Phase will consist primarily of a nondirective child-led play session. The therapist will structure the beginning of the session with a short 2–4-minute regulation activity which the child chooses. The remainder of the sessions will be child-led with a more nondirective approach implemented by the therapist. The child can explore and include the therapist in their play preferences. The therapist will meet every four to six sessions with the parent for a parent consultation.

- It is evaluated, discussed, and decided that the Structed Play Intervention Phase involve the child participating in a child-led nondirective approach facilitated by the therapist. The therapist will teach the parent how to have a modified nondirective special play time at home that will happen once a week between sessions times.

The length of the Structured Play Intervention Phase varies. How much time is spent during the Structured Play Intervention Phase will depend on the depth and number of therapy needs and goals of the child, the spectrum of presentation of the child (low needs or high needs), the progression of the child, and the level of parent/family involvement. Typically, the lower the needs and the more parent participation, will indicate the Structured Play Intervention Phase will progress more quickly. It is important to let parents know that there is not a set number of sessions for the Structured Play Intervention Phase. Neurodivergent children will move through addressing needs, processing, and conceptualizing at their own pace and this should be validated. Many case studies and clinical outcomes have shown that neurodivergent children have shown a marked improvement in initially identified therapy needs and goals after participating in AutPlay Therapy after six months. This does not indicate an end to the Structured Play Intervention

Phase but rather a guide to showing improvement and progress toward therapy goals.

Therapists should implement an evaluation process which periodically re-evaluates to make sure therapy needs and goals are being met and to assess for the need for any changes or additional therapy goals. One approach would be to have parents complete updated AutPlay inventories from the first session and compare parent ratings from the initial inventories and the current ones. As progression is made and therapy goals are being met, it may be appropriate to lessen the parent involvement and have more session times with the child. If parents have learned most of the techniques and approaches and are actively and accurately implementing the techniques and approaches at home, then session times with the parents may be limited to a once per month consultation until therapy is terminated. Meeting times (consultations of some type) with parents should continue on some level until therapy is terminated. Remember that the combination of parent training sessions and child sessions can be implemented in a variety of ways. Therapists may discover a unique way that child and parent involvement happens that works for their particular family. Also, therapists will decide initially and may adjust as therapy progresses, the level of parent involvement.

An exception to the three-phase process in AutPlay Therapy involves the AutPlay Follow Me Approach (FMA). This approach is defined in later chapters. The FMA is a nondirective based play approach to working with children and parents. It is most appropriate for children who have higher needs and/or co-occurring conditions and struggle with attunement, interaction, and communication. All children and parents would participate in the Intake and Assessment Phase. During this phase it if was established that the FMA would be a more appropriate approach, the child and parent would begin participating in FMA sessions instead of the Structured Intervention Phase.

Termination Phase

Kress and Marie (2019) proposed that when it comes to the actual process of termination, therapists can take many different approaches with clients. The interests and developmental level of child and the content of therapy should all be considered when planning termination activities. Termination is often an ideal time to incorporate active, engaging, and creative interventions that encourage children to engage in active learning and reflection upon the therapy process as a whole. Often, as termination nears, child engagement and enthusiasm in therapy may diminish. By using active and creative termination interventions, therapists can inject new enthusiasm into the last few therapy sessions. Children tend to more readily remember play interventions in which they are interactively involved. Regardless of the specific intervention used, termination is an ideal time to incorporate an optimistic, empowering and future-oriented approach. Therapists can compassionately empathize with children who are reluctant to terminate while concurrently encouraging them to see the end of therapy as a new adventure in which they can use the new tools they have learned throughout their therapy time.

The Termination phase will typically begin with the therapist initiating the transition. As the therapist becomes aware that therapy goals have been achieved and maintained, they should have a session with the child and parent to discuss termination of therapy. The Termination phase usually consists of three sessions. The first session introduces the idea to the child and parent to elicit a discussion about the readiness for therapy to end. The therapist can determine the appropriateness of having the child present or not for this session. The therapist should review the therapy goals and plan and point out/discuss that therapy goals have adequately been accomplished. The therapist should discuss to make sure there are no other therapy goals to work on at this time. It is important to note that the initial therapy plan will likely be updated by the therapist, child, and parent throughout the Structured Play Intervention phase with new goals being added as others are accomplished.

Termination phase begins with the therapist, child, and parent reviewing and agreeing that all therapy goals have been met and there are no new goals to accomplish. The therapist should then explain that therapy will be ending within the next couple of sessions. The therapist should review with the child and parent what they have learned and how to maintain the progress they have made. The therapist can emphasize with the importance of continuing to facilitate play times, interventions, and activities at home. The therapist should also emphasize the continued use of any coping and/or regulation tools that have been learned. Some children and parents may have a difficult time with the thought of therapy ending. They may have come to view the therapist and the therapy time as a type of self-care or steady support in their life. The therapist will want to be mindful of this and help the family transition out of therapy. For some families, it might be appropriate to have a few sessions once a month and gradually end the therapy time. If needed, the therapist can adjust the termination process to best fit the child and parent they are working with. The therapist should remain positive and encouraging throughout the Termination phase. The language and attitude should convey celebration for the completion of therapy.

Session two of the Termination phase can be a session with the child alone or include the parent. This is decided by the therapist and/or child. The therapist will remind the child that sessions will be ending, and the next session will be the final session. The therapist will review with the child all they have accomplished. The therapist will encourage the child to continue using the techniques they have gained. The therapist and child will plan the basics of the final session (graduation party), what they want to do to celebrate. The therapist can include the parents or give them the information after the session. Before the session is over, the therapist will complete a closing or termination intervention with the child. Kress and Marie (2019) identified three termination interventions that can be helpful for children:

> **Aloha lei (hello-goodbye) activity:** Counselors can explain to clients that the word *aloha* means both hello and goodbye. Counselors can then discuss with clients that every end is the start of a new beginning, as is the case with the end of counseling.
>
> For the activity, paper flowers can be cut out (clients can select the color of the materials to enhance autonomy). Clients can write effective coping skills, memorable counseling experiences, or other notable takeaways on the flowers. Next, punch a hole in each flower and thread them along the string. Family members or caregivers can also be involved in the process (with client consent), adding their own flowers to the lei. The lei can then be given to the client as a parting gift. This intervention involves creativity and metaphor in a way that summarizes the counseling experience while actively involving the client.
>
> **Building blocks:** This activity can be tailored to clients of any age. During the final session, counselors can bring a number of building blocks, LEGO bricks, Jenga blocks, or other toy blocks to session. Clients can then construct a tower or creation of their choosing. Each block in the creation can represent a powerful moment in counseling, a coping skill clients now possess, or another skill clients have learned during counseling.
>
> As the height of the tower increases, clients may become anxious, especially as the tower begins to lean. If the tower ultimately falls, the counselor can explain that, given the clients' fundamental skills—the skills they assigned to each block—the tower can be rebuilt. This intervention helps clients understand that even if they experience the inevitable "falls" of life, they possess the fundamental "building block" skills to rebuild. This intervention is a tactile and empowering activity for the end of counseling.

Goodbye letter: There are many variations of a goodbye letter that can be used as the counseling process comes to a close. Counselors can provide a letter template with certain blanks to be filled in, or they can simply provide a blank piece of paper on which clients can write their own letter. Adding prompts or sentence stems for clients to complete can add a degree of structure to the letter.

There is flexibility in terms of the letter's point of view. Goodbye letters can be written from client to counselor, from counselor to client, or even from the perspective of the process of counseling itself being personified. Possible writing prompts include "One thing I remember from counseling is …" or "The most memorable moment of counseling was …" Although counselor creativity can yield limitless possible prompts, it is important that the goodbye letter be narrowed to focus on the most relevant moments of the counseling process. It is also important to keep the activity strength-based (as is the case with any termination activity).

(para. 28)

Session three of the Termination phase is the final session which includes parents, child, and any other family members that the child would like to invite. This session is a graduation party (celebration) for the child. The emphasis should be positive, fun, and focused on how much the child has accomplished and thus, has now graduated from therapy. Typically, the party is held in the therapist's office, a play therapy room, or any space that is decorated with party decorations and balloons. A graduation cake or other dessert is provided, and other components may be included such as a small graduation gift, card, additional food, etc. The therapist, child, and parents should plan the party together. Proper goodbyes are given at the graduation party and child and parents are reminded that they may contact the therapist at any time if they have questions or need to resume therapy.

Goals in AutPlay Therapy

In AutPlay Therapy, the therapy needs and goals are specific for each neurodivergent child. This is typically conceptualized during the Intak and Assessment Phase of therapy. Any issue or combination of needs could include, anxiety reduction, addressing depression, sensory issues, trauma issues, identity issues, parent and child relationship strain, etc. Regardless of the specific therapy needs addressed, the following presents expected goal outcomes for children and families who participate in the AutPlay framework.

Goals for the Child

- Give the child a voice and opportunity to express their thoughts and feelings.
- Feel empowered in their neurotype. Learn that differences are okay and not bad, and they are valued as they are – without masking.
- Increase problem-solving, decision-making, and regulation tools.
- Increase self-worth and realize and value their neurodivergent identity.
- Eliminate presenting, troublesome needs that are interfering with the child's ability feel stable in their quality of life.
- Increase healthy relationship development between the child and parent.
- Learn self-advocacy skills.

Goals for the Parent(s)

- Increase their understanding and appreciation of their neurodivergent child.
- Decrease feelings of frustration with their child.
- Learn about neurodiversity paradigm and movement principles and how to advocate for their child.
- Increase positive relationship development with their child.
- Learn about their child's play preferences and how to support their child's play.
- Improve family fun time together.
- Strengthen the family unit and improve inter family supports.
- Increase appreciation for each family member and diversity of neurotype within the family.
- Increase confidence in their ability to parent their neurodivergent child.
- The phases of therapy in AutPlay are designed to help the therapist put forth the most mindful and beneficial therapy experience for the neurodivergent child and their family. The phases have an intentional fluidness that can be and should be shifted for each individual child. The phases present enough structure to guide the therapist in a direction while encouraging the therapist to pay close attention to the child in front of them. The neurodivergent experience is not the neurotypical experience and much of mental health theory and process has been based on the neurotypical experience. The AutPlay framework strives to change this – to place the therapist in a position of understanding the neurodivergent experience and reframing the

process to see, hear, value, appreciate, and truly help the neurodivergent child.

Case Example

Michael

Michael entered therapy as a seven-year-old autistic child. He had been given the diagnosis of autism a few years prior by a neuropsychologist who completed a psychological evaluation on Michael. He had recently transitioned from being in a private school that focused on working with autistic children to now being in first grade in a public-school setting for the first time. Michael had received an IEP and was participating in special education classes for the majority of his school time and in a few mainstream classes with the help of a paraprofessional. At the time Michael and his family began AutPlay Therapy, he was not participating in any other therapies. Michael's parents reported that he made substantial progress in increasing verbal communication and social navigation during the time he participated in the private school.

Michael's parents brought him to therapy due to transition difficulties with switching from the private school to the public-school setting. They described that he was experiencing social navigation struggles, dysregulation, and having challenges with some of the other children. Michael's parents stated that Michael had begun to make statements such as, "I am different from everyone else," "I do not fit in," and "No one at my school or in my family is like me." Michael's parents furthered that they wanted help in learning how to talk with Michael about autism to help him better understand himself and how to navigate issues and situations at school. They also wanted to see him improve his peer relationships and develop some positive friendships.

Michael lived with his biological mother and father and 6-year-old brother. Michael's paternal grandparents were also actively involved in his life and assisted regularly in caring for Michael and his brother. The family attended activities hosted by their church and participated in a local autism focused parent support group. Michael participated with his family in various church-related events and activities but otherwise did not participate in any additional activities outside of going to school. The family was unfamiliar with a neurodiversity affirming approach and had not heard of the term neurodiversity. The therapist spent time explaining the terms and process to the parents and providing them with additional information to read at home. The therapist explained that therapy goals would be established to address Michael's needs and therapy would be cognizant of Michael as an autistic child. It was explained that affirming meant there would not be a focus on trying to "cure" or erase Michael's autism, instead the focus would be on helping Michael understand and value himself and address any mental health needs that were creating problems for Michael.

The first three sessions were primarily assessment gathering sessions designed to gain more specific information about Michael, help Michael and his family build rapport with the play therapist, and help Michael feel safe and familiar in the therapy process. Michael participated in a child observation session with the play therapist and the play therapist observed Michael and his parents together in a child/parent play time. Both observations were conducted in a play therapy room. Michael's parents also completed three inventories: the AutPlay Social Navigation Inventory, the AutPlay Assessment of Play Inventory, and the AutPlay Emotional Regulation Inventory (child version). All inventories were provided to the parents to complete in the first session. The assessments helped identify Michael's needs, play preferences, and strengths. Michael's assessment sessions demonstrated that he was able to participate in some structed play interventions initiated by the therapist. Michael seemed most comfortable and interested in more nondirective play and too advanced instruction or activities seemed to trigger discomfort and dysregulation resulting in Michael not participating.

After the Intake and Assessment Phase was completed, it was decided that Michael and both his parents would participate in therapy sessions together. The sessions would integrate nondirective play with introducing simple structured play interventions. Therapy goals would focus on helping Michael increase a positive self-awareness, improve emotion understanding and expression, help with social navigation, teach the parents how to have play times with Michael, and address any advocacy needs related to school issues. Michael, his parents, and younger brother would meet weekly with the therapist and the whole family, including Michael's younger brother, (who Michael seemed to interact with and respond to positively) would participate in home play times between therapy sessions. Michael and his family attended therapy once a week for approximately ten months.

The integrated play sessions began on session five. The play therapist introduced the *Draw My Feeling Face* intervention to Michael and his family. This intervention involves the adult making a face to the child and showing a feeling. The child then draws the face on a piece of paper and labels what they think the feeling is that the adult was demonstrating. The child is then asked to make a face displaying a feeling, and then the adult draws the face and labels what feeling they think the child was showing. The play therapist chose this intervention for Michael to help him begin to connect and engage with others, begin basic learning about emotions, and participate with the therapist and parents in a fun and playful way. The play therapist explained the intervention to Michael and his parents and instructed the parents to watch as Michael and the play therapist completed the intervention. Michael had a difficult time engaging with the therapist. He was able to begin the intervention but seemed to become anxious about accomplishing the game. He struggled with identifying the therapist's feeling face, struggled with drawing faces, and struggled with making a feeling face himself. It appeared that Michael was concerned or preoccupied with accurately completing the activity without making mistakes.

After 15 minutes of working with Michael, the play therapist suggested that Michael and his younger brother try to complete the intervention together. Even though he was one year younger than Michael, his brother was intellectually gifted and played well with Michael, often functioning more like an older sibling instead of a younger one. The idea to have Michael and his brother complete the intervention was beneficial. They were able to complete the intervention several times during the session and seemed to have a fun time participating together. The structured play therapy intervention lasted approximately half the session, The reminder of the session was spent implementing a nondirective play time with Michael and his brother. The therapist facilitated the play time and the parents observed. It was discussed with Michael, his parents, and younger brother for Michael and his brother to play the intervention several times at home before their next session and for the parents to try and join in and play the intervention themselves with Michael at least four to five times before their next therapy session.

At the next session, Michael's parents reported that Michael and his brother played Draw My Feeling Face several times; they had also played the intervention with Michael, and he responded positively each time. The play therapist played Draw My Feeling Face again with Michael to assess if he would participate with the therapist. Michael completed several feeling faces with little to no struggle and displayed a positive playful attitude. This was a significant difference from the previous session. The therapist decided to teach Michael and his brother how to complete the play interventions instead of teaching them to Michael only. This formula was successful for the entirety of therapy. The experience of learning something new and feeling challenged in new ways was much more comfortable for Michael when he participated with his brother first and then generalized to his parents and the therapist.

During session six, the play therapist taught Michael and his family two more play interventions: *Together Balloons* and *Midline Mirror Moves*. In *Together Balloons*, the family is instructed to pair up and place their hands forward in front of them while holding another person's hands. A balloon is thrown in the air, and the pair has to keep the balloon from hitting the ground while holding each other's hands. They must work together to keep the balloon in the air and they cannot stop holding hands. They continue to play until the therapist says stop. This play intervention was chosen because Michael likes balloons. The play intervention was designed to help Michael become more comfortable interacting with another person, attuning to another person, and facilitate secure attachment between Michael and his other family members.

In *Midline Mirror Moves*, the family can play in pairs or as a whole group. The instructions are that one person goes first as the leader and the rest of the family follows all the moves the leader makes like they were mirroring the leader. The leader should make slow moves so all the family can follow and stay with the leader's movements. Also, the leader should make several midline crossing moves (body moves that activate the whole brain and cross over the right and left brain). After a few minutes the family can switch roles and there can be a new leader. They can continue to switch until each person has been the leader. This intervention was chosen to help Michael with engaging and attuning to others, helping with regulation, and opportunity to participate in a fun social game.

The play therapist taught both interventions to the family during the session. Both of Michael's parents, his brother, and Michael participated, and the session was a success. Michael's participation while teaching the interventions was somewhat reserved but he remained present and tried to participate throughout the session. The family was instructed to try and play both interventions at home four to five times before the next weekly play session. The remainder of the session involved Michael and his bother participating in a nondirective play time with the therapist. The nondirective play times usually involved a combination of Michael playing on his own and some playing with his brother. Michael's play in the nondirective times was typically some type of constructive play (building a train track, building with bricks or LEGOs).

In session seven, the play therapist reviewed with Michael's parents how the intervention play times were progressing at home. They reported playing both interventions several times as a family since the last session. They reported that the play times had gone well, and Michael seemed to enjoy them and appeared less anxious than he normally did when participating in activities with the family. They reported that family friends, who have a neurotypical son close to Michael's age, visited them. They introduced the *Together Balloons* game to the friend's son for him and Michael to play together: the play time went positively. In the past, when this family visited, Michael would not engage with the other child. He might do some parallel play but no other type of play engagement. This time, however, Michael played the *Together Balloons* games with him for approximately 20 minutes and then reverted back to more solitary play. The family reported that they had not seen this type of peer play from Michael before, and they were pleased.

After the update was complete, the therapist introduced a new play intervention to the family called *The Progressive Balloon Game*. There are four play levels with each becoming progressively difficult. The first level is hitting the balloon back and forth and keeping it from hitting the ground (participants can use any body part, including hands, head, feet, and knees). After about five minutes, the participants move to level two that involves continuing to hit the balloon back and forth (keeping it in the air) with the dominant hand behind one's back. After five minutes of level two, the participants move to level three that is the same goal only with both hands behind the back. After five minutes, the final level is played which is hitting the balloon with one's head only. The family is instructed beforehand that if the balloon hits the ground, to pick it up, and keep going. This play intervention was chosen for Michael and his family to help Michael learn to participate pro-socially in a group activity with others, help him with general regulation improvement, and provide his parents a tool to help Michael practice feeling comfortable in more social play. Michael and his family played the game together and the reminder of the session Michael and his brother participated in a nondirective play time with the therapist. The family agreed to continue to play the intervention at home before the next session.

The remainder of the play therapy sessions with Michael and his family progressed in the same formula; checking in with Michael's parents on interventions during home play times, discussing any questions and/or concerns Michael's parents might have, teaching Michael and his family new play interventions to complete at home, and facilitating nondirective play times with Michael and his brother. At around the tenth-month mark of participating in therapy, Michael's father was transferred to another state, and the family relocated. At that point in therapy Michael seemed much more regulated in general, was engaging with other children in group play to a moderate extent and had demonstrated improvement in his social navigation comfort level. He also showed less dysregulation when entering new social situations. The social and play gains helped improved Michael's transition to the public-school environment. He was participating with more children and had developed a couple of friends. Further, he seemed to display less anxiousness about going to school. Michael's parents reported feeling a stronger relationship with their child and more empowered to play with Michael. They also stated they felt they had several tools to help Michael work on his social navigation, regulating ability, and advocating for Michael. Overall, Michael's therapy time appeared to be helpful.

Reflecting on Michael's therapy, several pieces helped influence a successful therapy outcome. First, conducting a thorough assessment process (observations and AutPlay inventories) before entering into therapy enabled the play therapist to make informed decisions for a play approach and intervention selection. It was imperative that the play therapist first understand Michael and his family before implementing play interventions. Second, incorporating Michael's brother in the sessions, proved to be a valuable tool. Had the play therapist chosen to work with Michael individually, it is unlikely the same level of progress would have been obtained. Third, teaching Michael's parents about neurodiversity, how to build relationship with Michael, how to work with him at home between sessions, and how to advocate, showcased the importance of the family approach in AutPlay. Michael's parents also felt empowered and confident in supporting Michael throughout the day in multiple and diverse situations. Throughout therapy, Michael's parents regularly reported being in a public situation with Michael and referencing something they had been working on in one of their play interventions. Having tools to use in "real life" situations in real moments was valuable to them and provided a practical application piece for Michael.

References

Biel, L. (2014). *Sensory processing challenges: Effective clinical work with kids & teens.* W. W. Norton & Company.

Koehler, C. M., Wilson, B., & Baggerly, J. (2015). Play-based family assessment and treatment planning. In E. J. Green, J. N. Baggerly, & A. C. Myrick (Eds.), *Counseling families* (pp. 91–105). Rowman & Littlefield.

Kress, K., & Marie, M. (2019). Counseling termination and new beginnings. *Counseling Today.* https://ct.counseling.org/2019/10/counseling-termination-and-new-beginnings/

10
Parent and Family Involvement

Parents, Families, and Play Therapy

Family therapists tend to view the family as a system that is greater than the sum of its parts and believe that family members mutually influence one another. They do not see one person as the problem; rather, family therapists view problems as having circular causality, with all family members (adults and all children) involved to some degree in creating or maintaining the problem; thus, individual issues are often reframed as family issues (Gil, 2015). Several family and child therapists have specifically advocated for a family play therapy (the integration of family work and play therapy) approach and offered innovative family play suggestions (Ariel, Carel, & Tyano, 1985; Busby & Lufkin, 1992; Combrinck-Graham, 1989; Gil, 1994; Vanfleet, 2014). Play therapy and family therapy complement one another, and the integration of the two has a synergistic effect in meeting the goals of each. Play provides an important tool for assessing family systems as well as for helping to reach the range of possible family therapy goals (Gil, 2015).

The therapeutic powers of play and benefits of play in family work exist for all members of the family – the adults, not just the children. "Play provides an opportunity to experience what has been denied or ignored, in the safe, benign, fun world of pretend. The play experience lives in the twilight zone between cognition and emotion, where the defenses are not on alert" (Ariel, 2005, pp. 6–7). There are a number of reasons why the involvement of family members in a child's play is important and healthy for both child and parent. Not only is formal family play therapy valuable but supporting play in the home setting can be important in neurodivergent children's self-worth, social, emotional, regulatory, and cognitive development. As children grow

DOI: 10.4324/9781003207610-11

from young childhood to older children, imagination and creativity through play continue to be important for learning, exploration, expressing ideas, and communicating feelings. Thus, the private context of the home can offer toys, materials, objects, along with family members as play partners, which allow for continued development and consolidation of various growth avenues throughout the totality of childhood (Trotter, 2013).

Trotter (2013) discussed several reasons play is important to a child's health and wellbeing and why family play is instrumental for a myriad of family and individual growth and healing initiatives.

> When working with families and children, meaning is embedded in action and behavior, and play is a significantly ingenious and creative way to illuminate meaning through an action that constitutes the child's preferred way of communicating. Play is a powerful medium within to work with families and offers therapist and family members alike a myriad of wonderful techniques that range from family art therapy to family puppet interviews to spontaneous and meaning saturated storytelling. Play has many benefits. It creates feelings of well-being between players, helps to release emotions, is a natural way to express the self, facilitates positive interactions between parent and child, creatively and symbolically deals with concerns, allows processing to take place on a number of different levels, and allows family members to step outside the confines of well-rehearsed and problem saturated narratives. Family play therapy increases the potential for family members to laugh and have fun together and engenders creative expression in both problem formulation and solving.
>
> (p. 92)

Freeman and Kasari (2013) reviewed how parents play with their autistic child and examined which strategies lead to longer and more connected play interactions. They summarized the following:

• Parents of autistic children have difficulty playing within their child's zone of proximal development (the space between what a learner can do without assistance and what a learner can do with adult guidance or in collaboration with more capable peers).
• Parents of autistic children tend to be more directive during play (suggesting and commanding more often), which results in shorter play interactions.
• Children match their play level to that of their parents.
• Imitating (recognizing and joining play preferences) an autistic child results in longer play interactions/engagement.

(p. 159)

Lowry (2016) furthered Freeman and Kasari's work stating by helping parents follow their child's lead, play within their child's zone of proximal development, and imitate their child, therapists can promote positives in how children interact and communicate with their parents. Furthermore, and possibly more importantly, parents will discover new ways to connect and have fun with their child. Lowry identified several key points to keep in mind when helping parents of autistic children follow their child's lead as they play together:

- Parents might find play challenging – children with autism often have unique or repetitive interests, limited play skills, and/or lack of social engagement. As a result, parents sometimes find it difficult to start a play interaction or to keep it going. This is reflected in Freeman and Kasari's (2013) observation that parents of children with autism had difficulty playing within their child's zone of proximal development, and that they resort to commanding and directing their child in an attempt to get their child's attention. Helping parents find ways to engage their child during play by determining the right types of toys and the right play strategies can be a great first step in intervention.

- Parents should follow their child's lead – Freeman and Kasari (2013) showed that didactic-style interactions in which parents attempt to direct and "teach" their child result in shorter play interactions. This lends support for the AutPlay Follow Me Approach (FMA) and non-directive play therapy such as Filial Therapy, in which parents are taught to follow their child's lead and focus on relationship development. Teaching parents nondirective play times and skills can be a particular challenge when working with parents of autistic children, as there are competing approaches in autism which advocate a more directive style.

- Parents need to play within their child's zone of proximal development – parents had difficulty with this in Freeman and Kasari's (2013) study. Therapists should ensure that parents are not responding to their child at a play level that is too high (or too low). When parents match their child's play level, interactions last longer and joint engagement is promoted. Parents should also respond in ways that are slightly above (but not too far above) their child's play level, so that their child benefits from modeling within their zone of proximal development. In order for this to happen, we need to raise parents' awareness about their child's current play skill level. Having parents observe their child and complete the AutPlay Assessment of Play Inventory can help parents become aware of their child's play level.

- The power of imitation – the power of imitating is confirmed by Freeman and Kasari's (2013) observation that imitating the children resulted in longer play interactions. Imitation is also a useful strategy to use during direct intervention when faced with a child who has little social engagement and restrictive play skills. It can be difficult to let go of designated goals and intervention agenda. But taking a step back and imitating a child in order to establish an interaction can be a valuable first step in accomplishing other goals.
- Choosing toys that promote play – Freeman and Kasari (2013) didn't examine the impact of different types of toys on parents' and children's abilities to play together. The children in their study were verbal children (average language age 37–38 months) who engaged in some pretend toy play. Parents of children who struggle with toy play or are less verbal might find play even more challenging than the parents in this study. For children with less play skills, a good place to start can be with playing with people. This would be using toys for which the involvement of another person is necessary, such as bubbles, balloons, or wind-up toys. Because a play partner is needed to operate the toy or help the child in some way, these toys facilitate interaction.

(para. 10)

Gil (2015) described the research and results of Sori and Sprenkle's (2004) best practices to train family therapists to work with children. These practices present a guide for the family play therapist, the AutPlay therapist, and for those implementing an integration of family therapy and play therapy.

1 Include children in family sessions unless discussing sensitive issues such as sex.
2 Course content should include developmental issues, theoretical issues, methods to engage children and adults, both play and family therapy theories, and family therapy protocols to address child issues.
3 Therapist attributes are important, including being playful, humorous, and creative, and liking and joining well with children.
4 The therapist should participate in deductive and inductive training methods, including live supervision and an apprenticeship model.
5 Family play therapy techniques should be understood and may include puppets, storytelling, drawing, games, and nonverbal art techniques.

(p. 35)

AutPlay Therapy and Parents

AutPlay Therapy offers a great deal of flexibility when working with parents/caregivers and the parent partnering (training) component. In AutPlay, we identify the parent as being a co-change agent or partner in the process. This means the parent is considered an equal and important member of the therapy process. The parent's voice, opinions, and concerns are valued. The parent is considered the most influential and important relationship in the child's life. As such, the therapist will actively pursue the parent's insight and expertise on their child and family. VanFlett (2014) stated about Filial Therapy (a primary integration approach in AutPlay Therapy) that

> therapists welcome and encourage parent input at every step of the way. What parents think, feel, and say matters. Whether they are reflecting on their own play sessions of trying to determine the possible meanings of their children's play, parent's views are elicited and discussed. Therapists consider and use parent's perceptions, realizing that parents know the child's context much better than they, and that parent's ideas about the meaning of the play is significant.
>
> (p. 16)

The Filial philosophy highlights the AutPlay approach to working with parents. Although the level of involvement from parents may fluctuate, parents should always be conceptualized as parents in the process.

The term "parent" is applied loosely. In AutPlay Therapy the therapist works with the legal caretaker of the child. This may be the biological parent, or it may be another adult. This may be a foster parent, adoptive parent, grandparent, a residential facility case manager, or whoever is primarily involved with and raising the child. It AutPlay, we are also cognizant of and try to involve other family members or others who are active in the child's life. For example, if there is an older sibling in the family, then at some point, that sibling might be brought into the parent partnering (training) time and taught how to implement play interventions or special play times at home with the child. This could also be done with a grandparent, aunt, uncle, sibling, or any family member who is actively involved with the child.

Before involving various family members, it will be necessary to discuss with the parents and assess for appropriateness and benefits of involving other family members. The other family member will need to be someone who could be taught the play interventions and/or play times and would be capable and appropriate to work with the child. If it appears that the other family member in question would not work well with the child (possibly they are a trigger for the child), then that family member should not be incorporated into the partnering (training) process. Some reasons for not involving a family member might include the person does not know the child very well or does not spend much time with the child, the person does not agree with therapy or with neurodiversity affirming constructs, the person seems to have a negative relationship with the child, or the person seems not capable of learning the play interventions or special play times. When appropriate and possible, therapists should try to incorporate other family members as this will provide additional support for the parents, relieve some of the implementation responsibility from parents, and help the child generalize relationship development working on therapy needs with a variety of people.

AutPlay may involve working with one parent/caregiver or if there are two parents involved, then both parents can participate at the same time. Often, this involves logistic issues of scheduling. Sometimes, only one parent is capable of attending sessions. When working with separated or divorced parents, and one of the parents does not support the therapy process, the therapist should adhere to legal mandates, their licensure best practices, and ethical guidelines. If both parents want to participate, the therapist should try to offer two sperate sessions with the child – working with each home independently. As the therapist works with each home, this might involve working with step parents or significant others. The management of these constructs should be decided by the therapist determining what seems to be the best scenario to help achieve therapy goals.

Parents partner in the AutPlay Therapy process in a few possible ways. All parents are considered partners from session one to termination in being involved, working with the therapist, contributing ideas, providing feedback, and generally being a part of the therapy process in a number of ways. The parent's thoughts, feelings, questions, and feedback are important and wanted. Parents may also participate in sessions with their child and learn directive play therapy interventions and then continue to implement the interventions at home between sessions. Whatever play intervention the therapist is facilitating with the child, the parent is also a participant and learning the intervention. The parent and child are then instructed to continue to play the intervention at home.

Additionally, parents may participate by being taught how to have a special play time or a Follow Me Approach play time at home with their child. The therapist provides instruction to the parent helping them learn how to have these play times and supports and monitors for successful home implementation.

For therapists working in a school setting or other setting where access to parents may not be an option, trying to incorporate other professionals who could also work with the child is an appropriate alternative. Some examples might include a paraprofessional, another teacher, or an intern. The goal would be to include one or more people so the child could practice the play intervention or play time multiple times between meeting times with the primary therapist. Ideally there would be parent involvement, but if parent involvement is not possible, then incorporating other professionals to create additional play times and play intervention implementation would be appropriate.

As needed, it may be appropriate to incorporate into the parent training sessions traditional parenting skills training. The therapist may recognize that the parent needs parenting help or reframing. The parent may also ask the therapist for information and support. The therapist should plan to work this component into the therapy time – possibly scheduling one or two sessions to address these needs with the parent. Some examples of formalized parenting programs might include providing information from Love and Logic, 123 Magic, Nurtured Heart, or any parenting approach that would have elements helpful for the parent. It is important to be aware that many popular parenting programs are designed for neurotypical children and may have components that are ableist and/or not helpful or beneficial for an autistic or neurodivergent child. The therapist should fully understand both the neurodivergent child, the parent needs, and the parenting approach they are teaching to apply elements that would be helpful and affirming.

It is likely that the parent training sessions will cover some level of talking about and addressing behavior (this may include addressing discipline approaches). Constructs that could be covered include teaching the child and parent how to create and set up a weekly visual schedule for their child, developing routine and consistency, establishing appropriate consequences, and understanding the meaning of behavior. The AutPlay Situation Behavior Assessment (located in the appendix) can be completed by the therapist, parents, or others observing the child's behavior. This inventory can be helpful in identifying what might be causing particular behaviors and what might be implemented to help decrease the behaviors.

Therapists can also use the AutPlay Unwanted Behaviors Inventory (located in the appendix) to help identify what types of behavior issues are happening at home and at school. This will help therapists identify what the parent and/or school officials are referring to when they communicate there are behavior issues happening. It also helps illuminate possible reasons the behavior may be occurring. As a general rule, many "behavior issues" are a result of the child becoming dysregulated. It becomes important to focus on what is creating the behavior and/or what is the behavior communicating and address the core issue. Some possibilities may be sensory issues, anxiety responses, trauma, confusion, etc. Therapists should take special care to avoid labeling the child as defiant, oppositional, disobedient, doing the behavior on purpose, etc. This is very rarely the case with neurodivergent children. The therapist may need to help parents, school officials, and others understand this awareness of behavior.

Addressing Parent Hesitation and Resistance

A common issue echoed by AutPlay therapists is what to do when there is a lack of parent participation. For a variety of reasons, a therapist may encounter a parent who does not participate in implementing play interventions and play times at home. Parental lack of participation can manifest for a variety of reason including parents may be too busy, parents may have good intentions but live a very stressful life and have difficulty scheduling play times at home, parents may feel inadequate or not prepared to implement interventions at home, parents may believe the interventions will not help or it seems like a waste of time, parents may have never played as a child and may not play with their child and do not know how, parents may be dealing with their own neurodivergent needs or other emotional needs and cannot focus on their child, or a variety of other reasons.

Therapists should try to discover what is creating the lack of parental participation and support the parent to resolve the issue(s). The therapist should be encouraging (nonjudgmental) and attempt to work with the parent and empathize with their situation. If all else fails, and there is a lack of parent participation that cannot be resolved, therapists should continue to work with the child and try to make as much gain as possible toward the therapy goals. Therapists may try to incorporate other professionals to work with the child such as an intern or try to have multiple sessions each week with the child. Although the level can vary, parent participation is an important piece to fully implementing the AutPlay Therapy framework. It should be noted that there may be situations where there is no parent available to participate. This could be due to a termination of parental rights, a child living in residential placement or a child in foster or other type of care. The baseline is providing care for the child and if there is no parent to participate, the therapist should still work with the individual child.

Suggestions for Addressing Parent Lack of Participation

1 Provide empathy, encouragement, and support. Treat parents with respect and remember the goal is to have parents as partners and co-change agents in the play therapy process. The therapist's approach to addressing any parent hesitation or lack of participation should be layered in helpful and emphatic responses.
2 Gently address the lack of participation and try to assess what might be creating the lack of participation. Listen to parent's issues and concerns, brainstorm with the parent, and work with parents to rectify the issue(s) that are creating a lack of participation. Help parents explore potential problems and feel comfortable and safe discussing the issues. Remember that therapeutic relationship development should be happening with parents just as the child.
3 Educate parents about autism and neurodivergent children. Provide information to parents about the benefits (research supported) of including parents in the therapy process with their child. Remind parents that they do not have to be perfect and are not expected to understand how to do everything, but they are an important and valued part of the therapy process.
4 Educate about the importance of empowering parents to become change agents for their child. Make sure parents understand the value in learning lifelong tools to work with and help their child. Explain to parents that parent participation helps them learn tools, learn how to advocate for, and learn how to assist their child in the present and into the future.
5 Discuss with parents that typically the AutPlay Therapy process moves at a slower pace regarding the accomplishment of therapy goals when there is a lack of parent participation. This is not done to try and make

the parent feel guilty but to be honest. Clinical outcomes have shown that therapy goals are achieved, and therapy is progressed through more quickly when there is active parent participation.

6 Talk with parents about adjusting the level of parent participation. Help parents understand that whatever level they can commit to is okay and they should not overcommit. This might be reducing the at home play times, having parents just participate in sessions with no at home component, having periodic parent consultations, or some other established, workable involvement. It is better to have some level of parent involvement than to have nothing.

7 Consider starting with small parent participation steps. Introduce a simple level of involvement and then gradually increase parent participation. Consider providing a level of accountability for parent participation such as asking the parent to commit to a day and time at home to implement the play therapy intervention. Once the time is established, let the parent know you will call them a few minutes after the home play time is over to see how it went. Consider if you need to become more directive with some parents, providing more direction for setting up the home play times and the overall parent participation.

8 Discuss with parents the possibility of other family members participating in therapy in place of the parent. If the parent is struggling with active participation, explore the option of another appropriate family member who could attend sessions and implement play times at home with the child.

Teaching Parents Directive Play Therapy Interventions

AutPlay Therapy incorporates a parent partnering (training) component which teaches parents how to facilitate directive play therapy techniques at home. Parents learn the procedures and techniques and are shown how to implement techniques at home to help address therapy needs and goals. Around session five, the therapist will begin facilitating directive play therapy interventions with child and parent. This may be done by child and parent participating together in the same session and playing/learning the intervention at the same time. It could be done by meeting one week with the parent and the next week meeting with the child; or this may be done by having two sessions in one week – one with parent and one with the child. How the child and parent participate while introducing and facilitating a play intervention should be given careful consideration. There may be topics to discuss or explanations that need to be covered with the parent which would not be appropriate for the child to be present. It may enhance the therapeutic process by ensuring that the child and parent are together in the play time in a true family play therapy fashion. The arrangement will depend on several factors such as scheduling, but there should be some type of parent participation to adequately train parents in implementing play interventions at home.

Gil (1994) stated that family play therapy offers special insight into family dynamics. In assessing a family engaged in play activity, the therapist may observe how the family organizes and engages around a task, revealing its communication styles, hierarchy, and boundaries and exposing any coalitions. Play exposes who is in charge, whose ideas prevail, whose voices are being heard, and who might be marginalized. Gil (2015) proposed the following guidelines for observing the family's behaviors and interactions during family play therapy interventions:

1 The family's level of cooperation and organization as they approach a play task.
2 The ability to reach consensus, and the manner in which this was achieved.
3 The level of affective and physical contact.
4 The level of enjoyment in participating in the activity.
5 The level of spontaneous insight, such as seeing the play as a metaphor for their own reality.
6 The collective unconscious, where themes are developed individually and collectively, allowing families to communicate on an unconscious level.

(pp. 42–43)

As the child and parent engage in play therapy interventions together, both the process and content can be revealing. Process observations include noting how the family communicates and the nature of their interaction – noting awareness of others, nonverbal and physical interaction. Content refers to what is talked about and what is communicated or produced through the play, metaphor, symbolic presentation, and expressive presentation. As the therapist introduces and teaches a directive play intervention, they should be observing the process and content and providing constructive feedback. The therapist should feel comfortable with the child and parent continuing the play intervention at home between sessions. Any additional feedback the therapist needs to make should be given before the session ends and the family goes home to continue the play time.

Home play interventions should mimic what the therapist is doing with the child and parent in sessions. For example, if the therapist has a session with the child and parent and implements the feeling-focused play intervention, the child and parent participate in session and are taught how to continue playing the intervention at home. There is an expectation they will complete the play intervention at home between counseling sessions. When an intervention is taught to child and parent and sent home, it is most helpful to establish with the child and parent specific instructions regarding completing the intervention home. An example of a specific instruction might be asking someone to complete the feelings intervention three times before the next session, or complete the intervention once a day before the next session. Working with the child and parent to establish this type of expectation will give the family a better guideline to follow and they will be more productive in ensuring they complete the intervention at home.

As the Directive Intervention Phase progresses, the therapist will review how things are going at home and ask the child and parent for an update on any at-home play techniques the family has been implementing. The therapist will also discuss with the child and parent any new play techniques to begin at home and any adjustments to the home implementation. During the Directive Intervention Phase, it is common for the therapist to engage with the parent concerning their own process in parenting their child. Often, therapists will listen to and counsel parents regarding their own needs or questions in parenting a neurodivergent child. In some situations, this may be done with the child and parent together. In other situations, this may warrant scheduling a separate session to meet just with the parent. If this happens with the child and parent together, it should not consume the entire session. It is important that the child and parent sessions cover the play interventions that the child and parent are going to be doing at home. If it seems like the parents would benefit from, or need their own regular individual or couples counseling, then a referral should be made for such intervention.

In AutPlay Therapy, the ultimate goal in regard to parent involvement is to have parents become co-change agents with the child and therapist. Parents should be encouraged, supported, and feel empowered to work with their child in ways that will be productive to established therapy goals. The therapist is training the parents to implement directive play therapy techniques at home with their child. These techniques are typically chosen by the therapist (although the child and parent can participate in choosing techniques) as techniques to use to help add mental health needs and therapy goals. The therapist will continue to meet with parents and train parents on implementing play techniques at home until the therapy goals have been met. It may be appropriate, after a certain length of time, to reduce parent involvement to once per month, but parent meetings should continue at some level until therapy has been terminated.

Checklist for Teaching Parents Directive Play Interventions

1 Explain to parents that they will be participating in play interventions with their child, and they will be learning the interventions to implement with their child in the home setting.
2 Explain to parents that the play interventions are chosen to help address the identified therapy needs and goals.
3 Once the play intervention has been completed, explain to parents that they will be facilitating the intervention at home with their child before the next session, establish with the parent how often and when they will implement the intervention.
4 Explain to parents that home play interventions may look different than in session interventions. This is normal and to be expected. Play times at home may have a more casual and loose application. Make sure they understand the intervention and check to see if they have any questions.
5 When the child and parent return for their next session, begin by reviewing how the home play intervention went. How often did they implement the intervention? Did things go smoothly? Were there any problems? What were observed outcomes? Did the child participate and seem to gain from the intervention? Are there any questions?
6 Get an update from the child and parent on how things have been going in general.

7 Try to cover any issues or questions that the child or parent may have about the therapy goals, AutPlay, home behaviors, parenting strategies, school issues, and the home interventions play times.
8 Teach the child and parent any new play interventions to implement at home before the next session. Play and complete the intervention in session and facilitate a discussion of where and how often the family will complete the play intervention time at home.

Teaching Parents Relational Play Times

The AutPlay Therapy framework incorporates a parent partnering (training) component where parents are taught how to have nondirective relational play times at home with their child. Whether to teach child and parent directive play interventions or a nondirective relational play time will depend on the child and the therapy needs. The therapist should use assessment and discretion in deciding what approach would be best. The therapist may also do an integration of relational play times and directive play interventions.

When teaching parents how to have a nondirective play time with their child, the parents should first observe the therapist facilitating a nondirective play session with the child. Once the parent feels confident in implementing a nondirective relational play time, they can begin to have these play times at home. The therapist will work with the parent to teach them how to have these play times and will continue to support the parent as they implement the play times at home. These play times provide opportunity to improve the parent and child relationship, help the parent develop a better understanding of their child, increase engagement and connection, and improve communication. A nondirective relational play time would incorporate the following constructs:

• The play time should be introduced. This can be as simple as saying "It is time for our special play time, you can play with anything you want, and I will be here with you." The relational play time does not require any special toys or materials, this can be done with whatever exists at home.
• The child leads the play time, the parent follows the child's lead and does not try to direct the play time. This may be a challenge for some parents as they may be used to directing play with their child and/or introducing and facilitating the play.

- The play time is focused on the child's play preferences and interests. Whatever the play preference of the child, the parent should honor the preference and follow the child's lead in the play. The play interest may be technology play, constructive play, or playing with objects not considered toys – whatever the play, the parent does not try to change it, instead the parent stays attuned, accepting, and focused, essentially joining the child's play world.
- Tracking and reflecting statements can be provided by the parent. A tracking statement is periodically tracking what the child is doing. It communicates that the parent is present with the child. An example would be the parent saying, "You built that tower with blocks." or "You are done with cars and now you are playing with the puppets." Reflective statements reflect back what the child is feeling or expressing. An example would be "You feel proud of your painting," or "You are frustrated with that doll." Tracking and reflecting statements can be made periodically. Parents do not need to feel like they must be making a statement continuously. It is okay to have silent attunement and observation in the play time.
- The parent will primarily provide tracking and reflective statements but may also ask "can" questions. These types of questions include "Can you show me," "Can you teach me," and "Can you help me understand?" Can questions provide opportunity to empower the child and for the parent to learn more about their child. "Can" questions are appropriate during relational play times but should be used minimally.
- The parent follows the child's lead and does not direct but if the child invites the parent into their play, wants the parent to play with them, or gives the parent a role in the play – the parent should participate. The parent should remember that they are participating in the way the child wants and dictates. The parent should not use this as an opportunity to start trying to direct the play.
- The parent should have a positive and curious attitude during relational play times. The parent should be mindful of the time spent with their child and both child and parent should find enjoyment in the play time.

Checklist for Teaching Parents Relational Play Times

1 Introduce the concept to the parents and explain that they will be learning how to have a relational play time with their child. Explain the

benefits of a relational play time and how this will help address therapy goals.

2 Give the parents written material that explains the constructs of a relational play time. Read through the material with the parent and explain each of the components of a relational play time – what the parents will be doing and what they will not do. The concepts/skills include introducing the play time, being nondirective (following and joining the child's play preferences), making tracking and reflective statements, asking "can" questions, and joining the child's play when invited.

3 Conduct a relational play time with the child while the parent observes. End the play time after about 30 minutes and use the rest of the session time to again go over the basic concepts of the play time with the parents. Answer any questions the parent may have.

4 Conduct a mock relational play time with the parent (the child does not attend). The therapist will role-play being a child and the parent will practice having the relational play time. This session is an opportunity for the parent to practice before they begin having the play times with their child. Typically, there are 1–2 of these mock play sessions. How may will depend on how quickly the parent understands and implements the skills and when both the parent and therapist feel they are ready to start having play times with their child.

5 The therapist will establish with the parent when they will have relational play times at home, how often, for how long. The therapist will remind the parent to be flexible and adaptable with home play times, focus on enjoying being with their child. A typical arrangement might be one to two times a week for 30 minutes each time.

6 The parent will begin having relational play times at home with their child.

7 The child and parent will continue to have weekly sessions with the therapist. The therapist may conduct a relational play time with the child, may conduct a more formal CCPT process, or may implement directive play interventions with the child and parent. The therapist can integrate depending on the therapy goals and what seems to be the best process for the child. For example, the therapist may teach the parents to have a relational play time and get this established at home and then in sessions with the child, facilitate directive play interventions.

8 Regardless of what the therapist is doing in sessions, at each session the therapist should check in with the child and parent about the relational play times and how they are going. The therapist will want to support the family in successful implementation of the play times and answer any questions they may have.

Considerations with Home Interventions

The implementation of play times and/or play interventions at home is a critical piece of the AutPlay Therapy process. Some special considerations or issues may occur with home implementation. Being at home can provide a familiarity and comfort that might not be the same in a clinical office setting. While this can be positive, it can also present a challenge to implementing home interventions. Families may not take the interventions as seriously or value the home play times and interventions. This can result in the play interventions becoming less than or a watered-down version compared to the play times and interventions being implemented by the therapist with the child in a therapy session. This would be something to assess and take note of during check-in times in sessions when gaining feedback. If this is happening, parents should be encouraged to try and present the interventions fully and with a purposeful intention, possibly even adding a more formal piece such as establishing with the therapist exactly when, how, and where interventions are going to be done at home that week. The therapist might even follow up later that week to see how things have been going.

Another possible home consideration would be distractions and disruptions. The home environment will likely be less controlled than the therapist's office. Families may have other children or even other relatives in the home. There may be a challenge to finding space and time where the parent can exclusively focus on and implement a play time or intervention with the child. This is something the therapist would address with the parent and try to establish the best possible option with the least amount of distractions or disruptions. Therapists may also discover that parents are implementing the play times and interventions in an inaccurate version. This could be due to time restraint issues, not fully understanding the intervention when it was explained, not remembering the instructions, or a variety of other reasons. Therapists will want to address this issue and make sure parents are accurately implementing play times and interventions at home.

Occasionally parents may find that they have a more challenging time getting their child to participate with them in the play times and interventions at home than is experienced by the therapist working with the family in the therapist's office. This would be important feedback to acquire during check-in sessions and to discuss with the child and parent to discover what is happening at home. The therapist may want to address with the child and parent more formally explaining the expectation for participating in at home play times. The therapist might ask both the child and parent to start sharing in each session a favorite thing from their at home play times. The therapist can also try observing the child and parent during their play times – either having them record the attempts at home or have them complete a play time in the session while the therapist observes. It is important to try and troubleshoot any at home issues and support the child and parent in successful implementation of play times and interventions at home.

Parents may also have difficulty with providing materials at home that are needed to complete various play interventions. If parents are struggling to provide the needed materials, the therapist should try to provide interventions that require little or no materials or assist parents with ideas for acquiring the needed materials. Some AutPlay therapists keep tubs of toys and materials in their offices to lend to parents who are implementing home play times and interventions. This would be another way to support parents who are struggling with any materials that are needed.

Therapists may discover that play times and interventions are not being implemented at home. The therapist will want to discover why this is happening and focus on helping parents become successful with home implementation. This may require exploring parent hesitation and resistance mentioned earlier in this chapter. When introducing play times or interventions to parents, therapists should make sure to present the instructions and expectations in written form (provide a handout detailing the intervention or have the parents write down the instructions), verbal form (explain the play time or intervention), and practice the implementation of the play time or intervention with the child and parent. This will help ensure proper implementation and follow through in the home setting.

Checklist Prior to Home Implementation

1 Does the parent feel comfortable with implementing the play time and/or intervention at home? Do they need more instruction or practice?
2 How often will the child and parent have a play time and/or implement the play intervention?
3 When and where will the child and parent have play times and or implement the play intervention?
4 How do they play to manage disruptions?
5 Do they understand the importance in staying consistent with home times?
6 Do they understand that the play times and interventions may look differently from in office implementation? This is okay, and any questions that arise, should be discussed with the therapist.
7 Do they understand the play times and interventions may look differently due to the therapist not being present? This is also okay and again, any questions that arises should be discussed with the therapist.

Encouragement and Parent Self Care

I recall being at a large training several years ago. I cannot remember the venue or much about the trainer, but I do remember something he asked the audience. He said, "What do you think is the most important thing a parent can do for their child?" There were many responses and most all of them were very nice and seemed appropriate, yet the speaker continually stated, "That's a good thing but it's not the most important." Finally, he revealed that the most important thing a parent can do for their child is *take care of themselves.* The sentiment has stayed with me throughout my professional career and has rung most true in my work with parents of neurodivergent children.

Parents of autistic and neurodivergent children may find themselves in a life that requires a high degree of focus and attention with little or no respite or opportunity for some much-needed self-care. Often parents are the lead person in daily care, scheduling and getting to multiple appointments, dealing with various systems, advocating for their child, and just generally trying it parent. Some research has suggested that stress and anxiety levels of parents with an autistic child can equal the levels of someone with PTSD.

A common discussion during parent trainings involves discussing with parents the concept of self-care. Self-care is often defined as the ability of individuals, families, and communities to promote health, prevent disease, maintain health, and to cope with illness and disability with or without the support of a healthcare provider. In more practical terms, it can be thought of as the practice of individuals looking after their own health using the knowledge and information available to them. Some parents may understand the benefits and necessity of self-care and are already producing regular self-care into their lifestyle. Other parents (unfortunately many) may not understand what self-care looks like and how to implement self-care into their life. The AutPlay Parent Self Care Inventory (located in the appendix) can be useful in identifying self-care beliefs and needs for parents. Therapists should address parent self-care at some point and identify if parents currently have self-care resources and options in place, and if not, process with parents to establish some self-care resources and strategies.

For many parents, self-care must be understood on a micro level. I have talked with several parents who have explained to me that self-care is lying on a beach somewhere with nothing to do. While this may be true, this is not a realistic self-care plan for most of the families I work with in Southwest Missouri or across the United States. Even for those families who could take a break and go to a beach once or twice a year, healthy sustainable self-care must happen more than once or twice a year. Indeed, it needs to happen

Table 10.1 Self Care

Examples of Daily Self-Care Activities			
Read a book	Take a walk	Meditate	Take a bath
Color or paint	Draw	Relax in nature	Pray
Exercise	Listen to music	Do yoga	Deep breathing
Self-talk	Garden	Cook	Go shopping
Watch a movie	Journal	Take a nap	Play a video game
Talk to a friend	Get a massage	Knit	Lift weights
Go for a drive	Unplug from media	Go to a museum	Make a grateful list

weekly, sometimes daily. Therapists will want to help parents conceptualize how self-care can be a meaningful and active part of their everyday life. They may need to understand that simple, small, and even short interval activities can be self-care and can have big impact. Table 10.1 list provides several ideas for everyday self-care. The application of any type of self-care is always individualized. It must be something that the specific person feels helps them, rejuvenates them, gives them a break, etc. Sometime after the therapy goals have been established and therapy is well underway, the therapist should find a couple of sessions to meet with the parent(s) and discuss self-care.

Parenting the Neurodivergent Child

Ramesh, J., & Raghav, P. (2022). *Parenting at Intersections of Race and Neurodivergence*. (Excerpt shared and adapted with permission).

I would notice differences in them that made us do a double take as some of the things they did and said were unexpected for a child their age.

When they were 2.5 we moved into a bigger home. I was excited that we had wall space to hang a whiteboard on the kitchen wall at their level. I imagined them practicing letters or doodling on this whiteboard while I made dinner or sat and worked at the dining table. Instead, they knelt down at the wall and with their chubby fingers begin to calculate the number of seconds in a year with repetitive addition. I asked them what they were doing and in a thick honey voice of a toddler they answered, "I'm calculating seconds in a year mamma." I respond with an "Oh!"

I took pleasure in their curiosity, and I also begin to feel the rumblings of what I would later identify as a feeling called overwhelmed; how am I supposed to satiate this child? It would be untruthful if I did not claim the pride I felt in my child's abilities. And in that pride in my child's ability, I would come to recognize that as a parent I participated in something called humble bragging.

"Oh, I can't tell you how many books we have to keep getting!" someone in our social circle would say about their child. Or another parent would complain half-heartedly "We could not get her to leave the museum, she was so enthralled by the spider exhibit." And then I might add something to the effect of how my child continues to excel in math and what a struggle it is to find the right school system for us. Underlying all of these "complaints" was something else unspoken. Today I understand these conversations to be about pride in our children that is also rooted in ableist values.

And it is also historically rooted in being products of colonized cultures and immigrants. For those of us whose ancestors have been colonized, a value we have inherited is that our worth is connected to how well we perform and produce. We as adults were already on a capitalistic treadmill, which values bodies that produce. A subtle and insidious way we were inculcating our children on to this way of life was by talking about the ways in which they could perform.

Then there were the differences that would provoke concern, like how they played. And my worry would kick in right on cue. Was something wrong with them? What would the other parents say? My own desire for community and belonging would become a tug of war internally. Do I stay and talk to the parents, or do I leave and be with my child?

What I was not noticing was the faulty narrative I was setting up – that their differences were causing me (our family) to be more alone in the world.

A shift in my parenting started to take seed when I started critically looking at our own family dynamics and the impact of my own upbringing and how that was informing my parenting. My inclination towards social justice analysis would widen the lens of understanding to include how larger systems of capitalism, white supremacy, and ableism, have also informed how I was parented and how I was parenting.

And all of this was helpful to me in that it helped me to see my child more holistically, it helped me to move away from the ADHD diagnosis as something to be fixed, it helped me to see beyond just giftedness and it began to help me to see my own pain, my own longings and how I had swallowed wholesale the narrow narratives of success.

References

Ariel, S. (2005). Family play therapy. In C. Schaefer, J. McCormick, & A. Ohnogi (Eds.), *International handbook of play therapy: Advances in assessment, theory, research, and practice* (pp. 3–22). Jason Aronson.

Ariel, S., Carel, C. A., & Tyano, S. (1985). Uses of children's make-believe play in family therapy: Theory and clinical examples. *Journal of Marital and Family Therapy*, 11(1), 47–60.

Busby, B. M., & Lufkin, A. C. (1992). Tigers are something else: Case for family play. *Contemporary Family Issues*, 1(3), 246–255.

Combrinck-Graham, L. (Ed.). (1989). *Children in family contexts: Perspectives on treatment*. Guilford Press.

Freeman, S., & Kasari, C. (2013). Parent-child interactions in autism: Characteristics of play. *Autism, 17*(2), 147–161.

Gil, E. (1994). *Play in family therapy*. Guilford Press.

Gil, E. (2015). *Play in family therapy* (2nd ed.). Guilford Press.

Lowry, L. (2016). Play & Autism: More evidence for following the child's lead. *The Hanen Centre*. https://www.hanen.org/MyHanen/Articles/Research/Play---Autism--More-evidence-for-following-the-chi.aspx

Sori, C. F., & Sprenkle, D. (2004). Training family therapists to work with children and families: A modified Delphi study. *Journal of Marital and Family Therapy, 30*, 479–495.

Trotter, K. (2013). Family play therapy. In N. R. Bowers (Ed.). *Play therapy with families*. Jason Aronson.

VanFleet, R. (2014). *Filial therapy: Strengthening the parent-child relationships through play* (3rd ed.), Professional Resource Press.

11
The AutPlay® Therapy Follow Me Approach (FMA)

What Is the Follow Me Approach (FMA)

Directive play therapy approaches and techniques are utilized and important to the AutPlay Therapy process. With most directive play therapy techniques; the technique can be adjusted to be more simple or more complex depending on the child and family. The adjustment from simple to complex does not affect the quality of the technique in being effective for helping children and adolescents, it is simply individualizing the therapy process to the specific child. It is essential that the therapy process aligns with the child instead of trying to force a child into a therapy process.

For some neurodivergent children and adolescents, directive play approaches and interventions may not align with their needs, manifestations, and therapy goals. For some children a more structured or directive approach will be too directive, and the child will not respond well to the therapy process. In situations where it is more appropriate, beneficial, and needed, the AutPlay Therapy Follow Me Approach (FMA) will be implemented. This approach exemplifies a more nondirective play therapy approach. Often children and adolescents who have higher support needs or who are younger (preschool age) can benefit from participating in the FMA. Children (of any age) who may have a difficult time attuning to and participating in directive techniques even when the interventions are simplified would also be good candidates for the FMA.

The FMA is a nondirective family play therapy approach which is used with children who would benefit from a more nondirective play therapy process. It was created to provide a supportive and healing therapeutic play approach for children who have higher needs and for a variety of reasons are unable to participate in structured or directive play interventions. Axline (1969) described nondirective play as therapy that starts where the child is and bases

DOI: 10.4324/9781003207610-12

the process on the present configuration, allowing for change from minute to minute during the therapeutic contact. It grants the child permission to be themselves and accept that self completely, without evaluation or pressure to change. It offers the child the opportunity to learn to know themselves and to openly chart their own course so they may form a more satisfactory design for living.

Axline (1947) furthered that nondirective play therapy can be described as an opportunity that is offered to the child to experience growth under the most favorable conditions. Since play is the natural medium for self-expression, the child is given the opportunity to play out their accumulated feelings of tension, frustration, insecurity, aggression, fear, bewilderment, and confusion. When the child has achieved emotional relaxation, they begin to realize the power within themselves to be an individual in their own right, to think for themselves to make their own decisions, to realize selfhood. Axline explained that as a result of the nondirective therapy experience children are able to:

- Gain respect for themselves as an individual of value
- Learn to accept themselves
- Grant themselves permission to utilize all of their capacities
- Assume responsibility for themselves
- Gain a respect and acceptance for people as they are
- Gain responsibilities for making their own decisions
- Gain a belief in their capacities
- Understand a positive and constructive way of life

(p. 27)

Mittledorf, Hendricks, and Landreth (2001) discussed the merits of play therapy (primarily nondirective play approaches) with autistic children. They noted essential recognition of autistic children's play that support the use of nondirective play processes.

> Play is the most natural thing all children do, and autistic children engage in their own self-involved play through which they express themselves and communicate with their world. Although much of the play of autistic children is ritualistic, it is, nevertheless, play and is their way of declaring themselves. Play is the language of children, and when toys or play media are used, the item can become the words of children conveying vast resources of messages, which cannot be communicated verbally. Useful toys of play items are not necessarily what would be thought of in the traditional sense, but rather are any items that children use for play

or expressive purposes. Children can ascribe their own personal meanings to nondescript items. The therapist may not understand what meaning an item has for a child, but it does potentially possess some meaning to the child. The therapist's job is to make contact with autistic children through the medium chosen by the children and with which they are most comfortable. Once play is viewed as having meaning, the therapist is much more likely to sense the inner rhythm of the child since children's play activity expresses the inner rhythm of their emotional life.

(pp. 257–258)

The FMA creates space for the autistic and neurodivergent child to feel accepted and free to explore and express. The FMA is an integration and extension of established nondirective play therapy theories and approaches such as Child Centered Play Therapy, Child Parent Relationship Therapy, and Filial Therapy. Ray, Sullivan, and Carlson (2012) described that in nondirective play therapy approaches, the therapist seeks to understand the child in the context of their world. The therapist provides full acceptance to the child, offers unconditional positive regard, and sends a message of respect and safety to children to enable them to share their world freely. The FMA utilizes established nondirective play therapy processes and individualizes the processes to the specific neurodivergent child being sure to acknowledge the neurodivergent child's play preferences and interests as well as their unique strengths.

Implementation of the FMA would begin with the Intake and Assessment Phase, and through observation, inventory assessment, and feedback, it will become clear to the therapist if a child is a good fit for the FMA. If this is the case, then the therapist will begin implementing FMA sessions and teaching parents how to have these types of play sessions at home. Often FMA sessions become the primary therapeutic approach until termination. In other instances, FMA sessions continue for a period of time until more directive interventions can be implemented. The nondirective element of the FMA approach does have variation. Just like any process in AutPlay, the exact approach is individualized to the child. The best fit for some children will be conceptualized with primarily nondirective play sessions, while others may have more of an integration of nondirective and some directive play. This chapter will outline the skills for implementing FMA sessions and help conceptualize how to individualize the FMA for each neurodivergent child.

Relationship as the Agent of Change

The FMA focuses heavily on relationship development as the agent of change in the nondirective play process. Axline (1947) stated during play therapy, relationship is established between the therapist and the child that makes it possible for the child to reveal their real self to the therapist, and having their self accepted, and thus growing in self-confidence – the child is more able to extend the frontiers of their personality expressions. Knobloch-Fedders (2008) defined the qualities of therapeutic relationship as mutual trust, respect, and caring, general agreement on the goals and tasks of the therapy, shared decision-making, mutual engagement in "the work" of the therapy, the ability to talk about the "here-and-now" aspects of the relationship with each other, the freedom to share any negative emotional responses with each other, and the ability to correct any problems or difficulties that may arise in the relationship. Knobloch-Fedders (2008) furthered that the therapist's ability to communicate empathy and understanding to the patient is very important. Another essential component is the therapist's openness, flexibility, and willingness to adapt the therapy to the patient's needs. Skilled therapists actively solicit patients' input about the goals and methods of therapy, in order to facilitate collaboration.

Kool and Lawver (2010) described the therapeutic relationship as a key criterion in play therapy-effectiveness. As play becomes a creative outlet that blends imagination and reality, it becomes fun and absorbing; the therapeutic relationship is deepened in play. The child is afforded the freedom to abreact and displace the unconscious ideas on the play event, allowing them to be observed by the therapist. The relationship-focused play therapist recognizes that growth is a slow process, not to be pushed, prodded, and hurried along. This is a time when the child can relax, a place where growth takes place naturally without being forced (Landreth, 1991). It is the focus on relationship development with autistic and neurodivergent children which facilitates children becoming more comfortable and confident which promotes engagement gains. Landreth (1991) outlined the following for therapeutic relationship development in play therapy:

- Establish an atmosphere of safety for the child
- Understand and accept the child's world
- Encourage the expression of the child's emotional world
- Produce facilitative responses
- Produce reflective and tracking attention and statements
- Establish limit setting

(pp. 154–155)

Ray, Jeffrey, and Sullivan (2012) stated that there are six conditions that must exist for the therapeutic process to work effectively. All six conditions are based on the primacy of the relationship between the therapist and child:

1 Two persons are in psychological contact.
2 The first person (client) is in a state of incongruence.
3 The second person (therapist) is congruent in the relationship.
4 The therapist experiences unconditional positive regard for the client.
5 The therapist experiences an empathic understanding of the client's internal frame of refence and attempts to communicate this experience to the client.
6 Communication to the client of the therapist's empathic understanding and unconditional positive regard is to a minimal degree achieved.

(p. 162)

In FMA application, the AutPlay therapist and child participate in a typical (CCPT) playroom setup. The child is given no directive instructions from the therapist. The therapist introduces the play session and follows the child's lead, moving with the child around the playroom, focusing on the child and staying attuned with the child. The therapist transitions as the child transitions – as the child transitions from one toy or activity to another, the therapist transitions with the child and does not try to bring the child back to a toy or activity. The therapist provides space for the child to lead but occasionally attempts to get involved with what the child is doing – trying to engage with the child in whatever type of play they are expressing. The therapist is observant in looking for opportunities to connect with the child through the child's play and notice any engagements back to the therapist.

Throughout an FMA session, the therapist is periodically implementing reflecting and tracking statements and being mindful of the child's comfort level. In the FMA, it is important to not only share physical space with the child, but also share attention, emotion, and understanding with the child. Initially, autistic and neurodivergent children may find FMA sessions uncomfortable and the experience of a new place and someone trying to connect or engage with them intrusive. If a child starts to become agitated or dysregulated by the therapist's presence or attempts to get involved with the child's play, then the therapist should discontinue attempts to get involved and simply stay present with the child occasionally providing reflecting and tracking statements until the child feels safer and more regulated. Although the FMA consists of some elements that encourage the therapist engaging with the child, the primary focus is on relationship development through nondirective play. There are a few integrated directive constructs, but the therapist should be aware that the directive constructs are not interfering with relationship development goals.

The therapist is not only having FMA sessions with their child but is also teaching the parents how to implement FMA play times at home with their child. The therapist must be mindful of facilitating relationship development with the parents. When parents are taught the FMA, it will be helpful for them to watch the therapist conducting the FMA with their child in sessions. Parents should be observing the FMA sessions the therapist is having with the child. The therapist will not only be developing relationship with the parents but also teaching the parents about therapeutic relationship development in the FMA play times. When parents implement the approach at home, they are instructed to try and schedule a FMA play time for 25 minutes multiple times a week (whatever is realistic for the family). This is an ideal scenario, parents and therapist will need to be flexible with the length of time and the number of times that the play times can be implemented at home. When deciding how many play times to have and the length of the play times, consideration should be given to the child's needs and ability to participate. The therapist stays active and connected to the parents (continually developing relationship) as they are implementing play times at home. During therapist process times with the parents, the therapist will review with the parents how the FMA play times are going at home and address any questions or concerns parents may have. Parent training in the FMA is discussed further in Chapter 12.

As FMA sessions progress, the therapist stays consistent in recognizing therapeutic relationship development as the primary agent of change. As the child enters the FMA sessions, the child is given no directive instructions from the therapist. The therapist begins the session with a structuring statement such as "You can play with anything you want in here and I am going to be in here with you." The therapist lets the child lead but periodically attempts to engage with what the child is doing. The therapist transitions as the child transitions. The therapist notes when the child participates in engagement or connection with the therapist. If appropriate for the specific child and their therapy goals, the therapist may be continuously looking for opportunities to introduce more directive play therapy techniques. This is a testing-out time to see if the child is yet capable to engage in some directive play therapy techniques. If the child responds well, then the therapist could continue to introduce more directive techniques. If the child does not respond well, the therapist will continue with FMA sessions and keep looking for opportunities to introduce more directive play therapy techniques.

Integrating Directive Elements

The FMA focuses primarily on relationship development through nondirective play therapy processes. There is an integration of two directive elements that add to the nondirective skills that make up the totality of FMA skills implemented. Therapists periodically ask the child questions. The questions are basic questions that should make sense and be relevant in regard to the child's play or what is happening in the play session. For example, if the child is playing with a dog miniature, the therapist might ask the child "Do you have a dog?" Another example would be if the child is painting a picture, the therapist might ask "What is your favorite color?" The question asking should not be continuous and should integrate with the other FMA skills. Questions should not probe for deeper psychological context, be leading or invasive, or attempt to illicit therapeutic information. Questions are simple and relevant in the moment. The purpose for the question asking skill is to help further connection and engagement and begin social navigation processes. Some children (those with higher needs and little to no engagement) will likely not answer questions at first. If a child does not respond to a question, the therapist should move on and try another question at a later time. Over time, the therapist will notice and note as children begin to acknowledge the therapist's questions – this is a positive sign of relationship development and increasing engagement and connection.

Therapists will also periodically attempt to engage with the child in the child's play. This should also be done in an integrated fashion along with the other FMA skills. As the child becomes established in a type of play, the therapist may try to join the child in their play and see if the child will allow the therapist to join and if the child will accept the joining through a reciprocal play interaction. For example, the child may be filling up a bucket in the sand tray. The therapist would move over beside the child and the sand tray and take another shovel and see if they could help fill up the bucket. The therapist might get their own bucket and place it in the sand tray and fill up their own bucket doing a type of parallel play. The therapist might also hold out their hands over the child's bucket and ask the child if they could pour sand in the therapist's hands. There are multiple ways the therapist could try to engage in the child's play. The therapist should be respectful to not lead or change the play, be respectful of the child's ignoring of the therapist or desire to not have the therapist engage and be mindful of the child's limits or discomfort with the therapist's engagement attempts. It is likely that some children will not engage back with the therapist, and this is okay. The therapist should make an attempt and then back off of attempts until a later time and try again. It is the therapist's role to offer and the child's right to accept or reject. Engagement and connection should move at the comfort level of the child.

In some situations (due to the child's needs and therapy goals) the therapist may be looking for gains in moving toward the child being able to participate in directive play therapy techniques and approaches (the Structured Play Intervention Phase). Some children may stay in the FMA until termination of therapy. For other clients, the FMA may be a beginning approach to lead to the child to participating in more directive play therapy techniques. It is important to note that typically if a child is at a need level where the FMA is going to be implemented, it is likely that the child will need other concurrent therapies in addition to AutPlay Therapy. Such therapies might include occupational therapy and speech therapy. If this is the case, the therapist should make the appropriate referrals.

For situations where the goal is to eventfully move the child into the Structured Intervention Phase, there is progression from the FMA to the Structured Intervention Phase. The therapy starts with the FMA and moves to connecting games and then to the Structured Intervention Phase. Table 11.1 demonstrates the progression. Connecting games are a natural next step or middle step between the FMA and more directive techniques found in the Structured Intervention Phase. Connecting games are focused on engagement and reciprocal participation and consist of a set of several short, fun, engaging games between the therapist and the child. The therapist introduces the connecting game, and each game requires a simple level of instruction and participation with the therapist.

Connecting games should consist of several games or activities that last approximately 15–20 minutes. The activities should be short and simple and have a connection component. Activities will likely begin slowly with little or no response from the child. Therapists should continue with the games and look for the child to gradually increase their participation with the therapist. The therapist should have several connecting games to choose from and introduce to the child, as the child will likely respond more positively to

Table 11.1 The Progression from FMA to the Structured Intervention Phase The Progression

Intake and assessment phase ⇨ FMA phase ⇨ Connecting games ⇨ Structured intervention phase ⇨ Termination phase

some games versus others (depending on the child's play preferences). The therapist and child may play one activity for 30 seconds and another for five minutes. This will vary and depend on the child's interest. In the beginning of introducing connecting games, it is likely the connecting set time will not reach 15–20 minutes. The child may start by only participating with the therapist for one minute. The therapist can work toward building up to 15–20 minutes of connecting games.

Once the therapist identifies that the child is ready to start participating in more directive engagement with the therapist, the therapist will introduce a connecting game. The therapist should have some indication that the child is willing, interested, and/or capable of participating in a simple game the therapist introduces before the therapist would introduce a connecting game. For example, the therapist might introduce to the child to hit a balloon back and forth and work together to keep the balloon from hitting the floor. The first-time balloon toss is introduced, the child hits the balloon back once and then leaves the activity and plays by themselves. The next session the therapist tries the balloon hitting game again. This time the child hits the balloon back three times, by the fourth session, the child is hitting the balloon back ten times before becoming disinterested. During the fourth session, after the balloon game, the therapist immediately introduces a second connecting game; bubble blowing and popping. The child participates with the therapist blowing the bubbles and the child popping the bubbles for approximately five minutes. By the seventh session of introducing connecting games, the child is participating in approximately 15 minutes of connecting games with the therapist.

Connecting games do not have to be designated therapeutic games. The therapist has a wide range of options available when introducing a connecting game. The primary goal is to have the child participating with the therapist in a simple game that requires a level of following instruction, attunement, and acknowledgment. Some examples might include hitting a balloon back and forth, lotion games, thumb wrestling, playing hand games such as patty cake, feeding games, throwing, rolling, or kicking a ball back and forth, playing hide and seek, playing chase and catch, mirroring games, bubble blowing games, Play Doh games, movement games such as duck, duck, goose, and hand games.

Once the child is regularly participating in 15–20 minutes if connection games, the therapist can begin to move into the Structured Intervention Phase and implement more directive interventions that focus on therapy needs and goals. In this type of scenario, the FMA would be considered a beginning approach with the goal of moving into more directive interventions (the Structured Intervention Phase). Throughout the FMA, the therapist could be periodically "checking out" the possibility of moving into connecting games and then more directive interventions. Becoming more directive will likely be a step process with the child responding to the therapist to gradually and at their own comfort level.

Who Should Participate in the Follow Me Approach (FMA)

Anyone can participate in the FMA. If the therapist feels that this would be the best point of therapy for the child, they should move forward with the FMA. Technically, the FMA was designed for working with autistic and neurodivergent children and children with developmental disabilities that have higher needs and co-occurring needs. The basic description of the child would be a child who has little to no engagement or interaction. This may be a nonverbal or non-speaking child, may be a child who does not respond in any way to others, or a child in which the therapist assesses would likely not participate in directive play approaches or interventions.

The therapist would begin by assessing for appropriateness and best fit for implementing the FMA. Typically, this is done in the Intake and Assessment Phase. Through observations and inventories, the therapist should have an indication if the FMA is the appropriate avenue of therapy for a particular client. This would primary be based on the child's manifestation and presentation and the identified therapy needs and goals. Remember that there are fluctuating levels in AutPlay. A therapist may decide the FMA is the best avenue but also feel they could integrate in some basic directed play interventions. Another therapist may feel their client needs to begin exclusively in the FMA with a higher focus on nondirective play processes. This depends on the individualization of therapy for the specific client. Also remember that the child and parent are partners (co change agents) in the therapy process. They will also have a say in formulating what would be the best fit for moving forward with therapy.

To help conceptualize what types of clients would benefit from the FMA, the following simple vignettes presents some of the clients that would likely be good candidates for the FMA. This is not a complete presentation but assists the therapist in gaining a better understanding. These vignettes do not reflect judgments about children as many therapists will discover many strengths and capabilities of children as they begin to develop relationship with the child. These vignettes are simply provided to give a very superficial presentation of what children might be a good fit for the FMA approach. Remember a basic construct of AutPlay and being neurodiversity affirming is presuming competence.

- A three-year-old autistic child. Due to the child's young age, the FMA would be a likely approach.
- A seven-year-old neurodivergent child who displays little to no engagement or interaction with others. The child will not respond or acknowledge when addressed and seems to be in their own space not aware of others.
- A six-year-old autistic child with an additional diagnosis of intellectual developmental disorder, and a chromosome disorder. The child has limited verbal output and does not respond to others.
- A 12-year-old child who has down syndrome and intellectual developmental disorder and typically does not acknowledge others.
- A seven-year-old autistic child who has verbal and speaking ability and can interact with others but is strongly against directive instruction and will not participate in therapist introduced interventions.
- An eight-year-old child who has high support needs and multiple diagnoses and medical issues who uses a wheelchair and cannot implement fine or large motor skills. The child has little to no verbal output and seems to be non-responsive or aware.

A special consideration would be working with extremely limited or non-responsive clients. This can be a child of any age. Occasionally a client might have high medical and physical needs that prevent them from being mobile. They may have to stay in a wheelchair or similar accommodation all the time. Some clients in this category may be able to be mobile but they do not speak or seem to have verbal or other identified communication and do not respond to initiations from others. This could also be a client who has the majority of things done for them or require someone to help them such as eating, dressing, bathing, going to the bathroom, etc. These would certainly be children with high needs and co-occurring diagnose or issues. This would not be simply an autistic child or a child with only ADHD.

This is a client who will likely not initiate anything on their own. They will not engage in nondirective, or directive play on their own. With these clients, it is still appropriate to start with the FMA as a base, but the therapist will have to be more directive with the child. The therapist will likely have to introduce various toys, materials, activities to the child and assess for response that indicates a preference or interest. This might be a traditional toy, a sensory item, art, music, or technology-based play. The therapy session and process may look very differently from work with other neurodivergent children. There may be much less happening in the sessions and progress toward therapy goals may seem to move at a much slower rate. This would be expected and should not be something the therapist is surprised to experience. It may be an adjustment for the therapist who may not be used to this type of presentation and how to appreciate the process of sessions and moving toward therapy goals with a child with very high support needs.

In my work with children with this type of presentation I have often began with an exploration of introducing various things to see what the child might be interested in and respond to. I have discovered this to be technology games on an iPad (this has often been a positive result), baby dolls, sensory trays, puppets, and various other things. Once a play preference or interest was discovered, it facilitated the process of beginning to connect and engage together through the play interest. The FMA base is helpful in keeping the therapist in a space of building relationship, assuming competence, and looking for all ways possible to value the child's voice.

The Follow Me Approach (FMA) Skills

There are five primary skills in the FMA. These skills represent what the therapist is doing in each FMA session and ultimately what the therapist is teaching the parent to do. The nondirective play skill serves as the foundation for the FMA sessions. The other four skills should be implemented periodically during a session and at the therapist's discretion.

Nondirective Play Skill – The child leads the play in the session. The child is allowed to maneuver around the playroom and play with or attend to anything they like. The child is also allowed to switch from toy to toy or types of play as they like. The child leads the time, and the therapist follows the child figuratively and literally in the playroom. The therapist stays present and attuned with the child, paying attention to the child, and observing the child closely. The therapist does not try to lead the play or direct the child to participate in a play therapy intervention. The therapist is communicating presence and awareness and that the FMA session is a safe place for the child to be themselves and engage in play their way. The therapist is also building relationship with the child.

Reflective and Tracking Statements Skill – The therapist periodically provides a reflective and/or tracking statement. These statements communicate to the child that the therapist is present with them, sees them, and is attuning to them. These statements further help develop relationship with the child. Reflective statements in particular help the child identify and express their emotions. A reflective statement is reflecting to the child any emotion stated or shown by the child or that the therapist perceives is coming from the child. An example would be a child struggling to get a cap off a marker. The child is looking frustrated with their effort. The therapist might say "That cap is frustrating you," or "You are frustrated that the cap will not come off." Another example would be if the child says "This is my favorite" while tightly hugging a stuffed animal. The therapist might reflect "You really like that one," or "That one makes you feel happy." Additional examples include "Blowing the bubbles makes you feel happy" or "You don't like it when I move the cars." A note of caution. Because neurodivergent children can experience and express emotion differently from neurotypical presentations, the therapist will want to be careful about interpreting a feeling they see from the child. Unless the therapist feels absolutely sure they are interpreting a feeling correctly, they may want to reflect something more general such as, "It looks like something is happening with you," "Something is happening," "I'm noticing something," I'm noticing you and what is going on," or "You can't get the lid off and you might be feeling something."

Tracking statements are simply tracking what the child is doing. An example would be if the child is scooping up sand and putting it into a bucket, the therapist might say "You are putting the sand in the bucket," or "You are doing what you want with the sand." Another example would be if the child paints a picture and holds it up to show the therapist, the therapist might say "You finished the whole painting," or "You finished that and now you are showing me." Additional examples include "You are finished with the sand tray, and now you are playing with the doll," or "You are hammering that really hard."

Asking Questions Skill – The therapist periodically will ask the child a question. The questions are designed to communicate to the child that the therapist is present, to begin developing social navigation, and to help the therapist assess for engagement improvement. The questions asked should be in the moment and related to what is happening in the therapy session. An example would be the child painting blue on a piece of paper and the therapist asking, "Do you like the color blue?" Another example would be the child is building with blocks and the therapist asks, "Do you have blocks at home?" Additional examples include "Do you have any brothers at home,"

"Do you like to play sports," or "What color is that?" It is likely that many questions will not garner a response from the child. Many children may not even acknowledge they have been asked a question. The therapist is asking questions to identify when a child begins to answer questions and how well and often a child answers questions. When a child begins to answer questions regularly and fully, it is an indication the child is attuning more with the therapist and is moving toward being able to do connection games or directive techniques.

Engage with the Child Skill – Throughout an FMA session, the therapist is periodically trying to engage with the child in whatever the child is doing (the child's play). Remember that the child leads and chooses whatever the child wants to play with, and the therapist follows the child and tries to get involved with what the child is doing. The therapist should make attempts throughout the session to get involved in the play. How many attempts, in what ways, and at what time is left to the therapist's discretion. The therapist does not need to be constantly trying to engage. If the child responds and engages with the therapist, the therapist should continue with whatever is being done until the child is no longer interested. If the child begins to show irritation or dysregulation with the attempts the therapist is making to engage, then the therapist should stop trying to engage and move away from the child and simply make some tracking and reflecting statements for a period of time and then return to trying to engage with the child. Some examples of engaging with the child include:

- The child starts playing with the play dishes. The therapist sits beside the child and takes a bowl and puts it on the therapist's head and says to the child, "Look at my silly bowl hat." The therapist is trying to engage the child by having the child look at the therapist and notice the bowl on the therapist's head. The therapist might take a bowl or plate and put it on the child's head and say, "Look at the plate on your head." The therapist might ask the child to put a bowl or plate on the therapist's head and see if they can begin to engage in this activity back and forth.
- The child starts playing with the sand tray building a sandcastle. The therapist moves beside the child and starts adding sand to the castle or asks the child where to put the sand. The therapist might try pushing sand to the child to use for their castle. The therapist might also try building their own castle in a separate area in the sand tray.
- The child is shooting a basketball into the basketball hoop. The therapist moves beside the child and helps get the ball and hand it back to the child after they shoot a basket. The therapist might also try getting

another basketball and also shooting the ball in the basket. The therapist could try getting the child to take turns shooting the basketball or allow the therapist to pass the basketball to the child and then the child shoots it.

Being Mindful of Limits Skill – The therapist should be sensitive to the child's comfort, feelings of safety, and regulation level. Some sessions may be mostly tracking and reflecting statements if the child is displaying discomfort with the therapist's attempts to engage. The therapist should not engage or try to get involved with what the child is doing to the point where the child becomes fully dysregulated and has a meltdown. An example would be the child starts to play with rolling some cars around on the floor. The therapist sits down beside the child and starts rolling some cars with the child. The child grabs the cars from the therapist and pushes the therapist away. This is a clear sign the child does not feel comfortable with what the therapist is doing, or the child may be becoming dysregulated. The therapist should move away from the child and observe the child while periodically making some tracking and reflecting statements and try to engage with the child again when the therapist feels it would be appropriate.

Goals for the Child

The therapist will want to always be looking for some advancement or displaying of progress toward therapy needs and goals. Prior to beginning the FMA, the therapist, along with the parents and child (if appropriate), should identify and establish therapy needs and some basic attuning and engagement goals to work toward through the FMA. Some examples might include recognizing the therapist, responding to questions and/or asking questions, reciprocal communication (this can look many ways and does not have to be verbal), initiating with the therapist, engaging with the therapist, participating in reciprocal play, asking the therapist, etc. The therapist should take note of instances where the pre-identified goals occur and seem to happen more frequently, or the child has achieved the goal with the therapist. Accomplishment of these goals is another indication that the child is moving toward being able to participate in more directive techniques and the Structured Intervention Phase if this is warranted for the child.

Another goal of the FMA is developing empowerment vs dis-empowerment. Jeffreys (2021) described dis-empowerment as removing one's own or someone else's power. Usually, it is used to describe a power of self-care or emotion versus some violent self-defense action. Neurodivergent children are often dis-empowered. They are susceptible to others taking their power away in many shapes and forms. Much of this is driven by unchecked ableist practices. The FMA attempts to empower neurodivergent children. Empowerment encourages confidence, decision making, self-advocacy, and self-care. In the FMA, neurodivergent children can lead, use their voice, make decision, gain confidence, and feel empowered through the FMA skills. The therapist should be monitoring for gains in empowerment as children progress through FMA sessions.

A possible goal might be implementing the FMA as a beginning point for therapy to help the child progress to where they could participate with the therapist in more directive play techniques and approaches. This would not be a goal for every child but if it was, the therapist should periodically initiate and see if the child will participate in a more directive game or activity with the therapist. As the child begins to progress in this way, the therapist can begin to advance the games or activities and increase the child's level of participation.

There are some standard goals which apply to all children participating in the FMA. Standard goals for children include:

- Give opportunity for the child's voice to be heard.
- Increase the child's self-worth.
- Increase relationship development between the child and parents and others in the child's life.
- Empower the child in decision-making, identity, and self-advocacy.
- Help the child express emotions.
- Help the child develop problem-solving and coping skills.
- Promote positive social and relational dynamics for the child.
- Reduce and/or eliminate presenting needs/issues.

Pragmatics of the Follow Me Approach (FMA) Session Setup

Using a Playroom and Toys/Materials – A playroom or play space is recommended when implementing the FMA. A playroom with toys and materials provides the greatest environment for play preferences and interests expression and utilization for processing and growth. The playroom design is typically a CCPT playroom setup. Landreth (1991) stated that the atmosphere of the playroom is of critical importance because that is what impacts the child first. Ideally, the therapist would have a large enough space to have a variety of toys and materials available for access and space for movement. The toys and materials selected should reflect a variety of play preferences and interests with include pretend play, functional play, constructive play, sensory play, movement play, technology play, and expressive (art) play. The variety is important, but the playroom should not be overstocked. If the room is too full of toys and materials it can become overwhelming. The children should be able to easily access the toys and materials and consideration should be given to children who may have physical needs or accommodations and those with sensory differences. A recommended toys and materials list is provided in the appendix.

Starting and Ending a FMA Session – The practitioner begins by introducing the child to the playroom. The practitioner explains to the child that, "This is a playroom, and you can do whatever you like in here, and I will be in here with you." No rules or limits are established at this time. The therapist begins each FMA session with this structuring statement. The therapist gives a five-minute verbal and visual warning that the play session is almost over and again at the one-minute mark. The verbal statement can be "We have five minutes left of our play time and then it will be over for today," and again at the one minute, "We have one minute left of our play time today and then it will be over." The visual can be as simple as the therapist holding up their hand with five fingers and then one finger as they are giving the verbal warnings. When the session is over, the therapist states, "Our time is up for today" and leads the child to the take home (transition) item and then out of the playroom. In AutPlay, a transition item is used at the end of the session to transition out of the session. The transition item can be a sticker, small toy, balloon, a pebble, a LEGO piece, or it can be an activity – a game that is played as the therapist and child leave the playroom and exit the building. Transition items are used to provide routine to the session and ease the ending of the session and help with progressing on for the child.

Limit Setting – The limit-setting approach in the FMA is fairly simple. Many of the children that will be participating in the FMA may not understand limit setting models that are too verbal or too cognitive and they may need a more basic redirection. For most limit-setting needs, the therapist should simply redirect the child or remove the limit casing toy or material. The therapist could try implementing the CCPT ACT limit setting model. This may work for some children, but for others it will likely involve too much language and cognitive processing. The Act limit setting model was outlined by Landreth (2001). (A) Acknowledge the child's wants/needs (C) Communicate the limit in a non-punitive way (T) Target acceptable alternatives. For example, (A) "Sarah, I know you want to paint on the wall." (C) "but in here we cannot do that." (T) "You can paint on the easel or on this paper." The therapist decides what is a limit to set and limits should be set as little as possible. If the child did not respond to the limit, the ultimate action the therapist would take is ending the session time.

Therapists Guide for Implementing the Follow Me Approach (FMA)

The Therapist Should

- Follow the Child – The child leads, and the therapist follows the child figuratively and literally. The therapist lets the child move around the playroom and provides space for the child play with anything in any way they choose. The therapist moves with the child, sits by the child, and transitions as the child transitions.
- Make Tracking Statements – These are statements that the therapist makes periodically tracking what the child is doing. For example: "You are playing in the sand tray," or "You just shot the Nerf gun," or "You are looking around at all the toys in here."
- Make Reflecting Statements – These are statements that the therapist makes when the therapist notices a child displaying a feeling. For example: "That makes you mad," or "You feel sad that there is no more paint."
- Ask Questions – The therapist should periodically ask the child questions. The therapist should try to ask questions that are relevant. For example: The child picks up a basketball. The therapist might ask, "Do you have a basketball at home?"
- Attempt to Engage with the Child – The therapist should frequently try to engage the child or play with the child in whatever they are doing. For example: The child is playing in the sand tray. The practitioner might try scooping up some sand and pouring it on the child's hand or scooping up some sand and putting it in the bucket the child is trying to fill. Another example: The child is playing with some balls; the practitioner might pick up a ball and try to roll it or toss it to the child.
- Monitor for Dysregulation – The therapist should be sensitive to the child's comfort level especially regarding engaging with the child. If the therapist notices that the child is becoming uncomfortable or dysregulated by the therapist's attempts to engage, the therapist should discontinue making attempts to engage and move away from the child for a period of time and then try again.

- Be Mindful of Goals – The therapist is working on relationship development and increasing the child's comfort level being present with the therapist. The therapist is looking for ways to connect and signs of the child responding to or connecting with the therapist. This might be through verbalizations or playing together or in some way acknowledging the therapist. The therapist should never try to force engaging or a connection. If the child is showing they are not interested, then the therapist should do some tracking statements for a while and try engaging again later.
- Introduce Simple Connecting Games (if part of the therapy plan) – The therapist should periodically introduce a simple connecting game or activity to see if the child will participate with the therapist. This is somewhat of a "testing out" process to evaluate if the child is making progress toward participating in more directive interventions.

Autistic and neurodivergent children often find themselves in therapies and programs designed to dictate and "instruct the child in what to do and when to do it. Often children find little to no time in their life to control their process. The FMA provides children many opportunities that are not often present in their lives. The nondirective elements of the FMA promote empowerment and therapeutic relationship development – a key component for therapy. Relationship development is not only foundational and central to the successful implementation of the FMA but also with implementing directive play interventions. It is the relationship that gives the interventions, approaches, and the totality of the therapy experience its power and effectiveness.

References

Axline, V. (1947). *Play therapy*. Houghton Mifflin.
Axline, V. (1969). *Dibs: In search of self*. Houghton Mifflin.
Jeffreys, R. (2021). *You were made for this*. Empowerment Publishing.
Knobloch-Fedders, L. (2008). The importance of the relationship with the therapist. The Family Institute at Northwestern University. https://www.family-institute.org/behavioral-health-resources/importance-relationship-therapist
Kool, R., & Lawver, T. (2010). Play therapy: Considerations and applications for the practitioner. *Psychiatry (Edgmont)*, 7(10), 19–24.
Landreth, G. L. (1991). *Play therapy: The art of the relationship*. Accelerated Development Publishers.
Landreth, G. L. (2001). *Innovations in play therapy: Issues, process, and special populations*. Routledge.

Mittledorf, W., Hendricks, S., & Landreth, G. L. (2001). Play therapy with autistic children. In G. L. Landreth (Ed.), *Innovations in play therapy: Issues, process, and special populations* (pp. 257–269). Routledge.

Ray, D. C., Sullivan, J. M., & Carlson, S. E. (2012). Relational intervention: Child-centered play therapy with children on the autism spectrum. In L. Gallo-Lopez & L. C. Rubin (Eds.), *Play-based interventions for children and adolescents with autism spectrum disorders* (pp. 159–175). Routledge.

12

The AutPlay® Therapy Follow Me Approach (FMA) with Parents

The Importance of Parents

There must be a fundamental understanding that if you support neurodivergent children then you must support parents and families of neurodivergent children. Parents play a vital role in the life of any child but perhaps the relationship between the neurodivergent child and their parent is an extra significant one. Parents enter into the AutPlay Therapy process as partners (co-change agents) but parents often bring with them their own needs and issues that warrant attention. If these needs are left unaddressed, it can have a detrimental effect on the child and everyone in the family. Parents of autistic or neurodivergent child can look like and have the same issues as any family but there are some considerations and possible needs that may be specific to or at an extra level for these families.

- Financial stressors from services and therapies
- Social isolation
- Lack of respite care
- Sibling struggles
- Extended family members not understanding the child
- Waiting lists for therapies
- Mislabeled and misunderstood
- Worrying about the future after the parents are gone
- Education struggles, being kicked out of school
- 24/7 parenting attention, hypervigilance on prevention
- Highly scheduled and consistent routine
- Marriage stressors

Booth and Jernberg (2010) discussed that working with parents is often multifaceted. As you assist parents in developing healthy relationship, you

DOI: 10.4324/9781003207610-13

must be sensitive to their needs. You may need to discuss developmental issues while helping parents understand the meaning and communication of their child's behaviors. You may need to help parents with general parenting issues – how to provide appropriate discipline, helping extended family members who do not understand neurodivergence, addressing school related problems, etc.

Why are parents and families so important? The family unit is the foundation for children, it has the greatest impact on the child's development. The family is the main environment for a child, little else has the same influence as the family environment. What the parents do greatly affects the child and what children do greatly affects parents. Often individual therapy may not be addressing the "real" issues or not fully addressing the issues. Many presenting issues may have a root in what is happening in the family or issues are being exasperated by situations happening in the family.

Parents often need help as well as the child. Parents and anyone in the family unit may be having struggles that need attention. Siblings and extended family members matter. Family is not just the child and parent. Siblings often play a large part and so do extended family members that are actively involved in the child's life. Family is where the child's learning and development is modeled – from attachment to social navigation. Each family will possess their own unique family culture which carries influence into adulthood.

Stinnett and DeFrain (1985) identified six features of strong or healthy families, (1) Commitment – Family members were committed to each other's growth as individuals. (2) Appreciation – Family members told each other often how much they appreciated them, and were also specific about it. (3) Communication – Family members communicated frequently with each other, using good communication skills. (4) Fun Time Together – Family members spent time together, and some of that time was used for having fun together. (5) Spiritual Wellness – Strong families in the study felt that spirituality helped them keep a perspective, especially when times were tough. (6) Coping Ability – When times were tough, strong families would work to face the problems together. The family coming together in a family play therapy process such as the Follow Me Approach (FMA), has the opportunity to address a whole host of possible needs in a sustainable way. The family has the safe environment of the play sessions to process and explore and create strong and healthy features for their family.

An effective family play therapy approach strives to heal relationships so that all family members can engage with each other in a way that encourages safe, positive, and creative relating. In family play therapy, play is the vehicle for change, and it is a vehicle for engagement. It provides a context for both assessment and intervention and is the crux of therapeutic communication (Trotter, 2013). As child and parents enter into the FMA, the process will provide growth and empowerment for both, and as additional family members may become involved, they will grow as well.

Play engages both the adults and children in cognitive and affective processes where fantasy and symbology facilitate one's ability to organize information and entertain divergent thinking. It is far preferable to act aggression out through the play rather than actual fighting. Working through powerful emotions such as aggression while using a toy or play as a vehicle for expression, enhances one's capacity to process and regulate emotions as well as integrate them with cognitions (Trotter, 2013). Play benefits everyone in the family and can address both intrapsychic and interpersonal problems throughout the family system. It allows families to recapture the joy they once had as they laugh and play together, experiencing mutual delight in pleasurable activities (Gil, 2015).

Gil (2015) furthered that family play therapy holds a myriad of possibilities. It can help individual family member's shift perceptions of each other, break up old patterns of interaction and introduce healthier alternatives, foster attachment and breathe new life into families, open windows of opportunity to observe family interactions on a deeper level than achieved in traditional talk therapy, and can address the goals of individual children and adults, promote overall family functioning, and strengthen relationships.

When we consider involving parents and other family members in the FMA, we value them as partners in the process. If parents are struggling, we want to provide help for them. This may be in the form of offering counseling sessions just for the parents or referring them to another professional who can help. As parents participate in the FMA, it is important that they feel empowered, competent, and encouraged to work with, play with, and be co-change agents in helping their children. It is important that parents can be in a state of mind where they are celebrating their child and understanding their child through an affirming parenting lens.

A component of the FMA involves helping parents build health relationships and providing neurodiversity affirming messages to their child. Jeffreys (2021) stated that the healthiest parents are the ones who have unlimited pride in their children who struggle. They don't hide their children's limitations. They celebrate them and their success. They have thrown out society's scale of success and built their own.

The Autistic Self Advocacy Network (2021) created a parent's guide, *Start Here: A Guide for Parents of Autistic Kids*. Their guide provides many affirming pieces of information to help parents better understand their child. Although the guide focuses on autism, much of the information can pertain to all neurodivergent children. The guide highlights the need for parents to understand an affirming way to view and parent their child, proving direct suggestions for parents included the following:

> Your kid is still the same kid as they were before they got their autism diagnosis. All the things you love about them haven't changed. Your kid loves you, and they know you love them. Now that you know that they are autistic, you are going to be able to understand them better. Being autistic is a part of what makes your child who they are. Autism doesn't mean that your child will have a worse life than other children. Their life may be different than what you had expected. But your child can still have a great life. Part of building that great life for your child is learning how to support them as an autistic person... Your child is still the same child as before they got an autism diagnosis. They still have the same personality, likes and dislikes. You should still treat your child with the same love and respect as you did before. At the same time, now that you know your child is autistic, there are lots of things you can do to support them. Your support can help your child have an easier time in the world.
>
> (pp. 3–13)

Teaching the Follow Me Approach (FMA) to Parents

Many parents interact with, teach, and play with their children through a didactic directive style that they probably learned or experienced as a child. Certainly, there is a time and place (even in AutPlay Therapy) for a more directive type of teaching and playing but it is not the most natural way for children to learn and communicate. The nondirective attuned parent participating in an FMA type of play with their children provides the most successful environment for the child to express their natural language, heal, grow, and communicate. MacDonald and Stoika (2007) described this as a responsive approach which allows the adult to focus on the child's signature strengths and the interests the child currently demonstrates successfully, because the adult responds to what the child does instead of directing or insisting that the child does what the grown-up has in mind.

Landreth and Bratton (2020) shared that play is the most natural way children communicate. Toys are like words for children and play is their natural language. Adults talk about their experiences, thoughts, and feelings. Children use toys to explore their experiences and express what they think and how they feel. Landreth and Bratton (2020) furthered the benefits for parents and child when participating in nondirective play times:

> In special play times, you will build a different kind of relationship with your child, and your child will discover that they are capable, important, understood, and accepted as they are. When children experience a play relationship in which they feel accepted, understood, and cared for, they play out many of their problems and, in the process, release tensions, feelings, and burdens. Your child will then feel better about themselves and will be able to discover their own strengths and assume greater self-responsibility as they take charge of play situations. How your child feels about themselves will make a significant difference in their behavior. In special play times where you learn to focus on your child rather that your child's problem, your child will begin to react differently, because how your child behaves, how they think, and how they perform in school are directly related to how they feel about themselves. When your child feels better about themselves, they will behave in more self-enhancing ways rather than self-defeating ways.
>
> (p. 16)

VanFleet (2014) proposed that special play times format permits optimal relationship development and attention to the child's needs. VanFleet (1994) stated that when parents conduct nondirective play times with their own children it creates a safe and accepting environment which create opportunities for the expression of feelings, communication, and resolution of social, emotional, and behavioral issues. The process also helps shift parent's negative attitudes and beliefs about their children, helps parents cooperate more effectively with each other, reduces parental stress and frustration, and motivates parents to change some of their own behaviors.

As defined in Chapter 11, the FMA is a nondirective family play therapy approach which is used with children who would benefit from a more nondirective play therapy process. A significant piece of the FMA process involves teaching parents how to have FMA play times at home with their child. Parents are taught by the therapist how to facilitate and implement FMA play times at home with their child between sessions with the therapist. The therapist will teach parents the core skills for implementing an FMA play time which include nondirective play, making tracking and reflecting statements, asking questions, and attempting engagement with their child, and monitoring for the child's limits. Therapists will also guide parents on how to implement the FMA play times in the home setting. Parents will decide on a specific area in their home to have an FMA play time – preferably not the child's own playroom or bedroom. Parents should also collect some toys and materials to use during the FMA play time and the toys and materials should be boxed up and put away and only used for the FMA play times. Some autistic and neurodivergent children may be very attached to their toys and their space and they may not want the parent "intruding." Further, the FMA play times are therapeutic play times, not general play times like the parent might be already doing with their child. The separate space and toys provide a cleaner distinction between the two types of play times. There are always exceptions. Again, in the AutPlay Therapy framework, the process is individualized to the specific child. There may be situations where it would work best to have the FMA play time in the child's own playroom using their own toys – perhaps this is what the child prefers and how they respond best. It should be noted that general ideas shared in conducting the FMA play times are a guide, and adjustment and individualization for each child is supported.

Many parents have reported it beneficial to have the FMA play time in a different part of the home and to collect toys that are only used during the FMA play time. Parents have shared that this seems to engage their child more in the play times. Some parents have discovered that the FMA play time occurs throughout the whole house with the child moving from room to room and the parent moving with the child. Other parents have shared that they have their FMA play times outside in their backyard. Any of these variations are acceptable as long as the parent is able to apply the core skills of the FMA. The therapist should communicate to parents that the home implementation can look many ways and there may be a bit of experimenting to discover what works best for the child. A list of recommended toys and other materials is available in the appendix and can be shared with parents. Therapists should explain to parents that they do not need to acquire all the toys on the list. The list is a guide and parents should select just some of the toys and materials that the parents believe will be the most engaging for their child. The parents are free to acquire toys and materials that are not on the recommended list. The priority is collecting items that would be engaging for the child to play with.

General Session Outline for Teaching and Implementing the FMA

Sessions 1–4: Conduct the Intake and Assessment Phase in AutPlay Therapy. This provides opportunity to get to know the child and parents better, develop relationship, and assess for readiness and appropriateness to participate in the FMA. During session four, the therapist would discuss with the parents about participating in FMA sessions and provide a general overview about what to expect. During session four it would also be decided if one or both parents were going to participate in the FMA play times. This is largely up to the parents depending on what works best for them. It may be observed during the Intake and Assessment Phase that the parents seem to not know how to play with their child or have never played with their child. In this case, the therapist would take a couple of sessions to work with just the parents role-playing and teaching to improve their play ability with their child. This would be important to do before beginning the FMA sessions.

Session 5: Begin the FMA sessions. The therapist conducts an FMA session with the child and the parent observes the session. The parent can observe through a monitoring window or be in the playroom sectioned off in one corner. The parent is given a paper copy of the core skills to read and watch for during the session. They are also given some paper and something to write with so they can record any questions that arise. This FMA session takes about 30 minutes with the child. The rest of the session time is used to go over the skills with the parent. There may need to be arrangements made for the child to be watched or have something else to do while the skills are covered with the parent. The therapist should read through and explain each skill. The therapist should also point out each skill as the therapist demonstrated them in the session.

Sessions 6–7: The therapist conducts an FMA session with the child for about 30 minutes. The parents are observing the sessions and learning the core skills. The therapist is using the reminder of the therapy time to go over the skills and help the parents learn how to implement an FMA play time with their child. The therapist should be mindful to respond to any questions the parents may have.

Sessions 8–9: Once the parent and therapist agree that the parent has the skills learned and feel confident, the parent can begin conducting the FMA play times with their child (in the therapist's playroom/office) and the therapist can observe. This usually take two sessions of observing the parents to make sure they have the basic skill ideas mastered and are ready to start having the play times at home. If both parents are participating, they will need to have separate FMA play times with their child. If this is the case, then each parent should have two times they are conducting the FMA play time and being observed by the therapist. This would mean four total sessions instead of two. The parent will conduct the FMA session for 30 minutes and spend the rest of the time following up with the therapist. The therapist should provide positive feedback on what the parent did well and provide any feedback on any area to work on. The therapist should remain positive and encouraging while providing feedback and address any questions the parent has.

Session 10: If the therapist's observations went well and the parent feels ready, the transition to home play times begin in session ten. In this session the therapist will meet with the parents to discuss the home implementation of the FMA play times. This is a time to make sure parents are ready and everything is set up for successful home play times. In-home play time implementation is discussed in more detail later in this chapter.

Sessions 11-termination: At this point, parents should have conducted their first in-home FMA play times. The format of sessions 11 through the termination of therapy look very similar. The therapist begins by getting an update on the home play times. The therapist should provide parents copies of the *In Home Play Times Summary Sheet* (located in the appendix). The parents would complete the summary sheet after the play time and bring it with them to the therapy session. This is an opportunity for the parent to ask any questions to address any issues that may have come up during the in-home play times. Once the update has been covered, the therapist will conduct an FMA play time with the child and the parent will observe. The parent is expected to continue to have in-home play times between session times with the therapist.

If the FMA is the primary approach being implemented with the child and family, then sessions will continue in this way until therapy goals have been met and therapy is terminated. The therapist and parent should be discussing periodically what advancement is happening regarding therapy needs and goals. This should be an ongoing evaluation to assess that therapy goals are being met and when therapy has been completed. There is no limit on the number of sessions prior to termination. This will depend on each child and the specific therapy needs and goals.

If the FMA is a beginning approach with the goal to move into the Structed Intervention Phase, then the therapist and parents should be monitoring for changes and opportunities that move through the progression from the FMA to connecting games to the Structured Intervention Phase. The therapist, parent, and child will progress as appropriate and re-examine therapy needs and goals as they move through the progression. Once they are functioning in the Structured Intervention Phase, they will proceed toward completion of any identified therapy needs or goals until reaching the Termination Phase.

Teaching the FMA Skills to Parents

The following descriptions can be copied and given to parents to help them understand the FMA skills. Additionally, therapists can provide parents with a copy of *the Parent Guide for Implementing the AutPlay Follow Me Approach (FMA)* located in the appendix.

Nondirective Play Skill – The child leads the play in the session. The child is allowed to maneuver around the play time and play with or attend to anything they like. The child is also allowed to switch from toy or types of play as they like. The child leads the time, and the parent follows the child figuratively and literally in the play time. The parent stays present and attuned with the child, paying attention to the child, and observing the child closely. The parent does not try to lead the play or direct the child to participate in play the parent wants to do. The parent is communicating presence and awareness and that the play time is a safe place for the child to be themselves and engage in play their way. The parent is also building relationship with the child.

Reflective and Tracking Statements Skill – The parent periodically provides a reflective and/or tracking statement. These statements communicate to the child that the parent is present with them, sees them, and is attuning to them. These statements further help develop relationship with the child. Reflective statements in particular help the child identify and express their emotions. A reflective statement is reflecting to the child any emotion stated or showed by the child or that the parent perceives is coming from the child. An example would be a child struggling to get a cap off a marker. The child is looking frustrated with their effort. The parent might say "That cap is frustrating you," or "You are frustrated that the cap will not come off." Another example would be if the child says "This is my favorite" while tightly hugging a stuffed animal. The parent might reflect "You really like that one," or "That one makes you feel happy." Additional examples include "Blowing the bubbles makes you feel happy" or "You don't like it when I move the cars." A note of caution. Because neurodivergent children can experience and express emotion differently from neurotypical presentations, the therapist will want to be careful about interpreting a feeling they see from the child. Unless the therapist feels absolutely sure they are interpreting a feeling correctly, they may want to reflect something more general such as, "It looks like something is happening with you," "Something is happening," "I'm noticing something," "I'm noticing you and what is going on," or "You can't get the lid off and you might be feeling something."

Tracking statements are simply tracking what the child is doing. An example would be if the child is scooping up sand and putting it into a bucket, the parent might say "You are putting the sand in the bucket," or "You are doing what you want with the sand." Another example would be if the child paints a picture and holds it up to show the parent, the parent might say "You finished the whole painting," or "You finished that and now you are showing me." Additional examples include "You are finished with the sand tray, and now you are playing with the doll," or "You are hammering that really hard."

Asking Questions Skill – The parent periodically will ask the child a question. The questions are designed to communicate to the child that the parent is present, to begin developing social navigation, and to help the parent assess for engagement improvement. The questions asked should be in the moment and related to what is happening in the play time. An example would be the child painting blue on a piece of paper and the parent asking, "Do you like the color blue?" Another example would be the child is building with LEGO bricks and the therapist asks, "What do you think you will build?" Additional examples include "Is that interesting," "Do you like to play with blocks," or "What color is that?" It is likely that many questions will not garner a response from the child. Many children may not even acknowledge they have been asked a question. The parent is asking questions to identify when a child begins to answer questions and how well and often a child answers questions. When a child begins to answer questions regularly and fully, it is an indication the child is attuning more with the parent and is moving toward being able to do connection games or directive techniques.

Engage with the Child Skill – Throughout an FMA play time, the parent is periodically trying to engage with the child in whatever the child is doing (the child's play). Remember that the child leads and chooses whatever the child wants to play with, and the parent follows the child and tries to get involved with what the child is doing. The parent should make attempts throughout the play time. How many attempts, in what ways, and at what time is left to the parent's discretion. The parent does not need to be constantly trying to engage. If the child responds and engages with the parent, the parent should continue with whatever is being done until the child is no longer interested. If the child begins to show irritation or dysregulation with the attempts the parent is making to engage, then the parent should stop trying to engage and move away from the child and simply make some tracking and reflecting statements for a period of time and then return to trying to engage with the child. The following examples of engaging with the child can be shared with parents:

- The child starts playing with the play dishes. The parent sits beside the child and takes a bowl and puts it on the parent's head and says to the child, "Look at my silly bowl hat." The parent is trying to engage the child by having the child look at the parent and notice the bowl on the parent's head. The parent might take a bowl or plate and put it on the child's head and say, "Look at the plate on your head." The parent might ask the child to put a bowl or plate on the parent's head and see if they can begin to engage in this activity back and forth.

- The child starts playing with the sandtray building a sandcastle. The parent moves beside the child and starts adding sand to the castle or asks the child where to put the sand. The parent might try pushing sand to the child to use for their castle. The parent might also try building their own castle in a separate area in the sand tray.

- The child is shooting a basketball into the basketball hoop. The parent moves beside the child and helps get the ball and hand it back to the child after they shoot a basket. The parent might also try getting another basketball and also shooting the ball in the basket. The parent could try getting the child to take turns shooting the basketball or allow the parent to pass the basketball to the child and then the child shoots it.

Being Mindful of Limits Skill – The parent should be sensitive to the child's comfort, feelings of safety, and regulation level. Some play times may be mostly tracking and reflecting statements if the child is displaying discomfort with the parent's attempts to engage. The parent should not engage or try to get involved with what the child is doing to the point where the child becomes fully dysregulated and has a meltdown. An example would be the child starts to play with rolling some cars around on the floor. The parent sits down beside the child and starts rolling some cars with the child. The child grabs the cars from the parent and pushes the parent away. This is a clear sign the child does not feel comfortable with what the parent is doing, or the child may be becoming dysregulated. The parent should move away from the child and observe the child while periodically making some tracking and reflecting statements and try to engage with the child again when the parent feels it would be appropriate.

Additional elements that the therapist will want to cover with parents include how to start and end the play times, what to do when the child invites you into the play, and how to manage when both parents or additional family members participate.

Starting and Ending the Play Times – The parent begins by introducing the child to the play space. The parent explains to the child that, "This is our special play space, and you can do whatever you like in here, and I will be in here with you." The parent gives a five-minute verbal and visual warning that the play session is almost over and again at the one-minute mark. The verbal statement can be "We have five minutes left of our special play time and then it will be over for today," and again at the one minute, "We have one minute left of our special play time today and then it will be over." The visual can be as simple as the parent holding up their hand with five fingers and then one finger as they are giving the verbal warnings. When the session is over, the parent states, "Our time is up for today." If the parent is having difficulty with the child ending the play time, they should repeat the ending statement and give the child some time to process. If the child refuses to end the play time, the parent can try implementing a transition item. This would be a small or simple item the child gets at the end of the session, a treat such as going to the kitchen with the parent and getting a snack, or a special game that is played as they transition out of the special play time.

When the Child Invites the Parent into their Play – Children may more readily involve their parents in their play. If the child invites the parent into the play, the parent should accept the invitation and join in the play. The parent will need to remember that they do not take over the play or start leading the play. The parent should think of themselves as the actor and the child is the director. The parent stays in the role the child gives them and changes only when the child changes it.

Setting Limits – The limit setting approach in the FMA is fairly simple. Many of the children that will be participating in the FMA may not understand limit setting models that are too verbal or too cognitive and they may need a more basic redirection. For most limit setting needs, the parent should simply redirect the child or remove the limit causing toy or material. If the therapist feels it would be helpful, they can teach the parent the Child Centered Play Therapy ACT limit setting model. This may work for some children, but for others it will likely involve too much language and cognitive processing. The Act limit setting model was outlined by Landreth (2001). (A) Acknowledge the child's wants/needs (C) Communicate the limit in a non-punitive way (T) Target acceptable alternatives. For example, (A) "Sarah, I know you want to paint on the wall." (C) "but in here we cannot do that." (T) "You can paint on the easel or on this paper." The parent decides what is a limit to set and limits should be set as little as possible. If the child did not respond to the limit, the ultimate action the parent would take is ending the session time. If parents are setting a lot of limits or struggling with limit-setting, the therapist should practice with the parent and/or observe a parent/child play time to discover and help with any issues that may be occurring.

In Home Follow Me Approach (FMA) Play Times

Before parents begin to conduct FMA play times at home with their child, there are some elements that need to be established. The therapist will typically have a session with the parents around session ten (before the in-home play times begin) to go over the following:

1 When and where will the play times happen? This includes how long and how often the play times will occur. Parents should be realistic about how many play times they believe they can do each week. A once a week play time is fine but if the parent wants to commit to more play times this is also acceptable. The primary consideration is not over-committing. The parent will want to try and stay consistent with whatever they plan to do. Typically, the play time would be 30 minutes. Some children may not be able to have a play time that lasts that long, and some parents may find that they go over this time. It is about what works best for the child. Some parents have discovered that they are most successful with a morning 15-minute play time and another 15-minute play time in the evening. The parent should think about what day(s) and where in the home the play times will occur. This can be adjusted as special play times begin to be implemented at home.

2 How will the play space be set up? There are many options available to the parent and it will likely be established by what works best for the child. It is often recommended that the parent collect some toys and materials they believe the child would enjoy and keep those items put away and bring them out for the FMA special play time. It is also recommended for the parent to think about a space or room in the home to have the FMA play times. Inevitably, things can deviate from these recommendations. Parents sometime find the play time is a roaming throughout the house play time or an outdoor play time, etc. The space and materials used are not as important as the parent being able to implement the FMA skills. The skills are versatile so many parents find it easy to follow the lead of the child with their play preferences and still be able to implement the skills.

3 Will in-home play times look the same as in office sessions? The home setting may bring more challenges than the office setting. The therapist should explain this to parents and be prepared for parent questions. The therapist will want to help parents find a way to work through any home challenges and be successful with their special play times. Typically, the home play times will not look as structured or flow as smoothly as office

sessions. This is okay, and the therapist should prepare parents for potential differences.

4 Do parents have to be perfect? It is important to communicate to parents that they do not have to be 100% effective in their home play times. It will take some time and practice for parents to feel confident in understanding how to implement the FMA and get into a comfortable rhythm. Parents may miss a planned FMA play time, this is okay, and they should get back on track as soon as they can. Parents are not becoming therapists. They do not have to know everything or do things like the therapist. The therapist should ensure the parent is producing an acceptable level of FMA skill and provide encouraging feedback to the parents.

5 Can both parents participate? Both parents can be involved in the FMA and having play times at home with their child. It is recommended that each parent has separate play times with their child. Children may become overwhelmed from multiple people trying to engage with them or even multiple people in the room making tracking statements. Parents may also talk over each other or get into each other's way. Parents should have separate play times; this creates a better experience for the child and benefits the parents as one parent does not become overwhelmed with being responsible for trying to implement all the play times.

6 Can other family members participate? Other family members can be involved in implementing the FMA. It is best if the therapist can meet with the family member who is going to be involved and having a FMA play time with the child and make sure that family member understands how to implement the approach. There are some important benefits to involving other family members. First, it provides support to the parent. Parents of neurodivergent children are usually doing a lot and having other family members be able to support with some of the tasks is extremely helpful to parents. Second, it helps generalize the child's connecting and relationship skills. The child can benefit from working with multiple people, not just one person. Before other family members participate, the therapist should ensure they are appropriate to work with the child, understand the FMA skills, and are someone who does not trigger the child.

7 Can the in-home play times lead to other things? Many parents discover, as they begin the FMA special play times, that they start to generalize new ways of engaging and interacting with their child throughout the entire day. This generalization is not unusual as parents tend to find a new way of interacting with and understanding their child and discover

an improvement in relationship development with their child. Also, parents often find that other issues or therapy goals begin to dissipate and correct as the progress through the FMA play times.

8 What happens if the in-home play times are not going well? Sometimes parents will share issues or problems happening with the in-home play times. If needed, the therapist can ask the parent to record the special play time and bring in the recording to watch or ask the parent to conduct the FMA play time with their child in session while the therapist observes. The therapist will want to try and discover what is happening and help the family correct the situation.

9 Are the in-home play times that same as other play times? The in-home FMA play times are therapeutic play times. They are different from regular play times the parent may be having with their child. The parent can continue to have their typical play times while they are implementing the FMA play times. The design of the FMA play times will help the child understand the difference.

10 What happens when the special play times are over? The FMA play times are designed to end at some point because they are a therapeutic process. As the FMA play times are ending, the therapist should help the parent generalize and transition their FMA play time to other time spent with the child. The parent should switch to a less formal play time but continue to have regular play times with their child which should provide some child- led processes. As the goals are accomplished and the special play times are drawing to an end, the children are usually ready to move from the structure of the FMA special play times to a less formal play time with their parent.

Goals for Parents

There are some standard goals which apply to parents participating in the FMA. Goals can be shared with parents and include:

- Strengthen the parent–child relationship.
- Increase and or develop play times and the level of playfulness and enjoyment in the parent–child relationship and help them recognize the importance of play.
- Help parents understand and value their child's play preferences.
- Increase parents understanding of neurodivergence and their neurodivergent child.

- Decrease parent's feelings of frustration with their children.
- Help parents understand their child's regulation and communication system and develop appropriate parenting practices.
- Increase parent's confidence in their ability to parent and advocate for their child.
- Increase parent's feelings of warmth and care toward their children.
- Address presenting therapy needs and goals.

Providing Continuous Support to Parents

The majority of parents are fully capable of learning the FMA skills and implementing the FMA play times with their children at home. Many parents may lack confidence, feel insecure, or worry they are not doing something correct. The AutPlay therapist will want to provide consistent support to parents, encouraging them in their parenting process, and as a co-change agent in working with their children. The AutPlay therapist will also want to respect the parent as an expert on themselves and their child and value their voice in the therapy process. Some potential issues that may arise include parents feeling inadequate to implement the play times at home without the therapist's presence, handling issues that come up at home during the play times, being hesitant to participate in therapy, struggling with their own fears and questions about parenting their child, and being overwhelmed. At the end of the FMA process, an empowered, educated, and confident parent is a great success.

References

Autistic Self Advocacy Network. (2021). *Start here: A guide for parents of autistic kids*. The Autistic Press.

Booth, P. B., & Jernberg, A. M. (2010). *Theraplay*. Jossey-Bass.

Gil, E. (2015). *Play in family therapy* (2nd ed.). Guilford Press.

Jeffreys, R. (2021). *You were made for this*. Empowerment Publishing.

Landreth, G. L. (2001). *Innovations in play therapy: Issues, process, and special populations*. Routledge.

Landreth, G. L., & Bratton, S. (2020). *Child-parent relationship therapy (CPRT): An evidence based 10-session filial therapy model* (2nd ed.). Routledge.

Macdonald, J., & Stoika, P. (2007). *Play to talk: A practical guide to help your late-talking child join the conversation*. Kiddo Publishing.

Stinnett, N., & DeFrain, J. (1985). *Secrets of strong families*. Berkley Books.

Trotter, K. (2013). Family play therapy. In N. R. Bowers (Ed.), *Play therapy with families*. Jason Aronson.

VanFleet, R. (1994). *Filial therapy: Strengthening the parent-child relationships through play*. Professional Resource Press.

VanFleet, R. (2014). *Filial therapy: Strengthening the parent-child relationships through play* (3rd ed.). Professional Resource Press.

13

The AutPlay® Therapy Follow Me Approach (FMA) Case Examples

Case Example "Mallory" by Robert Jason Grant

Mallory was 3-years old when she first entered the playroom with her biological mother and father. Mallory had been diagnosed with autism spectrum disorder six months earlier through testing and evaluation conducted by a psychologist. She was described as having limited verbal output (communication), sensory needs, and dysregulation struggles. At the time Mallory began play therapy, she was participating in speech therapy, occupational therapy, and on a waiting list for intensive in-home therapy. Mallory's parents sought play therapy to improve their relationship with Mallory and help Mallory improve regulation ability, gain social and play interaction with peers, and feel comfortable participating in group play with others.

Mallory lived with her biological mother and father. Mallory had one younger brother and was involved with other family members, specifically her paternal grandparents. Mallory's parents reported they had positive family and community support in place and were active in various support groups. Mallory was participating in several therapies throughout each week but was not involved in any extracurricular or play/social activities.

The first three play therapy sessions were designed to help Mallory build rapport and become more comfortable with me and being in the playroom. Following the AutPlay Therapy Intake and Assessment Phase protocol, the first three sessions were also used to further assess Mallory's strengths and therapy needs. I conducted a child observation session with Mallory and a parent/child play observation session with Mallory and both her parents. Mallory's parents also completed four inventories: the AutPlay Emotional Regulation Inventory, AutPlay Social Navigation Inventory, AutPlay Connection Inventory, and AutPlay Assessment of Play Inventory. Mallory was observed in a playroom. She presented around 75% nonverbal and did not appear to

DOI: 10.4324/9781003207610-14

have any obvious communication preference. She would periodically speak words, but they were not comprehensible. She would occasionally say a word that was understandable, and it seemed to be used in appropriate context and she would occasionally give an appropriate one-word response to a question. Most of the time, Mallory would not respond to my presence in the playroom; she would not respond to any verbal prompting; and she seemed to not pay attention to me or my efforts at engagement. Mallory played primary with one toy (the dollhouse) repeatedly and performed the same action with a person miniature entering and exiting the dollhouse door repetitively. At the end of the assessment period, the AutPlay Follow Me Approach (FMA) was identified as the therapy approach. This approach was used due to Mallory's age and her lack of interaction and engagement ability. Both Mallory and her parents would participate in therapy with the goal of teaching the FMA to Mallory's parents to implement in the home setting. Goals for therapy included increasing play interaction between Mallory and her parents, increasing engagement (relationship development) with another person, and decreasing regulation struggles. Further, it was discussed that the FMA would help Mallory gain the presence to be able to participate in more structured play therapy interventions – interventions that would require a greater level of attunement and engagement than she was currently displaying.

During the fourth session, I provided Mallory's parents an outline to review the FMA and described the process to them. At the fifth session, I conducted an FMA session with Mallory as her parents observed from the corner of the playroom. The purpose of the session was to further develop relationship with Mallory and demonstrate a FMA play session to her parents to help them begin to learn how to conduct play sessions at home. The play session lasted about 20 minutes. I demonstrated tracking and reflecting skills, letting Mallory lead the play and following her as she transitioned from toy to toy and making attempts to try and engage with her in her play preferences. Mallory seemed to be comfortable with my presence and attempts to engage her. It is important to note that about 90% of engagement attempts were not acknowledged by Mallory. She did seem to notice me during play time with a toy car and answered a question that I asked. This was the only overt engagement piece that occurred during the play session. At the end of the 20 minutes, I reviewed the play time with Mallory's parents and answered any questions they had about what they had observed. They were most curious about how often to try and engage Mallory and in what ways. I discussed the engagement attempts that I made and gave examples of other options that could have been attempted. Mallory's parents were instructed to review the written FMA skills they had been given and during our sixth session they would observe me demonstrating another FMA play time and have the opportunity to ask questions and clarify the process.

During the sixth session, Mallory's parents observed me conducting a play session with Mallory that lasted approximately 25 minutes. After the play session demonstration, I processed the session with Mallory's parents and discussed any questions or observations they had. The session time progressed similarly to session five, except that Mallory seemed more interested in exploring the playroom and she played with a greater variety of toys. She also seemed to be making more attempts to communicate with me verbally although much of what she was saying could not be understand. Mallory's parents were again instructed to review the written outline they were given describing the FMA skills and think about the observation they had watched. In the next session, they would have the opportunity to practice the FMA approach.

During session seven, each parent felt comfortable to try facilitating an FMA play time with Malory. Mom went first and Dad went second and each FMA play time lasted approximately 15 minutes. Both parents seemed to understand the approach and successfully implemented the skills throughout the session. Mallory's parents were instructed to practice the FMA at home with each other in a role-playing scenario, and during the next session, the therapist would again observe each of them having a FMA play time with Mallory.

The next session began with Dad having a FMA play time with Mallory while Mom and I observed from the corner of the playroom. Dad's session lasted approximately 15 minutes and then Dad and Mom switched places with Mom having a 15 minute play time with Mallory and Dad observing. After Mom's play time, I processed through the experience with the parents and discussed some observations giving them mostly positive feedback and a couple of things to work on for the next play time. Overall, both parents were efficient and seemed to have a solid grasp on how to have an FMA play time. Mallory's parents were very good at playing with her and seemed to have a natural instinct about children's play. They were instructed to begin having FMA special play times at home with Mallory. It was established that they would try to have a 20-minute play time four times before the next session. Mom and Dad could have separate play times so each of them would plan on having two play times before the next session. I also discussed logistical issues of where the play times would be at home, what toys they would use, and when they would try to have the play times.

During the next session, Dad was unable to attend, so I gathered from Mom an update on how things went with the play times at home. They had each conducted two play times with Mallory and they went well. I then observed Mom having a FMA play time with Mallory. Their play time lasted approximately 25 minutes. The remainder of the session was used to process the session with mom and go over details for continuing play times at home. In this session with mom and Mallory, there was a marked change in Mallory navigating around the playroom and playing with a greater variety of toys than previous sessions. She also made several verbal comments to her mom and invited her mom into play and engaged in some play with her mom. I encouraged mom to make more reflective statements as there were several times Mallory displayed emotions. I also encouraged her to continue to look for opportunities to try and engage Mallory in her play time as this seemed to be improving each play time. Overall, the play session and home implementation were a success.

The next session began with a check-in with both mom and dad on how the play times had gone at home. Things seemed to be progressing well and they did not have any questions. After the check-in, each parent conducted a play time with Mallory for about ten minutes while the other parent and I observed. These two play times seemed to be the most positive and productive to date. Both parents executed the protocol, and Mallory responded well to her parents. Mallory continued to display more verbal interaction, and her parents attempted to engage with Mallory in her play several times – the majority of those times Mallory reciprocated back. This reciprocal engagement was the most I had seen from Mallory to date. Mallory's parents noticed the advancements and seemed pleased with how the FMA play times were going. They were noticing an improvement in Mallory's reciprocating play with them, overall engagement, and overall increases in Mallory seeming more regulated. They expressed that the play times at home had been successful.

Sessions 10–20 continued with Mallory's parents having four to five FMA play times at home between sessions and processing the home play times during weekly session with me. During the weekly session with me. I would conduct an FMA play time with Mallory while the parents observed. Mallory continued to progress in becoming more engaging during her play times. Her parents reported each session improvement in engaging with them, acknowledging and attuning to them, some increase in verbal statements, and that overall, she seemed more regulated. Mallory's parents also reported they were now having additional play times with her that felt more natural and enjoyable. Around session 16, it was discussed to introduce more structured group games with Mallory. Her parents introduced games to play during their special play times such as hitting a balloon back and forth or blowing and popping bubbles. The games were simple connection/participation games.

Mallory responded to the introduction of the games well and participated with her parents. Around session 17, Mallory's parents began to involve the grandparents in the FMA play times and teach them how to have the play times with Mallory.

By session 20, Mallory was having play times once a week with her grandparents. She was also having play times with her parents and actively engaging with them in games that they were introducing to her that required her to attune to them and follow instructions such as "Ring Around the Rosie" and "Duck Duck Goose." During session 21, original therapy goals were re-evaluated and identified as accomplished. New therapy goals were established for Mallory and her family that involved integrating more structured play interventions. By session 21, Mallory had made great progress toward relationship development and engagement goals. She was also more verbal and interactive, seeming more comfortable being around and attending to others. She had also made improvement in being less dysregulated and was able to participate in more directive play therapy approaches that focused on specific interventions where this was not possible for her at the beginning of therapy.

Case Example "Alex" by Elaine Hutchinson

Alex was referred for therapy when he was 7.5 years old. He lived at home with both of his parents and his younger sister. His mother referred him because she wanted additional support for him to develop his emotional literacy. Prior to the referral, Alex was assessed for autism and ADHD, but his mother was told he "Didn't quite tick enough boxes" to meet the threshold for either diagnosis. The school's Education and Health Care Plan (EHCP) application was made before therapy started but was not finalized and additional provisions not provided at the time therapy began. His mother felt the school was not adequately meeting his needs, which had a significant impact on his education in relation to peer interactions and his ability to access the curriculum.

There was a family history of autism on both his mother's and his father's side. Alex's mother had an older brother and a father with an autism diagnosis, so she had an in-depth, personal understanding of neurodivergence. While wanting to support Alex in his uniqueness, she also felt he needed additional life and social understandings. According to his mother, Alex was a sensory seeker. He would easily get emotionally flooded, leading to regular "massive meltdowns" that often occurred several times a week at school and home.

Noise was a key trigger for him, so the noisy classroom and after school care environments didn't help him cope well at school. School also appeared to have trouble supporting him positively when he became dysregulated. The restrictions due to the Covid-19 pandemic have had significant implications for Alex in managing his school environment effectively, and his 1:1 support had been removed, leaving him without a supportive and familiar key adult.

Alex's mother and I completed the intake paperwork after an initial telephone conversation. She prepared Alex for coming to see me by using the video tours on my website to help familiarize him with the setup. We also had a "hello" call over Zoom so he could meet me without a mask. We shared an informal introductory session before starting face-to-face therapy so that Alex had an opportunity to come and meet both me and my therapy dog (Orca) and spend some time becoming familiar with my room.

The AutPlay Therapy Intake and Assessment Phase was completed along with the assessment and inventory paperwork. In completing the initial intake assessment, Alex's mother noted that he struggles with varied play, any change to his routine, stereotyped and repetitive mannerisms and abnormal functioning regarding his empathy for others. The initial assessment of play showed that Alex chooses to play mostly using sociodramatic play with some rare functional and representational play. Alex's mother noted that play at home is primarily sociodramatic. Alex and his sister like to reenact scenarios from TV programs. However, a large part of Alex's play is concerned with directing his sister, organizing the setup, and establishing the ground rules rather than interacting in play.

The initial social navigation inventory indicated that Alex's mother felt that most of Alex's social navigation involved struggles, with most of her scores listed as 2 or 3. Those indicated at a 4 or 5 were all linguistics-based skills. The initial emotional regulation inventory showed that Alex's mother felt that he struggles to verbalize or express emotion and understand emotion in others. At home, Alex tended to demonstrate "big emotions" that are hard to handle, including shouting, hitting, biting, and running away, even though both parents stated they and his sister correctly model emotions. The initial connection inventory revealed that relationships were challenging for Alex, with most connect components getting scored at a 2 or 3. Alex's mother stated that he has little awareness of personal space and when he would hug others, he can hug hard to the point of pain in the other person and then not release the hug when asked.

In completing the initial unwanted behaviors assessment, Alex's mother noted that he has sensory issues around oral behaviors (licking inappropriate things, biting people); an apparently high pain threshold, "he doesn't seem to feel pain often;" both a need for and overstimulation by loud noise and a need for heavy contact – bashing into people, leaning hard against them, and hugging overtly hard. When Alex would become overloaded, flooded, or experience a meltdown, Alex's unwanted behaviors included becoming uncontrollable, throwing, pushing, hitting, and biting. If he feels he is being disciplined, then his behaviors become even more extreme, with Alex appearing "manic" for up to 24 hours after the event. At school, he bashes into children on the playground, making peer friendships hard and, if triggered, will run off so adults cannot help address him. Alex's mother stated he will not listen to instructions, including those linked to his safety. He can be a danger to both himself and others. He is regularly threatened with exclusions at school with little effect.

During the child/parent play observation, Alex's mother demonstrated clear boundaries for her son and a warm, loving, and nurturing approach toward him. When playing together, she connected with him verbally and physically, often putting her arm around him if he came and leaned against her or dropping a kiss on the top of his head. Both these actions made him smile or say something positive to her in return. As they played, she recalled other times they have enjoyed playing together. She seemed to facilitate his success, would whisper cues to him when he was off task, giggled with him, noticed him and was curious about his play. She seemed to delight in his knowledge and competence, and clearly enjoyed sharing dialogue and questions with him and complemented him appropriately without going over the top, which again, he seemed to delight in.

At the end of the intake and assessment phase, it was agreed by Alex's mother and myself that Alex would begin with a series of sessions that were nondirective and using the FMA. The therapy goals would include increased social navigation needs-reciprocal play. After this, the second phase of more structured therapy would begin with therapy goals that would consist of Alex gaining in emotion identification and regulation awareness and his ability to feel more fulfilled in his connections with others.

A Goodman's SDQ (strengths and difficulties questionnaire) was completed at intake by Alex's mother, a common UK practice for play therapy and some NHS mental health screening. The SDQ scores showed Alex had significant issues with hyperactivity, conduct, and peer relationships, scoring 24 out of 30 possible difficulties and correlating to the AutPlay intake paperwork findings. However, what is interesting is that Alex failed to score for any prosocial behaviors on the SDQ but that some were evident and noted on the

AutPlay intake paperwork and seen during observations. One of the things I reflected on as a therapist is how I gather information on clients during the intake phase. Now I ask a lot of AutPlay based questions at intake for all clients, which benefits my understanding of them.

Alex initially presented in FMA sessions as a controlled but chaotic player. As is often the case with a child in the early stages of therapy, there was a great deal of room familiarization in the early sessions as he went through multiple activities in a short space of time. Throughout therapy, Alex was delighted when Orca met him at the door at the start of sessions. He spent a few minutes grounding himself and managing the transition by engaging with her, either by fussing her, giving her a treat, or throwing her ball. He would then transition to other play preferences. He did not seek her out in the main part of therapy sessions but would engage with her if she came to him.

At the end of each session, part of Alex's ending ritual was to acknowledge Orca and wish her a good week. He liked dogs, but he did not have one at home. Session endings were particularly hard for him, even with plenty of notice, time remaining warnings, and an ending count down. I had to be consistent with him about ending every time, but in some sessions, he found it much harder than others, possibly in reaction to days at school that had not been so positive.

From his first FMA session Alex was drawn to small world play, using figures on the table or the floor or create a "team" for him and for the adult who was playing with him. Often, he would not designate any team to the adult at all. Instead, he would instruct both his mother and me about the complexities of every team member. The briefing would include each character's role, strengths, and weaknesses, how they interacted with their team, and their role in challenging the other team. This detailed briefing would often go on for the entire session with no genuine desire to play it out, just to clarify and instruct. Sometimes Alex would give a demonstration between two character's combat so that the adults could see "how to do it properly," but there was no desire for reciprocal play on his part. The play was always socio-dramatic, with Alex re-enacting combat from TV series like Pokémon, Yu Gi Oh, and Power Rangers, which were his only real viewing interests.

Early on, sometimes the teams would battle it out on the table, the floor, or in the sand tray. However, regardless of location, the same formulaic socio-dramatic play was always used. Occasionally when Alex's concentration wavered, he would deviate to enclosure schema-based play, investigating lockable houses, jail cells, and treasure chests that I have in my room.

Over the course of a session, 80–100% of the session time would be team/combat based. Whenever the adult made reflections, they would be ignored. Often the use of his name would bring no response either. If Alex's attention was needed, it required physical touch and an "Alex, please give me your attention" type comment from either adult to get his attention. Alex would then break from his imaginary world and commentary, but he would then briefly make eye contact and acknowledge the adult before going back into his play.

In session five of the FMA, Alex made an interesting change to his setup. Everything on both teams had to be precisely matched in terms of relative size and placement of characters and symbols. This placement and organization would link to a Pokémon battle setup or using a Yu Gi Oh card deck, both of which were familiar to Alex. A fascinating development was that he could break from his setup dialogue to discuss it when I reflected on the need for symmetry. Another intriguing aspect of this was that once he had set it up, where it had to be "perfect," it was OK for someone else to move around characters or symbols on their side, and he felt OK with that. If his team came out of their planned alignment, it made him feel "yukky" in his body. Alex's comment would suggest a sensory whole-body response to his need for symmetry and order in that instance, but not necessarily an OCD based response, as it is the only occurrence of a need for symmetry that his mother can recall.

Something was definitely going on for him in this session because he lost the slight sense of personal distance he had retained until that point and was leaning hard against me as he was explaining the setup and needing to be up super-close to talk to me. Later, when Alex's mother and I reflected on the session together, we felt there had been a positive shift in Alex's process relating to his comfort level. Alex's mother could also think of no reason why Alex's need for symmetry had been triggered in that session, but we both acknowledged that didn't mean there hadn't been something he was responding to in the session. It is worth noting that symmetry is not essential at home for him, either before or after that session. It did not emerge again in therapy sessions, and Alex attended over 20 more sessions.

It was definitely a pivotal moment for Alex in his therapeutic process. For the subsequent eight sessions, his play and process completely shifted. He changed to playing board games in most sessions, with some very occasional painting and puppet work. Again, the setup and the rules were more important to him, perhaps reflecting his need for control and mastery still, but just in another skill set. However, he was capable and willing to engage in reciprocal play, turn-taking, engaging, and game-related conversations. Alex's change of activities in sessions could have aligned with changes to UK lockdown restrictions and rules at school. Perhaps the playroom changes reflected changes in his wider world, with his need for control reflecting the uncertainty of the new lockdown restrictions outside of the playroom environment he controlled.

Chess became important to Alex at this point, potentially echoing his need for rules and control in other areas of his life. When we played, he coped exceptionally well with losing pawns early in the game and other critical pieces as we played without any hint of frustration or annoyance. Outside of the playroom, he struggled at this stage with hyperactivity and following rules in school. However, Alex's behavior in the playroom did not reflect this.

At session 14, Alex looped back around in his play to the team-based small world play. This looped revisiting process showed a more mature approach to his play that was now far more independent and less reliant on the adult. Previously the teams had been based exclusively on fantasy figures and natural symbols. They now occasionally morphed into battle play with soldiers and tanks, but Alex's play was still fantasy-based for most sessions. The need for two teams has receded with often only one team being set up, sometimes, but not exclusively, enclosed in the safe confines of an armchair. The chair was situated next to my fantasy figures, so it could merely be a coincidence and a handy spot to play, but it is worth noting Alex didn't previously use it.

Following the change in his process for board games, Alex was much more likely to respond to reflections. However, he would only respond if he considered the reflections or comments worth answering. Alex's selective answering could be funny as he would pretend to ignore anything that he thought was not worthy of comment. He would acknowledge me more readily in conversation, right from greeting me at the door. He would now share jokes with me appropriately and laugh at me when I make a joke in return. Orca chasing her tail had him in fits of laughter, whereas previously, he looked bemused. Overall, Alex just felt lighter in himself and more assured in the playroom.

Sessions paused for the Easter holiday at session 18. Alex's mother and I agreed to use the break as a chance to move into the structured phase of AutPlay. We spent several sessions before the holiday discussing the change with Alex and showing him the sort of activities we would be working on together. Currently sessions are organized with set activities and games for the first half of the session. Once these are completed, the remainder of the session is FMA, as he still clearly needs a self-directed element to therapy.

Alex's mother has reported that he is much calmer at home, with meltdowns now a rare event in response to a specific trigger rather than a way of communicating a need. School is still a source of recurrent outbursts for Alex, with no real improvements there, mainly because he still is not getting the support he needs. However, Alex's mother is feeling more empowered by the therapy process. She thinks that she has a better understanding of Alex and his needs. Consequently, she feels able to be more assertive about requiring Alex's needs to be met in school and that she can ask for support and equipment from a place of authority and understanding.

It is clear that Alex still has some therapy goals to achieve. It is anticipated that he will graduate therapy within a year, probably after he has used sessions to support him to settle into a new school year with a new teacher.

Case Example "Melody" by Jen Taylor

Melody began Autplay Therapy services at age 5, a few weeks after she was diagnosed with autism spectrum disorder by a local psychiatrist. When Melody and her mother arrived at the office, the mother was carrying the child who was actively attempting to escape from the mother's arms. The mother reported that Melody was often extremely aggressive toward her, often hitting her or slapping her when she was frustrated. At other times, Melody was overly clingy and often refused to attend Kindergarten. The mother had to physically carry the child to the classroom and remain there for 30 minutes or more because Melody had such a difficult time transitioning from the car to the classroom. During class, Melody was struggling academically, isolating herself from other children and often refusing to participate in any activities.

Melody refused to communicate with this therapist during the initial interview. She spoke in a very low whisper during the few instances where she spoke at all. She would not answer questions directly and often whispered answers into the mother's ear instead of answering out loud. Melody would frequently hide behind the mother's back or bury her face into the mother's shoulder or lap. She was not interested in visiting the playroom and would not go anywhere in the office without holding onto the mother's leg or clothing.

Melody's mother did not have a positive experience with the psychiatrist and was resistant to any medication recommendations. She felt that Melody was "too little" and was worried that medications would result in potential side effects. She was using homeopathic vitamins but was not noticing a change in behaviors and wanted to explore other therapy interventions. During the completion of the initial AutPlay screening assessments, she was honest and forthcoming but very anxious about the use of the term "autism spectrum disorder" or any variation of those terms. She provided history of her own childhood where she had similar (although not as excessive) struggles and was able to learn how to manage those symptoms as she got older. Through the intake and assessment process, a history of delayed speech and toilet training and social/emotional needs were reported. In play observations, Melody seemed to have areas of concern in communicating wants/needs, parent and child interactions, dysregulation, and shyness/anxiety in social settings, lack of awareness of danger, and continued toileting issues, general anxiety, and difficulty with transitions.

Therapy began using the FMA due to the child's separation anxiety and refusal to participate in any play therapy without the mother in the room. In addition, the intensity of behaviors and the mother's own anxiety about the child's diagnosis created a strain in the parent–child relationship that could be addressed using this intervention. The next two sessions consisted of the therapist, mother, and child spending the entire session in the playroom and allowing the child to choose activities. The therapist gently reflected on the child's closeness to the mother at the beginning of the session and allowed for the child to take as much time as necessary in choosing any play materials. The focus of the sessions was on building a therapeutic rapport and reducing conflicts and power struggles with the child.

The next six sessions were spent allowing the mother time to practice the FMA in the office playroom under the supervision of this therapist. The mother initially struggled with allowing the child time to choose and frequently offered suggestions or encouraged specific play. Over time and with additional practice at home, the mother became more competent in accepting the child as she was and felt more comfortable allowing the child to choose what toys to play with and in what manner during these practice sessions. During this time, the therapist noticed that the child enjoyed racing cars across the table. The therapist and the mother were able to copy these play behaviors and encourage joint attention and shared play with Melody. Melody liked to push the cars off the table or watch them crash into each other. The therapist began introducing emotional regulation by identifying the feelings expressed during these races and by engaging the child in contests to see who could get closest to the edge of the table without going over the edge.

During future sessions, the therapist was able to use these cars in the waiting room to "race" to the door of the playroom. The child would often crash them into the walls and laugh or push them so they went very far past the entryway. However, throughout this practice, the child became less anxious about separating from the mother and more capable of entering the playroom independently. The degree to which the child was able to stop the car in front of the playroom doorway improved over time and appeared to be indicative of the ease with which the child was able to separate from the mother. At home, the mother and child practiced various emotional regulation games including Red Light, Green Light, Simon Says, and playing a card game known as Slapjack. The child's ability to name her emotions improved. In addition, she was able to control impulses better and was becoming less aggressive toward the mother.

Despite this success in the therapy setting regarding the separation anxiety and communication issues, the child was still struggling with transitions outside of the therapy session. She refused to walk to her classroom and would get extremely distressed if there was any change in the routine throughout the day. During the next session, the therapist worked with the child using the AutPlay intervention *Same Plan, New Plan*. In the session, the child decorated two signs made from popsicle sticks, paper, and arts and crafts materials. One sign had an "S" indicating "same plan" and one sign had an "N" to indicate a new plan or change in expected plans. The child and therapist used play to rehearse activities using the signs as a way to provide a visual cue to the other about what was going to happen next. This set of cards remained at the office and the mother and child made additional sets for home and for the car.

Upon arrival at the office for subsequent visits, the therapist would ensure that the cars from previous visits were available in the waiting room and hold the cards "S" and "N" when the child arrived. The child would indicate "S" if she wanted to race the cars as usual or "N" if she had a new idea for how to get to the playroom. She would practice coming up with her own new plans during the session and would sometimes walk in slow motion, hop, or bear crawl to the office instead of racing cars. Inside sessions, the therapist would interrupt the FMA by using the "N" new plan card to introduce a directive play intervention addressing emotional regulation or social needs. Melody was observed to be able to transition from non-directive to directive activities more readily using this technique. The mother practiced at home as well and found that it was effective in helping the child transition to and from the car on school days. The resistance toward entering the classroom had subsided and the child was walking, hopping, or skipping to class on most days.

Melody continued to participate in Autplay Therapy for nearly one year. She and her mother implemented the play interventions at home during structured practice for 20–25 minutes per day. The mother's own anxiety about her ability to manage the child's behaviors was significantly improved. She reported having more joyful interactions with her daughter and fewer power struggles. Melody continued to improve over the course of one year until the family moved out of the area and discontinued therapy.

In working with Melody and her mother, it was important to model acceptance for the mother's own anxieties and perceived shortcomings. The normalization of the mother's fears and insecurities created a model for the mother to accept her daughter's neurodivergent strengths and needs with less judgment. The use of child-centered play using the FMA allowed the child to feel less rushed, more competent, and reduced the power struggles in the relationship. The child became more verbal and emotionally expressive, and the parent and child had fun together and often laughed and giggled together. The use of more directive AutPlay interventions were critical in helping the child outside of the playroom. This specific practice provided the child with coping skills to manage transitions successfully.

Case Example "Lottie" by Lily Wake

This case example is set in my private practice, in a small village in the Southwest of England where I am lucky to have a large fully equipped play therapy room. Mum initially approached me as she had heard I offered a model of support and therapy for neurodivergent children. An initial intake meeting was conducted with Mum, to explain the process of Autplay, and get some background information.

Session one was an intake meeting with Mum, who shared that Lottie was 3 years old, and at the time was pre-verbal, and had significant developmental delays. Lottie was with a foster family for the first ten weeks of her life who nurtured her through neonatal opioid withdrawal, before being adopted by a couple who, for the purpose of this case study, I refer to as Mum and Dad. In addition to Lottie, this year her biological parents had another baby, who Lottie's Mum and Dad also adopted. The baby sister was 5 months old at this stage and was neurotypically developing, responsive, and engaging, although she was also born with neonatal abstinence syndrome – Mum and Dad have three children of their own, one has grown up and left home. However a teenage son and daughter live at home.

Mum shared that Lottie had autistic presentations of repetitive/indiscriminate patterns of play and narrow focused interests, little social communication ability, and poor emotional regulation, although there was no formal diagnosis of autism. Lottie attended a specialist communication pre-school five mornings a week, where they worked in conjunction with a speech and language therapist (SLT) to start introducing Lottie to the first stages of the pictorial exchange communication system (PECS), within a total communication environment. Mum reported that Lottie was oblivious to the other children unless irritated by their sounds and the school was also working on social interactions.

One of the most problematic behaviors at home and preschool was seen to be Lottie's obsessive throwing of objects. Mum described this behavior as having started when she was very young, and it has caused many breakages and the house to be turned into a projectile-free space. Which is hard to maintain with six people living in a small four-bedroom British terrace house, particularly with a new baby in the home. Mum shared the pressure this put on normal family social experiences, as Lottie cannot discriminate between acceptable projectiles, and presents this behavior wherever they go.

Another challenge Mum presented was that Lottie has no sense of awareness of her surroundings or safety. Lottie would run at any given opportunity, without seeing any hazards. Lottie will hold a hand for short periods of time – from house to car – car to her preschool building – but would attempt to break free beyond that. For her safety, Lottie was restrained in a buggy when they went out and about, particularly with the new baby as Mum could not chase Lottie and manage the new baby.

Lottie's diet was described as being limited, preferring bland unthreatening familiar foods, not engaging with food out of these food groups. She was noise-sensitive, particularly to her baby sister, who she did not acknowledge was there, unless she made a noise. Mum also described a lack of response from Lottie to her name being called, or any initiated engagement that was not on her terms.

Noise was often a trigger for dysregulated behavior like throwing things, shouting, crying, screaming, and rarely, but occasionally hitting. Other triggers were when she was tired, overwhelmed, or in an unfamiliar environment, when she needed to sit still, change of routine, and if she was excited or frustrated. The frequency of these sensory and impaired semantic and pragmatic responses, and subsequent dysregulation, was continuous at different levels throughout the day. Lottie also appears to need very little sleep, averaging 5–7 hours a night.

The initial three sessions were child-led, and child and parent/child observations were conducted, using Autplay observation forms. Session four involved meeting with the parent. Observations, Autplay inventories, and information received at intake were assessed, and informed my clinical decision to work with Lottie and the family using the FMA. Her age of 3 years old and her assessed needs in emotional regulation, connection, social safety, and her inability to participate in any directive play techniques, making the FMA the most developmentally appropriate place to start. I began working with Lottie and Mum, implementing sessions on a weekly basis, for 40 minutes each.

The first time Lottie came to the playroom, I met her and Mum in the car park, to show them the way in. Lottie grabbed my hand and walked with me, with no discrimination or concern that I was a stranger. When we entered the playroom and I dropped to my knees in front of Lottie and introduced myself, using spoken word, sign, and gesture to tell her "Here you can play with anything, and I will be with you." She ran around on her tiptoes looked at everything for a few moments, before heading to the fruit and play food. I followed, and she picked items up and threw them on the ground. I put my hands out for her to pass them to me, but she ignored me and continued to throw them on the ground. Her attention was lost after around two minutes, and she ran on to explore the doll's house. I verbally tracked and noticed, as I moved myself alongside her again "Now you're exploring the doll's house." She opened and closed the door, and the front panel, exploring the hinge motion, I said "Open, and close," and we made eye contact for the first brief moment.

She soon ran on from the doll's house to the sand symbols which are all displayed on shelving. I had to limit-set very quickly. Directing her hand with the first symbol in it, naming it, and said "On the shelf" before she could throw it, and showed her how to put it back on the shelf. She soon moved on again. Next, she discovered the drums. I sat alongside her, matching her, a beat and tone lower than hers, and for the first time I had engagement. She clearly observed and noticed our musical connection and started giggling every time I mirrored her beat. This exchange continued for about three minutes, which was the longest her attention had been held on an activity so far. As I saw her moving off, I pulled the draw of musical instruments out into view and reach. She almost fell in the tub headfirst as she eagerly pulled everything out, one at a time, shook it, explored it, and threw it over the other side.

Next, Lottie went and threw herself on the sofa with Mum and "Cuddles the Koala," a HUGE man-sized Koala. I sat on the other side of Cuddles, closed my eyes and pretended to snore. Lottie came to explore my antics, engaged, and intrigued she touched my arm. I pretended to wake up and said and signed "Ooh, good morning, Lottie," which made her jump a little and giggle, while looking at me. I repeated the action and this time she pushed Mum as if to tell her to go to sleep as well. We both snored and woke up with a jump and an excited "Good morning Lottie" when she touched us. She dissolved into a fit of giggles, delighting in the engagement. It was a lovely, nondirective piece of engagement work. This was an activity Mum was able to easily introduce to Dad and older siblings, to start to build all of their bonds of engagement and connection with Lottie at home.

Lottie established this circuit on that first session, and she would loop around the playroom engaging with the different objects, in the same order, at least seven times per session. From this first session, at various points through the loop, she would acknowledge my presence alongside her, matching her movement, energy, and pace, and gently, verbally, and through sign tracking some of her movements and actions. This was in line with FMA integration of Axline's (1958) child-centered play therapy foundations.

The acknowledgment of my presence increased over the sessions, little by little, with Lottie actively engaging with Mum and/or me, in nearly all aspects of the loop. Sometimes seeking our engagement, other times delighting in engagement initiated by us. Lottie started verbalizing on the second session. I would verbally and through sign label the food as she threw it down, I would pick it up and name the item again, and she watched my mouth and repeated, for example: "Banana, pear, cake," and many more words. Mum was thrilled with this development, and reported she was also starting to label items and objects at home by the third session.

After the initial assessment phase of three weeks, which mum was present for and observing, we were able to establish some therapy goals. We agreed I would teach mum the FMA, to empower her to become a co-change agent for Lottie's outcomes. I would spend the first 25 minutes conducting a FMA session, while Mum observed. The remainder of the session Mum would practice, and we would process and review the FMA session and answer any questions Mum had. Mum had taken the principles of the FMA on board quickly. I observed Mum was able to be alongside Lottie, and maintain the level of attunement, curiosity, and engagement needed to effectively implement the approach at home. After four weeks of practice (session seven) we had a review without Lottie present to create a plan for implementing the FMA at home. We discussed when and where the set playtime would take place, and she decided it would be in Lottie's bedroom, after the baby was in bed. This is where the majority of her toys were located and there would be the least disruptions. We considered how often would be feasibly practicable to maintain consistency, and Mum felt four nights a week would be manageable.

By session eight Lottie started to place the sand symbols in my hand voluntarily, wait for me to name, and she would repeat, and then take them from my hand and place them gently back on the shelf, in the correct position, unprompted. She would then turn to me, clap and cheer, along with me clapping and celebrating "Yay on the shelf." Playing musical instruments together was a particularly engaging and connecting experience. Lottie evolved in this play as well, and enjoyed the sound of me playing the harmonica, and Mum playing the guitar, while she ran across the room and back listening to the different pitches of the harmonica and moving with it. She would take them away from us, and then give them back and say, "Thank you," and run across the room, and say "Ready, steady, go," and we would start to play as she ran back. The loop had also diversified and evolved over time, with Lottie's confidence in exploring the playroom and our relationship now secure.

Lottie discovered the tea set at around session eight and quickly integrated it into the loop. She enjoyed setting up the plates, cups, and saucers, and quickly began to match the colors in their sets. In session ten I wondered if she wanted water in the tea pot and I took the lead in filling it up to offer. Once she understood the concept of pouring water, she quickly mastered it with careful, precise filling of the teacups – rarely overflowing them, and then tipping it back into the tea pot. She did not drink the water, but did pass me a full cup to drink, watching, smiling, and looking at me until I had finished it. Mum shared that she bought Lottie a tea set for Christmas, and she had been making everyone cups of tea daily.

We had now conducted 24 sessions, and Lottie was beginning to develop a sense of awareness of herself, both as an individual, and in relationships with others. Lottie regulated her emotions positively in the FMA sessions, as there were no obvious demands. An emerging theme had been focused on an observable, intrinsic desire to develop her expressive language. When we began sessions, Lottie was not verbally communicating at all – beyond screaming or crying. Lottie was now labeling dozens of objects throughout each session, intensely engaged with Mum and I, watching our mouths, waiting in anticipation for us to repeat and confirm.

Her vocabulary had grown, and Lottie was beginning to make concrete connections, generalizing songs learnt at pre-school and home, and initiating them in the playroom. For example, at Christmas I had a felt Christmas tree on the wall with Velcro decorations and a star on top. Lottie took the star down and started to say "twinkle, twinkle." I started to sing, and she was so excited, flapping her hands and bouncing up and down, and intensely looking at me. I reflected to her that she was excited that I knew twinkle, twinkle little star, mirroring her expressions. She had started to vocalize singing "baba black sheep," "itsy witsy spider," "I'm a little tea pot," and other nursery rhymes. She would regularly request them by handing me symbols (spider, sheep, tea pot) and saying one word.

Lottie appeared to be better connected, able to process, and generalize information received visually through objects and sign, alongside spoken word. The intensive interaction nature of the sessions allowed me to be a mirror to Lottie and provided her with the opportunity to rehearse these new skills of expressive language and connection. We delighted in all achievements, and Lottie glowed with confidence and joy.

Lottie was developing connection gains at a rapid pace, and I had been able to start to introduce more directive Autplay techniques such as *Perspective Puppets* puppet show, with two puppets. In this intervention puppets are used to display a story where each puppet has a different thought and/or feeling about the same thing. Mum, Lottie, the puppets, and I tried different play foods, and responding in different ways, each with a different thought or perspective. I also introduced a balloon into sessions, and into the FMA at home, passing it to each other, building anticipation and bringing connection. Sessions were typically fluid with Mum and I always seeking opportunity to engage and make new connection opportunities, and respond to signs of development – keeping her in her zone of proximal development as much as we could.

Lottie had a complex matrix of needs and presented with atypical pattern of receptive and expressive language development, which was often the cause of frustration and dysregulation. Lottie presented with repetitive concrete play, a lack of imagination and flexibility and limited understanding or awareness of the world around her. Lottie received a diagnosis of autism in January 2021, at age 4 after a multidisciplinary meeting to review all evidence, including my report with the outcomes from the AutPlay Autism Checklist Revised. A pre-school review celebrated Lottie's progress in all areas over the last eight months, but most notable in her connection ability, her tolerance and curiosity of other children, and the beginnings of side-by-side play developing.

Lottie, Mum, and I had established a strong therapeutic relationship and alliance, Lottie was engaging very well with the FMA process, and we were developing to the next stages, starting to weave more focused Autplay structured play techniques into sessions at the clinic and home. We secured funding to continue sessions for another six months. This allowed Lottie to continue to grow in the now well-established therapeutic relationship within the FMA, continue to make and rehearse gains, and offered Mum the ongoing support in implementing the FMA at home. Mum was consistently implementing the FMA at home around four nights a week, creating a 20 minute "Lottie play time," after the baby had gone to bed. The other children were also being taught how to use the FMA with Lottie and were all starting to notice more connection and interest in relationship from her.

Being a parent is never easy but creating the time and space to have a joyful and connected interaction brings rewards that help heal the pain of the battle for services and provision for children. Each neurodivergent child or young person I have worked with in education, or as a play therapist over the last 12 years has one thing in common. They are a child first and foremost, and they want and need connection, social validation, and emotional fulfilment. The FMA not only helps the child develop these fundamental elements, but helps to support often frightened, inexperienced parents who have not had experience with neurodivergence, or are feeling isolated and out of their depth to engage with their child in a new and more purposeful and meaningful way.

Case Example "Steven" by Daysi B. Onstad

Steven, age 3, was referred for receiving Autplay Therapy with this therapist. His biological mother was the adopted daughter of his current foster grandmother, who had her custody and brought him to see me. Family history noted her mother smoked and drank alcohol during the pregnancy. Steven's mother was diagnosed with bipolar disorder, posttraumatic stress disorder (PTSD), reactive attachment disorder, and persistent depressive disorder. Steven's father was diagnosed with autism spectrum disorder, ADHD, cognitive delays, and other substance abuse disorders. Steven's grandmother reported Steven was exposed to domestic violence, and he suffered verbal, emotional, and physical abuse as a baby and toddler. She also suspected he was sexually assaulted due to several sexualized behaviors. These included rubbing his penis when feeling upset, stimulating his private area on the floor when feeling distressed, and touching other people's toes when encountering new stressful situations. Steven's grandmother indicated she realized Steven was not reaching his developmental milestones at 8 months old, so she looked for further testing and additional services in the community.

By collateral information, Steven's mother used to give Steven alcohol and Nyquil to get him to sleep. It was also suspected that sometimes his mother would give him other types of medications to make him "sleepy."

According to Steven's grandmother, Steven was challenging to handle from the beginning. Steven would run in circles, throw things around, he struggled with low-frustration tolerance, difficulties with mood regulation, and poor social navigation. Steven was often unresponsive to others at daycare, especially other children, and he rarely noticed other people. When being redirected by daycare staff due to inappropriate or unsafe behaviors, he would punch, scratch, pinch, and self-stimulate to decrease high levels of anxiety. Steven often grabbed people's jewelry, eyeglasses, scarves and flung them across the room. He would often display aggressive behaviors when something new or someone new was introduced. Steven would also repeatedly drop small objects in front of his eyes to decrease anxiety. However, once he was done, he would throw these objects across the room.

Steven was diagnosed by his pediatrician with autism spectrum disorder with accompanying language impairment and needing substantial support. It was also suspected Steven met the criteria for ADHD and chronic PTSD. Steven started receiving occupational, physical, and speech therapy. However, his progress was little, and it seemed to plateau due to high levels of dysregulation. His grandmother also found extra resources in the community, and he was enrolled in the Early Childhood Intervention (ECI) in the town that provided additional support for Steven and his foster family. Even though his grandmother was vastly involved in his care, he still showed little progress in multiple areas and sometimes no progress at all.

Steven was unable to form any words or sounds that made sense. He made no effort to communicate with others and was often oblivious to others. Steven's grandmother communicated with him through sign language and sensory input, such as singing songs or gently rubbing his belly or head. She indicated it was difficult in the beginning even to get his attention. However, with time he seemed to respond positively to these forms of communication. His favorite toys included dinosaurs, cars and trucks, bubbles, and sharks.

Steven's therapy goals were established to decrease dysregulation (aggressive behaviors) toward himself and others, reduce unsafe self-stimulatory behaviors in public places, and increase relationship development. Steven's grandmother completed AutPlay assessment inventories and play observations and agreed to participate in Steven's healing process. It was discussed and decided that therapy would involve the FMA with some integrated connection interventions. In the beginning, Steven was significantly dysregulated, displaying aggressive behaviors toward his grandmother and this therapist (e.g., biting, scratching, throwing things, breaking toys, slamming doors, running in circles, yelling, and so forth). After removing multiple toys and sensory tables in the second session, Steven could only access ten of his favorite toys. It seemed to help with overstimulation. Since Steven was accustomed to having his grandmother around when engaging with other people, we decided to have them both in the playroom while the FMA was implemented for four sessions. The FMA concentrated on selected activities that the therapist planned for the day, allowing Steven to access and chose from those materials. Bilateral music in the background was also incorporated to decrease anxiety because his grandmother already had a repertoire of calming songs that were utilized for regulation. When implementing the FMA, we utilized his likes and strengths to modify some of the basic FMA activities due to his lack of verbal language. Some main components were introduced one at a time to improve communication – music and sign language.

Steven participated in the play interventions, but his engagement was limited. For the most part, he would display high levels of dysregulation as evidenced by self-stimulatory and aggressive behaviors. Steven's grandmother was also learning the play interventions and following AutPlay Therapy protocol by implementing the play interventions at home.

Steven participated in multiple connection interventions in the first six sessions. Due to high levels of anxiety, the activities proposed were modeled for the most part. He would engage in them in subsequent sessions from 25 to 35 minutes. Sometimes, his grandmother would help us with the setting of the activities. Steven loved bubbles, and the *Body Bubbles* intervention was one of his favorite activities. In this intervention one person blows bubbles while the other person has to try and pop them with a specific body part. I began by blowing bubbles and tying to pop them myself with a specific part of my body. I tried to call for his attention in two sessions, and he would only observe the bubbles drop to the floor. He would glimpse with the corner of his eyes, and at one point, he decided he wanted to be part of it.

Ring Around Me was also one of his favorites. In this intervention the adult holds the child's hand as they walk around the adult. The baby shark song was added to address connection and decrease anxiety at the beginning of our sessions. When this activity was introduced, Steven had difficulty holding my hand, so we added a teddy bear that he would bring to the session, and we both held its hands while Steven would walk around me. Little by little, Steven was able to get used to holding my hand and walking around an ABC rug in circles. Later, the *Obstacle Course* play intervention was implemented, which helped Steven and this therapist connect. In this intervention the child puts on a blindfold and the adult leads the child around the room avoiding obstacles. He seemed, for the most part, present and focus on collaborating to reach the end goal. The first time his grandmother and this therapist engaged in this activity and shortly after, Steven was able and willing to let this therapist touch his shoulders and redirected when needed. In the beginning, Steven seemed anxious to let this therapist grab his shoulder without facing me. However, with the help of a teddy bear and then grandmother, he fully engaged in the activity. It was a success.

By session seven, Steven started engaging in the *Iguana Walk* activity, allowing me to "tickle" (using his grandmother's words) his arms. In this intervention the adult uses their hands to press down on the child's arms (moving up and down their arms) like a lizard walking on their arms. In the beginning, Steven would copy me to use this intervention on a dinosaur stuff animal. Slowly, he allowed me to use a dinosaur puppet and clamp it onto his hands, his arms, and later his legs. The *Break Out* activity was also applied to address attunement and regulation. In this intervention the adult uses a soft paper like crepe paper and wraps different parts of the child's body (such as hands) and then the child breaks out. First, the therapist wrapped a dinosaur who needed to set itself free. After this demonstration, Steven allowed me to wrap his legs, and he burst out of it. He asked me to wrap his legs and arms as we did with the dinosaur in a second attempt. He burst out again, letting in a big smile and a big hug, which completely changed his comfort level with this therapist.

In subsequent sessions, Steven engaged in additional connection interventions. He was able to participate in the proximity and frequency of positive touch actively. All these connection activities were also practiced at home with his grandmother and grandfather. They reported good progress toward positive touch, attunement, and engagement.

During therapy, Steven's grandmother became a foster parent of two younger children, 1 and 2 years old. Steven's progress was jeopardized due to his grandmother's divided attention to his needs and high anxiety levels due to this new life transition. Steven needed extra time to engage in new activities, so we repeated some previous techniques. Slowly, Steven was able to engage in new activities with less preparation time. Despite all these new challenges, Steven continued his Autplay therapy sessions very consistently. Steven excelled at socializing with these new foster siblings in his home, and he was able to regulate, learn new words, and improve the recognition and implementation of social cues, such as interacting and taking turns. The therapist kept working on connection activities: *Hands, Hands, Hands* helped with positive touch toward his siblings. In this intervention several ideas are written down that two people could do together that involves touching hands. *Soft Touches* was also introduced with the help of his grandmother. In this intervention several soft items such as cotton balls and feathers are selected and then one person closes their eyes, and the other person touches them with one of the objects and they must guess what object it was. Steven collected some sensory items to touch his grandmother smoothly and brought them to the playroom. The younger siblings were also part of this activity in the following session. Steven showed better interaction with this therapist, his grandmother, and his siblings during these activities.

Steven showed significant improvement by session 30. His interactions were assertive in multiple settings with this therapist and other professionals in his different therapies. He was able to use over 20 words in the correct form. He started using sign language for longer phrases. He was able to recognize emotions with sign language and visual aids. Due to the COVID-19 Pandemic, our sessions moved to a telehealth modality after assessing his readiness. We completed eight more sessions while reviewing the central core of his therapy goals. At the same time, this therapist would help Steven's grandmother implement or modify several home activities with or without Steven's new foster siblings. Social navigation interventions were also implemented, reviewed, and changed at home involving Steven's siblings. Most of them were role-played by this therapist and his grandmother. At the same time, Steven would witness appropriate social cues for boundaries and touch. Steven successfully graduated therapy after meeting his therapy goals.

Case Example "Jace" by Daysi B. Onstad

Jace and his younger brother were removed from their mother's care due to neglect, emotional, and physical abuse and placed with a biological aunt. His social caseworker referred Jace to see me when he was 7 years old, due to an increase of self-harm behaviors. The first three play therapy sessions followed the AutPlay Therapy protocol for the Intake and Assessment Phase. In this first phase of therapy, assessment procedures were implemented to gain more specific information about Jace and designed to help Jace and his aunt build rapport with me.

During the intake process, Jace's aunt reported that in the three previous months, Jace became more challenging to manage after school, and his outbursts increased in frequency and intensity with transitions. Lately, his supervised visitations with his birth mother exacerbated these issues at home and at school. According to Jace's aunt, Jace usually felt irritable without an apparent reason. Jace displayed dysregulated behaviors in situations where he was not in control or in cases where he was expected to follow implicit rules that may or may not be to his liking. His biological father was never involved in his life since birth. During the first interview, Jace reported that his brother was "annoying," and they did not get along. He stated that he sometimes got along with his aunt and uncle, and he missed his maternal grandmother, who used to take care of him.

Jace had multiple motor delays for which he was receiving occupational therapy during the school year. Jace indicated he enjoyed watching cartoons but could not think of anything not going well with him at home or at school. He recognized he was very competitive and wanted to know things right away. Overall, Jace struggled with a change in routine, sensory issues, patience, and frustration tolerance.

By his aunt's reports, his mother struggled heavily with substance abuse, and she also had a long history of trauma. Jace witnessed his mother being physically abused by her partner. He described how his mother would sleep so deeply and breath so slow after drinking that on multiple occasions, he would think she was "dead." It was reported that Jace would take care of himself and his brother by cooking and getting help to resuscitate his mother, who usually was under the influence of illicit drugs or large amounts of alcohol. Moreover, Jace described his little brother being thrown across the room multiple times due to "his whining." Jace had a long history of family psychopathology, including depression, anxiety, PTSD, and ADHD. Jace also had significant mental health history due to self-harm tendencies, toileting problems, and aggressive behaviors in previous placements. During a psychological evaluation, Jace's scores fell within the low average range with a FSQI of 83. He also scored very low in social navigation. He was diagnosed with PTSD and autism spectrum disorder, requiring substantial support and accompanying language impairment.

Jace was attending first grade in a small public school, where he qualified for an IEP for reading, social interaction, and communication. His teacher reported Jace enjoyed math but was quickly frustrated when he did not understand it very well. He did not enjoy music class and "hated" children's music. Jace's aunt added he experienced communication issues, cognitive inflexibility, and difficulty transitioning. He reportedly experienced social difficulties with peers due to his inability to play well with others and take turns. Jace was also receiving school counseling, but it was mostly unsuccessful. The school environment was a massive source of anxiety and dysregulation for Jace. He was often getting in trouble due to poor emotional and mood regulation, low frustration tolerance, aggression, and lack of friends.

Jace would become overly aggressive toward his peers or engage in self-harm behaviors when he felt he was misunderstood. For instance, he would punch himself or others, scratch his face, arms, or legs when feeling extremely upset. He would also bang his head in the wall and pull his hair out. Jace would scream, yell, and throw things at peers if they would get close to him. Moreover, Jace would hide under tables or build a fort around himself when teachers would try to help him or talk to him. Jace was frequently sent to the principal office to de-escalate, and his aunt would pick him up. Jace started receiving some special education services, but his behaviors were still a significant concern.

Overall, Jace's aunt brought him to receive AutPlay Therapy due to Jace's inability to connect with them and others, poor regulation, and social concerns. Jace and his aunt participated in a child observation session while utilizing multiple toys in the playroom. Jace's aunt completed four AutPlay Therapy inventories: the AutPlay Social Navigation Inventory, the AutPlay Emotional Regulation Inventory (child version), the AutPlay Connection Inventory (child version), and the AutPlay Assessment of Play Inventory. All inventories were provided to identify strengths and needs for Jace in social/emotional, regulation, connection with others, and play preferences. Jace's assessment sessions indicated that Jace was able to participate at a limited level in directive play instruction. Advanced instruction or activities beyond his limited skill level-triggered discomfort resulting in Jace withdrawing and shutting down. It was also observed that Jace lacked interactive social engagement and the ability to engage in reciprocal play. Moreover, Jace seemed to not enjoy pretend or functional play and did not want to participate in interactive play.

After four sessions, therapy goals were determined to help Jace identify and label emotions, connect with caregivers, and build positive peer connections. The play therapist utilized the FMA in order to address engagement ability and attunement. The FMA was chosen to help Jace feel safe and comfortable in the play sessions and build relationship with the therapist. It also provided the opportunity to increase the relationship between Jace and his aunt.

Jace participated in a typical play therapy room with my assistance. At first, he was timid and would not utilize any toys, objects, board games, etc. Slowly, Jace was able to ask if he could touch a toy/object. Gently, this therapist explained multiple times that he could use and play with anything he may want or need. Slowly, Jace was able to go around the playroom and started playing with some action figures. This play therapist followed Jace's lead, but he soon would become overwhelmed and withdraw. Then, he would walk to another part of the room and engage with a new toy. The therapist would come around and ask additional questions about his play or the object. Jace continuously became extraordinarily anxious and would leave the toy he was playing with. As Jace transitioned from one toy or activity to another, I took every opportunity to engage but being very mindful of his limits.

In session seven, Jace still found it challenging to initiate play or interaction with this therapist. Throughout the session, Jace found new toys that he would ask the name of or its purpose. He would often touch or manipulate toys he did not realize were there the previous week. The therapist used tracking and reflecting statements to encourage Jace to engage or explore. Jace found it challenging to share space, emotion, and attention due to high anxiety and lack of agency. Jace would make statements such as "I just want to play by myself, can I just play with it – I don't want to share, I don't like taking turns," and so forth. Most of the time, Jace would share his uneasiness about being followed around the playroom. However, within the next couple of sessions, he would demonstrate parallel play, letting me sit down next to him or actively participate in his exploration of the playroom.

These sessions lasted around 30 minutes, and the remainder of the sessions were utilized to process them with Jace's aunt. She indicated that Jace reported enjoying coming to play with this therapist. Moreover, Jace seemed to like the variety of the toys and the rhythm of our sessions. On the other hand, Jace mentioned that he still preferred playing by himself.

In session ten, Jace invited me to play a board game he used to play with his aunt at home. He was able to explain the rules and show me some "tricks of the game." He mentioned he liked coming to my office, and he would like to bring some of his toys. The following session, Jace brought a puzzle he was working on at home. He then allowed this therapist to arrange all the pieces facing up on the floor to complete the puzzle "faster." After he completed his puzzle, the therapist asked him if he would like to play with bubbles. He indicated he loved bubbles and balloons. The therapist explained the *Together Balloons* activity, which Jace completed with interest, assertiveness, and good attunement. In this intervention two people face each other and hold hands. They must hit a balloon and work together to keep it in the air while their hands are held. We were able to keep the balloon in the air for over five minutes, which demanded a lot of Jace's patience and social interaction to describe his subsequent movements and/or needs. This session was the doorway toward an integrative and more directive FMA.

I would prepare multiple activities for him per session, and he would pick one. Jace would also have the opportunity to decide if his aunt would participate in these sessions. In session ten, Jace was still timid and unable to engage with his aunt during conjoint sessions. On the other hand, he followed my lead once he picked up an activity, game, or toy. Later, Jace would teach them to his aunt and redo them with his brother or uncle. *LEGO Emotional House* was implemented with multiple modifications in three sessions. In this intervention the child is instructed to build some type of house out of LEGO bricks and different colors or pieces will represent feelings the child has about their home and family. LEGOs provided a positive sensory experience, and he would modify it with some assistance. First, I explained that we would be building some houses, cars, or robots to identify multiple feelings. Jace picked to build a house with different colors that represented different feelings. While building, he would describe his feelings or situation where he displayed those feelings (usually frustration and sadness). For the first time, he was able to express his feelings of sadness regarding being in foster care and his sadness regarding his inability to live with his mother and help her when needed. Second, he wanted to keep working with LEGO's, so we worked on cars while he helped this therapist to work on a specific model. Third, he worked on a school building, which allowed him to describe his frustration at school with schoolwork and peers. Jace not only succeeded at this technique but was able to teach it to his little brother at home with his aunt's assistance. Jace utilized this technique to describe one feeling per day at home with his aunt when he had a rough school day.

Bean Bag Toss was also implemented. In this intervention the adult and child try to toss bean bags into a bucket. Each bean bag has a feeling word written on it. Whatever bean bags/feelings get in the bucket, the person has to share about the feeling. Jace was very competitive, and he was good at it. Again, he modified this technique, and it was utilized throughout the subsequent three sessions. I wrote six basic emotions and the ones Jace picked on ten bean bags while he arranged the playroom to his liking. He shared situations for the feeling bean bags he got into the bucket. He then came up with the option of acting out those feelings. Later, he asked his aunt to join us, and she was also instructed to share situations where she felt those emotions.

In session 15, Jace wanted to play *Feelings Don't Break the Ice* which allowed him to differentiate positive from negative feelings. In this intervention the board game Don't Break the Ice is used, and the child has to talk about a feeling each time they knock one of the pieces of ice out. He also modified this activity, including his aunt and his little brother. We also participated in various sand tray play because Jace loved sand. He connected with me and utilized multiple social tools when requesting more water, sand, or pebbles.

In order to address his social navigation needs, *What I am?* was implemented. In this intervention the child has to guess what is on a card they have been given without looking at it. The adult has seen it and answers the child's questions about what it could be. Jace could utilize index cards to ask this therapist questions to guess what was written on the cards. He invited his aunt who was able to join us in the following session. *Interview Me* also helped to address his social needs. In this intervention, the child creates a list of question and interviews another person. The therapist introduced the technique while Jace was able to interview me. He decided to add more questions to the original format and invite his aunt to the playroom in the following session to ask his unique questions.

Great improvement was shown in session 25. Jace no longer showed self-harm behaviors, aggressive behaviors decreased, and overall, emotional regulation and social navigation improved to healthier levels to keep everybody safe in the playroom and at home.

We completed the implementation of the FMA until session 30. Jace was able to engage in more directive play interventions without displaying self-harm behaviors such as punching his head, banging his head on the wall, scratching his arms or face, squeezing his face and nose until he turned another color, and so forth. Jace successfully graduated by session 40 as he had met all his therapy goals. Later, Jace was able to engage with his school counselor to address more specific school-related goals.

Case Example "Lio" by Canace Yee

Lio began play therapy at age 4 and participated in eight sessions (first phase) and then stopped therapy for more than 1.5 years due to Covid-19. She then returned to therapy and started a new phase of 16 sessions (second phase). She lived with her parents and had one younger sister. At age 4, Lio was diagnosed with an autism spectrum disorder. Her first speech assessment was completed around age 4, which demonstrated that her language comprehension skills were satisfied but vocabulary and concept understanding was weak. Pronunciation and language expression was also weak, but word utterance was satisfactory.

It was difficult for her to assimilate into the social occasions, especially in environmental adaptability and interacting with others. She had difficulty engaging in play with peers, she needed a long time to adjust and feel comfortable in public and school situations. Lio also appeared to struggle with emotional regulation capability, she would become anxious frequently in different social settings. She would hide her face, lower her head, and sometimes would cry when she noticed her parents/caretakers were not around her. She showed limited ability to manage in interacting with people. Her parents brought her to play therapy because they expected Lio to improve her social navigation and functioning, relationship development and connection, and reduce anxiety levels.

I first met her in a two-week social class when she was age 4. She became highly anxious and cried seriously when her parents would say goodbye to her. She needed my full attention to comfort her, and it took some time for her to enter into the playroom during that two-week social class. From the social class, she was referred to have individual play therapy sessions with me. Our first phase was in 2019 and I applied the FMA primary focusing on Child Centered Play Therapy methods to build relationship in order to help her in reducing her anxiety level. I found Lio to be timid, she would speak very little, would not ask questions, and showed no confidence in getting any toys from the shelves. I tried to move some toys (such as LEGO, miniatures, and doll house) closer to her. She seemed to be more comfortable in this arrangement and began engaging with me to a higher degree during the first eight sessions.

Therapy goals for the second phase involved working on improving Lio's separation anxiety, building trust, improving emotion regulation, and building on social competence. I implemented an integration of Child Centered Play Therapy, the AutPlay Therapy FMA, and EMOplay as this seemed to best algin with Lio and our therapy goals.

The first five play therapy sessions followed a more nondirective FMA and Child Centered Play Therapy protocol. In the first two sessions, Lio needed the door to be opened to ensure her mother was there. She focused on LEGO play and this was used as the intermedium to help reduce her anxiety levels. She was very persistent that small LEGO bricks should be on a small LEGO baseplate, and she worked on creating a LEGO animal world. She seemed to regularly seek encouragement in her play. In session three, she still wanted her mother near the door, but I advised her mother to stand a few steps back and Lio did not notice the distance had changed. She continued to play with LEGO bricks but also started playing with cooking toys and preparing meals. In session four, I tried to ask Lio if the door could be closed because we could be having a proper and quiet cooking time and she agreed. It greatly improved the connection and relationship between her and I as she felt more comfortable and ease in the playroom. In session five, I continued with the FMA and Child Centered Play Therapy. Lio entered the playroom happily and let the door close behind her, she continued to cook and prepare meals and she started to focus on things being done in the "right" and "wrong" way. She showed an increase in comfort with myself and the environment, she started to enjoy playing more, often laughing and making connection with me. Her level of anxiety was decreasing significantly, and her parents also notified her changes.

From session six to eight, structured play therapy interventions were implemented, with the aim to further increase engagement, connection, and relationship development. I introduced a role-play game that utilized Lio's play interest in cooking. We took turns being a customer ordering food or the chef cooking and serving the food. I showed Lio how we could design funny names for the food dishes. Lio would laugh when I created some silly names for the dishes, such as "tall-boy takeaway," and "Lio's clumsy kitchen chicken." I encouraged Lio to create funny names for the dishes and design dishes by herself. With minor assistance from me, Lio happily designed dishes and created some funny names for the dishes, and most importantly she showed less concern on things being "right" or "wrong" and simply created and enjoyed herself. This two-way collaborative play process further affirmed Lio's strengths, self-esteem, and helped reduce fear and anxiety.

An integrative approach of Child Centered Play Therapy, the AutPlay FMA, and EMOplay, were implemented during sessions nine and ten with the goal to focus on emotional regulation and enhancing social navigation. The AutPlay FMA was continuously applied in these sessions as Lio continued her cooking menu play for "Lio's clumsy kitchen" and I would join in her play. Her level of connection, communication, and social navigation were greatly improving. Lio began shifting her play to the dollhouse, and she began to express her feelings more through these toys. The dollhouse people would display feelings and I would reflect the feelings back. In session 13, I introduced EMOplay bean bags. There was a total of nine bean bags and each of the bean bag carried two feelings (positive and negative feelings). I placed the bean bags under a whiteboard and Lio boldly suggested to throw some sticky objects on the whiteboard (which would gradually roll down and fall onto one of the bean bags). I demonstrated to Lio that when it fell onto one of the bean bags, we would share that feeling. I modeled how to share a feeling with the emotion displayed on the bean bag. Lio and I took turns to sharing stories when the sticky objects randomly fell on the bean bags. With this integrative play approach, Lio learned how to recognize and understand different emotions, how to express feelings in a fun, playful way. Her emotional regulation ability began to increase significantly. I discussed

Lio's progress with her parents and encouraged them to play with Lio at home in ways that supported her therapy goals. They were excited to witness the positive changes in Lio, especially in the areas of relationship connection and the social/emotional growth. It was discussed with the parents and agreed to further work on the parent/child relationship to help in building Lio's self-confidence and self-esteem.

Session 14 displayed a new play for Lio – she played in the sand tray moving her hands around the sand and feeling it in her fingers. She displayed joy while playing in the sand tray and periodically looked at me with an excited expression. She began talking a lot about a sand game she was going to create and play in a future session. After she had finished with the sand tray, I introduced the EMOplay Capsule Machine with about 15 minutes left of the session time. The machine contains basic rules for families to interact (play) together, different missions to complete as a family, and feeling expression and rewards cards. Lio consented to invite her mother to the playroom and taught her how to play the capsule machine game. They promised each other to complete the missions at home within a week and they would share with me their progress and feelings in the next session. This play intervention was implemented to further help improve the parent–child relationship, feeling expression, and social navigation. The EMOplay Capsule Machine was used in session 15 and 16 as per Lio's request. Lio and her mother proactively involved Lio's younger sister in the game and they all completed different missions at home. This mission exercises strengthened the parent–child relationship and self-empowerment by guiding Lio in a manner that encouraged her belief in her own abilities and potential for positive growth. This further allowed Lio to rely on her inner strength and sense of self-belief to meet and overcome difficulties. This helped create a strong foundation for Lio to believe in her ability to overcome personal challenges and struggles in the future.

Lio seemed to progress more quickly with her therapy goals after 16 lessons. Her engagement ability and social navigation were more present and advanced. I suggested that Lio decrease her individual play therapy sessions to bi-weekly with a focus on helping her maintain social/emotional support and growth. I further encouraged her to join group play therapy with three to four other children to continue to develop her social and relational navigation and sense of competence. Lio progressed well in her play therapy time. The integration of the AutPlay FMA, Child Centered Play Therapy, and EMOplay was a positive fit for Lio and created a play experience that aligned with her individual presentation and therapy needs.

14
Social Navigation Interventions

Social Navigation

The term "social navigation" actually functions as an umbrella term, covering a wide scope and variety of social related awareness, strengths, needs, and experiences which range from simple to more complex (Grant, 2017). A person's social navigation is often interpersonal, specific behaviors that permit an individual to interact with others in an environment. The extent to which an individual would be considered to have social navigation needs has often been determined by others. This is especially true for neurodivergent children and adolescents as they have often been judged by a neurotypical standard and expectation.

Historically "social skills work" has been devaluing and harmful to neurodivergent individuals. Some programs and methods have used the term "social skills" to implement protocol that has not valued differences and forced neurodivergent children to try and become something they are not, which has produced poor self-worth, depression, and anxiety. When implementing a group or individual therapy focused on social interaction and work/needs, it is vital to check your process and make sure it is always affirming of the person of the child and their ways of being, preferences, and differences.

Autistic and neurodivergent children can have true social related needs. Helping children with social related needs can be an important component of play therapy. If needs are left unaddressed it can create a myriad of additional issues. Some constructs for play therapists to consider when addressing social navigation needs include:

- What is considered social (skills, expectations, norms, navigation) will vary from family to family, city to city, region to region, country to country, and culture to culture. It is a subjective construct.

DOI: 10.4324/9781003207610-15

- It is an invented construct by someone or a group who decides what is and is not okay. It has historically been someone in power who determined the "right way" to navigate.
- It is important to remember children should not be forced to perform a certain social "skill" because it is what has been deemed the norm. Much of this is based on a neurotypical construct which has not valued differences or a different way of navigating.
- Often the issue is an inflexible, unkind, and rigid environment or person the child is experiencing. It is not an actual social problem with the child, the problem is with others and there may need to be advocacy implemented on behalf of the child.

Social situations can be confusing as the social rules or expectations can vary from one person to another, environment to another, culture to another. Often there are hidden rules – things that are understood by many in a particular environment but would not be clear to someone new to the environment. Often social expectations can seem contradictory and do not make logical sense, for example, telling a child to work on "not ignoring others" and the very next day to work on "ignoring a particular child." Many social expectations involve a great deal of nuance which can be confusing. Many neurodivergent children get labeled as not understanding "social skills." Often this is due to a conditioned expected performance and if that is not demonstrated, the erroneous belief is that the child must not understand and needs to learn/change.

Many neurodivergent children do understand social navigation. Typically, if there is a true cognitive lack of understanding or awareness, there is a cognitive issue such as intellectual developmental disorder or a traumatic brain injury. Conversely, any child, neurotypical or neurodivergent, can have specific social needs. A child's specific social needs should be carefully assessed and always addressed through a neurodiversity affirming process. If possible, the child should have a clear voice in communicating what they believe their social needs are and what they would like to work on. Consider the following four questions.

1 Does working on the social need help the child better get what they want?
2 Does working on the social need address an issue/struggle the child is having?
3 Who's need is it, the child's, or someone else's?
4 Does the therapeutic process implemented clearly stay affirming for the child?

Bailin (2019) stated that we should not pretend that autistic and neurodivergent children don't have needs. But we also don't assume that neurological and behavioral differences are always problems. For example, there's nothing inherently wrong with disliking social activities. Not wanting to socialize is different from wanting to participate and being unable to. Both are possibilities for autistic and neurodivergent children. One requires acceptance, the other requires assistance. Play therapy interventions, whether addressing social navigation or any therapy needs, should always be scrutinized to avoid ableist concepts such as masking and code switching. Interventions should always be affirming in their message and application.

The AutPlay Therapy framework can help address the social navigation needs a child may be experiencing. Structured play therapy interventions can be used to address the child's specific needs while honoring the child's play therapy preferences. Children are first assessed to understand their strengths and needs. Assessment is done by having parents and other caregivers complete the AutPlay Social Navigation Inventory, parent and child reports, and by therapist observations. Once a child's social navigation needs have been identified, directive play therapy techniques that align with the child's strengths, play preferences, and interests can be implemented.

Social Needs Cross Off

Therapy Needs: Social navigation

Level: Child and adolescent

Materials: *Social Needs Cross Off* sheet, and a plastic chip

Modality: Individual, family, and group

Introduction

Neurodivergent children and adolescents may struggle with one or more social navigation needs. *Social Needs Cross Off* is an easily individualized play therapy intervention (game) that can be played to help address a variety of possible needs. The cross-off component of this play intervention provides a fun and engaging way for children to explore their needs while creating a game format to follow until the cross off sheet (or game) has been completed. It can also be replayed.

Instructions

1   The therapist explains to the child that they are going to play a game and explore some possible social needs/questions.
2   On a piece of white paper, the therapist and child will create a 6–12 space grid (see example in the Appendix).
3   The therapist and child will work together to think of and write down some social needs that child may be having. One need is written in each of the spaces.
4   The therapist may write some of the needs specific to the child's social goals, but the therapist should ask the child for suggestions and listen to the child's voice regarding what they feel they have questions about or need help with.
5   The therapist and child take turns flipping a plastic chip or a penny onto the grid. When a social need is landed upon, the therapist and child can talk about, explore, and/or role play the need.
6   Once it has been covered, the child crosses that need off the grid.
7   The therapist and child keep playing until all needs have been addressed and crossed off the grid. When the grid is completed, the child can earn a small prize for finishing the game.

Rationale

Social Needs Cross Off helps children and adolescents address a variety of social related needs. The needs that are written on the grid can be any social related need the child has or wants to place on the grid. If the game is played repeatedly, the needs can be changed each time the game is played. The needs can also start out basic (a four space grid sheet) and become more complex as a child plays the game (creating a six or nine space grid sheet). Parents can be taught how to play the game and given ideas for needs to write on the grid. Parents should try to play the game at home periodically and involve other family members. The more the child can address the needs, the more likely they will be able to implement them in real situations. A sample *Social Needs Cross Off* sheet is provide in Appendix at the back of the book.

Social Navigation Pick Up Sticks

Therapy Needs: Social needs, emotion expression, and connection

Level: Child and adolescent

Materials: Pick Up Sticks game and social needs sheet

Modality: Individual, family, and group

Introduction

This play therapy intervention provides an engaging game format to help children and adolescents address various social related needs. The common game of Pick Up Sticks is used with an additional element designed to explore social and emotional needs. Therapists are encouraged to create individualized social need sheets for each child to address the child's specific therapy goals and highlight the child's interest.

Instructions

1 Using the game Pick Up Sticks, the therapist creates a sheet of paper with each pick up stick color listed and several social and emotional needs to discuss, explore, and practice under each color (see example in the Appendix).
2 The therapist and child play a game of Pick Up Sticks following the normal Pick Up Sticks rules.
3 When the child or therapist picks up a stick of a certain color, they must look at the paper and pick one of the social/emotional needs listed under that color to discuss and/or practice.
4 Needs should not be repeated, and play continues until all the sticks have been taken and/or all the needs practiced.
5 It is important to note that some children will have trouble picking up some of the sticks without moving them. The therapist should be lenient on this as the point is for the child to acquire a stick so they can explore a social/emotional need.

Rationale

This play therapy intervention helps address social needs, emotion expression, concentration and focus, and fine motor skills. *Social Navigation Pick Up Sticks* can be played several times and the social need sheet can be changed as needed to work on new or more complex goals. The therapist should create the social needs list that matches the stick colors prior to the child beginning their session. Parents are taught the intervention, given a copy of the social needs sheet, and encouraged to purchase a Pick Up Sticks game. They are asked to play at home with their child between sessions. Parents and child can create their own social needs sheets as they like. A sample *Social Navigation Pick Up Sticks* guide is provided in the Appendix at the back of this book.

Magazine Minute

Therapy Needs: Social navigation, emotion expression, and connection

Level: Child and adolescent

Materials: A variety of magazines

Modality: Individual

Introduction

Neurodivergent children and adolescents can often experience high anxiety levels associated with social navigation and often this can lead to children trying to avoid social situations. This play therapy intervention focuses on helping children identify and explore various social situations and address any situations that may be creating anxiety or dysregulation.

Instructions

1 The therapist explains to the child that they will be using magazines to play a game that focuses on social situations.
2 The therapist provides the child with several magazines. It is best to have magazines that display a lot of people doing different things. Also, the therapist will want to monitor to make sure the magazine contents are appropriate for the child's age.
3 When the therapist says "go," the child will have one minute to go through the magazines to find and describe examples of someone doing something social. The child can find and share anything they want – it does not have to be positive or negative.
4 The therapist keeps track of how many examples the child presents in one minute.
5 The therapist also pays attention to the examples the child shares.

6 After the minute has passed, the therapist can ask questions about any of the examples and/or process anything the child shared.

7 The child can have several turns to see if they can increase their number each turn.

8 The therapist and child can also switch roles with the child timing the therapist and the therapist finding the social examples.

9 The switching of turns provides the therapist with the opportunity to model and talk about various social situations, especially ones that the child may be struggling with.

Rationale

Magazine Minute helps address a variety of possible social navigation needs or questions, especially helping children to identify and talk about social situations. If the child is struggling with finding examples and seems unsure, this intervention may be too abstract or advanced for them. A variation of the play intervention is used to work on emotion identification. Instead of finding social situations and explaining them, the child tries to find examples of someone showing an emotion and explain what is happing. Parents can be taught this game and encouraged to implement the play intervention at home.

Action Identification

Therapy Needs: Social navigation

Level: Child and adolescent

Materials: None

Modality: Individual

Introduction

Children and adolescents may struggle with understanding expected and unexpected behaviors in various situations or contexts. *Action Identification* is a fun and interactive game that helps children recognize expected versus unexpected behavior to do in certain situations and provides the opportunity to practice responses. Many children get mislabeled as "bad" and given consequences for behavior that others are not wanting to see from them. This intervention takes the judgment out of behaviors and gives the child a safe space to explore and learn about their own behaviors.

Instructions

1 The therapist and child write various behaviors/actions on index. These can be anything from running out of a room to playing a video game. They do not have to be "negative" behaviors. If the child cannot write, the therapist can ask them to think of a behavior.
2 The therapist and child try to not show each other their cards. They take turns acting out one of the behaviors on one of their cards and the other person has to guess what the behavior is.
3 For example, the therapist acts out an action such as running, talking, reading a book, playing a video game, eating, etc. The child has to guess what the action is and then share in what situations it would be expected to do that action and in what situations it would be unexpected to do the action.
4 The child would go next and act out one of their actions (yelling, picking your nose, bouncing a ball, sleeping, taking your shirt off, and playing with friends) and the therapist would guess and share when (what context) it would be expected and when it would be unexpected.
5 The therapist and child take turns and can go through several different behaviors/actions. If the child cannot identify the expected versus the unexpected places and situations to do the behavior, the therapist should help the child think if ideas. For example, the child had the action of hitting another person but could not think of a context where it would be okay. The therapist might share it would be unexpected to hit your brother because he was bothering you, but it would be expected to hit another person if you were a boxer, and you were competing in a boxing match.
6 Their may be an action or behavior that would never be expected or unexpected. In this case, the therapist would have a conversion with the child about this and explain there would never be a context where this would be okay.

Rationale

Action Identification helps address possible social navigation issues by exploring behaviors as expected or not expected in different contexts. Children enjoy acting out the action component and they can think about and process their own behaviors through a nonjudgmental lens. The actions that the therapist selects (writes down on their index cards) should include actions that the child currently has difficulty with. If the therapist is unsure, then asking the parents for suggestions would be appropriate. Parents are taught this technique and are instructed to play the technique at home each day focusing on a few specific actions/situations that the child is having difficulty with.

Social Needs Bag

Therapy Needs: Social navigation and connection

Level: Child

Materials: Paper bag, art decorations, markers, paper, and scissors

Modality: Individual and group

Introduction

This play therapy intervention provides a child with repetitive practice of social needs they may be wanting to address or are having trouble with. The social needs can be related to anything such as making friends, decreasing social anxiety, or generalized to any social desire the child is wanting to explore.

Instructions

1 The therapist explains to the child that they will be using a paper bag to make a social navigation bag.
2 The therapist gives the child a small paper bag and instructs them to decorate it anyway they like and try to include things on the bag that describe themselves.
3 Once the bag has been decorated, the therapist and child work together to write on seven strips of paper (one for each day of the week) different social goals that the child needs or wants to address.
4 After they have been written, the strips are put into the bag. If there is time remaining in the session, the therapist and child can practice some of the social needs.
5 The child is instructed to take the bag home, and each day they will draw out one of the strips of paper and practice that social goal three different times that day (child practices with parents).

6 In the next therapy session, the child, parents, and therapist review how the practice time went at home. The social goals practiced will be chosen by the child and therapist and the therapist may have to help the child translate the goals into something that can be practiced. Goals may be something like – I need help standing and waiting in line or there is a child I would like to talk to, but I don't know how.

Rationale

This play therapy technique is designed to work on a variety of possible social navigation goals. Parents are involved in this play intervention and should be taught how the social needs bag works and instructed on how to play and practice at home. It is important that the parent and child try to practice the goal around three times each day. The more practice, the more it will help the child accomplish their goals. If a child wants to continue this play intervention at home addressing the same goals, then the same bag can be practiced for another week or more. Also, a new social needs bags can also be created at any time to work on more social goals. A variation of this play technique is an emotion bag which would focus on one emotion such as worry, and the strips of paper would each have instructions on how to process and express worry. The same process would be followed with the child drawing one strip of paper out of the bag each day and practicing the idea for how to express their feelings of worry.

Friendship Universe

Therapy Needs: Social navigation and connection

Level: Adolescent

Materials: Paper, markers, and a pencil

Modality: Individual and group

Introduction

Autistic and neurodivergent adolescents may struggle with accurately identifying what constitutes a friend. Some adolescents might label a child at school that they have spoken to once as a good friend. Others might consider someone a friend, who is actually bullying them and treating them poorly. *Friendship Universe* helps adolescents learn about and understand different levels of relationship, how well a person is known, how the person treats them, and what to expect from a friend. It provides the opportunity for the therapist and adolescent to discuss current friendships in the adolescent's life and serves both as an assessment and social navigation intervention.

Instructions

1 The therapist explains to the adolescent that they will be doing an activity that identifies the adolescent's current friendships.
2 The therapist and adolescent draw planets on a piece of paper (see example in the Appendix).
3 The adolescent writes their name in the largest circle of the planet system. Each planet in the system will represent different friends in the adolescent's life.
4 The adolescent will write the names of the friends who are closest (emotionally) to them in the planets closest to the adolescent. The friends who are not as close to the adolescent will have their names written in the planets that are farther away from the adolescent's name. Friends can include family members.
5 Once the adolescent has finished, the therapist and adolescent will talk about what the adolescent has created and the different levels of friendships (close friends versus acquaintances).
6 The therapist will likely have to spend time discussing how well the adolescent knows some of the people they have written down and conceptualizing what constitute a close friend.
7 The therapist can also discuss how to know if someone is a friend and how to know if someone is not treating you well.

Rationale

This play therapy technique focuses on addressing social navigation related to friendships and relationships. This play technique can be shared with parents so they can further discuss with their child friendships and help reinforce the concepts. It is not a play technique that needs to be practiced at home throughout the week. It can be revisited in sessions with the therapist. The therapist may have the adolescent create a new friendship universe periodically to see if there are changes. A sample *Friendship Universe* work-sheet is in the Appendix at the back of this book.

Playful Role Play

Therapy Needs: Social navigation

Level: Child and adolescent

Materials: None

Modality: Individual, family, and group

Introduction

Children and adolescents can sometimes benefit greatly from role-playing through situations they might be struggling with. Therapists can try to iden-tify situations where a child or adolescent may need help with different so-cial scenarios or issues. Role-playing should be about the child and their need, not something that the therapist has decided they want for the child. Role-plays should also be designed to be fun and engaging and can include props and other people.

Instructions

1 The therapist explains to the child that they are going to role-play some social situations.
2 Ideally the therapist and child would discuss social situations the child would like help with or would like to practice how to navigate.
3 The therapist and child will decide on various social situations to role-play and how the role-play will be conducted – what props, toys, or ma-terials are needed.
4 Some examples might include recognizing when someone does some-thing on purpose or accident, how to respond when winning and losing, how to ask a teacher a question, how to respond to a bully, how to tell someone you like them, etc. Role-plays should be practiced several times throughout a session. Repetition and practice will help increase under-standing and application. The more the child can role-play situations, the more likely they will be able to manage during a real situation.

Rationale

This play therapy technique helps address social navigation needs through a role-play. The therapist and child can work on a whole variety of social goals. One of the best ways to work on social navigation for children is through role-play. The therapist can pick any scenario and role-play through it with the child and explore how to act, respond, or handle the situation. When doing a role-play, it is best to avoid working in a metaphor or an approximate to the child's situation; instead focus should be on directly talking about the child and what they are trying to accomplish in a situation. Role-plays can be taught to parents and parents can practice the role-plays at home with their child. Parents can also role-play any situation that comes up and that they feel needs attention. Some common role-play scenarios are listed below but the therapist should caution to listen to the child about what they want help with and not decide for the child.

Common Role-Play Scenarios

- How to respond when winning and losing a game
- How to communicate needs
- How to ask a teacher a question
- How to notice an unsafe situation or person
- How to navigate eating at a restaurant
- How to order your own food in a restaurant
- How to self-advocate
- What is safe and unsafe to do in car
- What to do when your sibling makes you mad
- How to ask someone for help
- How to recognize when someone is being mean to you
- What to do if someone is being mean to you
- How to navigate when you are getting your hair-cut
- How to navigate when you are in the doctor's office
- How to tell someone you like them
- How to take care of a pet
- How to play with other children
- How to navigate waiting in a line
- How to handle peer pressure
- Understanding and recognizing humor

Candy Kindness Activity

Therapy Needs: Social navigation and connection

Level: Child

Materials: Paper, aluminum foil, markers, art decorations, and glue

Modality: Individual, family, and group

Introduction

This play therapy intervention offers a fun and expressive way for children to recognize how to be kind to others and practice acts of kindness. Children can sometimes be unsure how to express their feelings of care and kindness to someone else. This play intervention helps children recognize what a kind action toward another person would look like and gives the child the opportunity to implement kind actions.

Instructions

1 The therapist explains to the child that they are going to be making pretend candy and learning about ways to show kindness to other people.
2 The therapist and child write on small pieces of paper various kind things the child could do for or to other people.
3 The child then creates and decorates candy wrappers out of other pieces of paper, aluminum foil, or any material.
4 The small pieces of paper with kind things written on them are placed inside the candy wrappers (one for each candy wrapper).
5 The therapist and child can make as many of the kindness candies as they want, but at least seven should be made (one for each day of the week).
6 The child takes the candies home and unwraps one a day and will try to practice/do that kind thing that day. The therapist will explain the intervention to the parents and the parents will help the child with execution at home.
7 The child will report back to the therapist at the next session how they did with implementing the kind actions and process any questions or feelings they may have.

8 This play intervention can be repeated several times with new kind actions being created or repeating previous ones.

9 The therapist will likely help suggest kind ideas that the child could do but should ask for the child's input. If the therapist is providing suggestions, they should make sure the kind actions are appropriate for the child and the child approves and is okay with the action. The child has veto power. This is not a space where the therapist exerts their personal morals or values onto the child.

10 If there is any remaining time left in the session, the therapist and child can practice the kind actions.

Rationale

Candy Kindness Activity helps explore the concept of being kind especially toward other people and doing something kind for them. This play therapy technique is explained to parents, and the parents are instructed to participate in unwrapping one candy per day and helping their child implement the kind action. If the child wants to continue to play this intervention, they can practice for another week or more. Also, new candies can be created in session or at home to conceptualize new ways to show kindness. The actions placed in the candy wrappers do not necessarily have to directly involve another person, they can focus on animals, the earth, etc.

My Safety Wheel

Therapy Needs: Social navigation

Level: Child and adolescent

Materials: Paper and a pencil

Modality: Individual and group

Introduction

There can be a great deal of concern and need for neurodivergent children and adolescents to learn about safety. Research indicates that neurodivergent children can be easily victimized in various ways and they are typically not sure how to handle themselves when they are in unsafe situations.

Some autistic and neurodivergent children may have a difficult time recognizing unsafe situations. This play therapy intervention presents a visual representation of safe and unsafe people, things, and places that the child can take home and keep as a reminder.

Instructions

1 The therapist explains to the child that they will be completing an activity focused on safety issues.
2 The therapist and child divide a piece of paper into eight quadrants (see example in the Appendix).
3 The quadrants are labeled: safe places, safe people, safe activities, safe objects, unsafe places, unsafe people, unsafe activities, and unsafe objects.
4 The child can decorate the quadrants if they would like. The therapist asks the child to identify safe/unsafe things or people for each quadrant.
5 The child writes the safe/unsafe things down in each appropriate quadrant.
6 The therapist talks to the child about the meaning of "safe" and "unsafe." The therapist may need to help the child if they are not familiar with who and what is safe and unsafe.
7 It is likely the therapist will add things to each quadrant, but the child should write everything they can think of first.
8 The therapist may have to keep explaining the concepts of safe and unsafe and the therapist may have to do the writing if the child cannot write – picture examples can also be used.

Rationale

This play therapy technique helps develop safety related social awareness and will likely look different for children versus adolescents in terms of content. The therapist should make sure that safe/unsafe things and people are covered adequately. If the child leaves something out, then the therapist should add it to the quadrant. This play technique should be taught to parents, and parents can periodically reinforce the concepts at home by going through the safety wheel with their child. Children will gain the most benefit from this intervention if they revisit it periodically and continue to practice learning what is safe and unsafe. A sample *My Safety Wheel* worksheet is in the Appendix at the back of this book.

Conversation Bubbles

Therapy Needs: Social navigation and connection

Level: Child and adolescent

Materials: *Conversation Bubbles* worksheet and a pencil

Modality: Individual

Introduction

Conversation Bubbles helps children and adolescents practice what to say and how to say things in certain situations. It also provides the child with a written narrative to take home to help them remember what to say in certain conversations. This play intervention can address general reciprocal conversation but can also be targeted toward a specific type of conversation that the child may want help navigating.

Instructions

1 Using the *Conversation Bubbles* worksheet (template provided in the Appendix), the therapist begins by writing something in the first conversation bubble to begin the conversation.
2 The child will then write a response in the next bubble.
3 The therapist then writes a response to what the child wrote in the next bubble. This goes on until an appropriate end occurs.
4 Once the conversation has ended, the therapist should process through with the child how they felt being in the conversation and address any areas that need to be discussed further.
5 The therapist and child can then begin a new conversation with the child going first.
6 If the child is having difficulty coming up with a response, then the therapist should help the child by giving them some examples.
7 The conversations can be about anything but are most helpful if the conversations are covering real situations that the child is needing help with.
8 *Conversation Bubbles* in not designed to teach a child to communicate in a neurotypical manner. They should be implemented to help child navigate to get something they want or need. This can even include how to self advocate.

Rationale

This play therapy technique works on helping children navigate in social conversations. If the child can write, it also works on fine motor skills and handwriting skills. The therapist and child can complete as many *Conversation Bubbles* worksheets as they want, covering many topics. Parents can also be trained in the play technique and given a copy of the *Conversation Bubbles* worksheet. Parents can periodically practice with their child at home especially covering any new situation the child may experience. The completed worksheets can help the child gain confidence and feel more prepared to address and communicate their needs. A sample *Conversation Bubbles* worksheet is in the Appendix at the back of this book.

What to Say? What It Do?

Therapy Needs: Social navigation and emotion expression

Level: Child and adolescent

Materials: Index cards and a pencil

Modality: Individual

Introduction

Social related anxiety issues can be a need for many autistic and neurodivergent children and adolescents. Feeling unsure about what to do or say and how to navigate can become very dysregulating. This play therapy intervention provides the opportunity to discuss and practice a variety of social related needs that a child or adolescent may want help in navigating. The therapist can individualize this play intervention and address specific situations that are known to be challenging for the child.

Instructions

1 The therapist explains to the child that they are going to explore various social situations that may be troubling for the child.
2 The therapist writes down several brief story scenarios on index cards (this may be done before the child arrives for their session or be done with the child in the session).

3 The therapist reads one of the stories to the child. The child has to answer one or two questions about the story; "What would you say?" and/or "What would you do?"

4 The stories should focus on scenarios that relate to the child's life. An example might be: One day a boy named Daniel (the client's name) was walking down the sidewalk. An older boy ran up to Daniel and told him he had to smoke a cigarette (a real situation that happened that the client did not handle well). The child will try to answer what they would do in this situation and/or what they would say?

5 The therapist will address any responses or struggles and help the child learn how to decide things to do and say in various scenarios.

6 The therapist and child should go through multiple stories discussing the child's responses. If the child is having a difficult time thinking of a response, then the therapist should help with ideas and encourage the child.

Rationale

This play therapy intervention can work on a variety of social needs and should be focused on empowering the child in navigating social situations that are anxiety-producing, confusing, etc. The therapist can address interactions, emotional responses, and connection elements with this intervention through the stories that are created. The therapist can write several stories before the session but should try to include the child and see if they can think of stories to explore. An additional element to this play technique would be to role-play out the scenario after it is read and responded to with the child showing what they would say or do. Parents can be taught this play technique to implement at home and practice periodically with their child.

Bubbles Social Interaction

(Adapted from Liana Lowenstein's Technique – *Bubbles* found in *More Creative Interventions for Troubled Children & Youth*)

Therapy Needs: Social navigation and connection

Level: Child

Materials: Bubbles

Modality: Individual

Introduction

Children can find themselves in all types of social situations that are confusing and anxiety-producing. Often children can feel confident and empowered in social situations when they have the opportunity to practice scenarios and responses. This play therapy intervention uses bubbles to engage and provide sensory input as a child practices various social scenarios that are relevant for the child's needs. Several different social "scripts" or situations can be created using the intervention bubble blowing process.

Instructions

1 The therapist explains to the child that they are going to work on addressing social situations while blowing bubbles.
2 The therapist begins by creating a script to use with the bubbles.
3 The therapist reads the script to the child and tells the child that they are going to practice implementing the script using bubble blowing.
4 Some examples include: (1) Playing with another child – The therapist and child take turns blowing bubbles, one turn blowing the bubbles for each person. The therapist starts by blowing the bubbles, the child then says, "Can I play with the bubbles?" The therapist says, "Yes, I will share with you" and hands the child the bubbles. The child says, "Thanks." The child then blows the bubbles once, and the script is repeated back and forth. This will likely continue several times for practice. (2) Telling others you don't like something and hearing them tell you they don't like something – The child blows the bubbles; the therapist then says, "I don't like bubbles, please don't blow them by me." The child says "Sorry, I will blow them over here." Then the therapist says, "Thanks." (3) Some other ideas might include handling a bully, communicating a feeling, and asking the teacher for help.
5 The therapist should create scenarios that are real social navigation needs for the child. The therapist should also ask the child if they have any examples they want to practice.

Rationale

This play therapy technique helps children navigate various social situations. Parents can be taught *Bubbles Social Interaction* to practice with their child. Parent and child are encouraged play *Bubbles Social Interaction* at home practicing any scenarios the child would like to address. The therapist will likely need to help conceptualize different scripts and teach the scripts to the parents, making sure the scripts are scenarios that match the child's needs.

The Social Brick Road

Therapy Needs: Social navigation

Level: Child and adolescents

Materials: Paper, markers, index cards, and candy

Modality: Individual

Introduction

The *Social Brick Road* is a fun and creative way for a child or adolescent to work on addressing social navigation needs. The therapist can design the intervention to address specific needs and repeat the game anytime to address new needs. Providing a small prize at the end of the play intervention can create extra incentive for the child to participate.

Instructions

1 The therapist and child create five to seven pieces of paper drawn like bricks.
2 The therapist and child then discuss some social situations that are not going well for the child and write those on the back side of the brick paper.
3 The therapist and child then discuss a way to address, react, or respond for each situation and write them on the back of the corresponding brick.
4 The therapist then places each paper brick on the floor around the playroom; the bricks should be placed in an order with a starting point and an ending point.
5 The child is instructed to walk up to the starting brick and pick it up and read the social situation and the suggestions for addressing it.
6 The therapist and child will then role-play a scenario experiencing and addressing the social situation. The child then moves on to the second

brick and repeats the process until they get to the final brick where a small prize waits for them.

Rationale

This play therapy technique can help address various social navigation needs. The therapist should focus on social situations that the child needs help with and provide encouragement for the child as they role-play scenarios. This play intervention can be played several times with new social situation bricks. Parents can be taught this technique and encouraged to play the game at home several times. The prize at the end of the brick road should be something that the child would enjoy earning such as stickers, a piece of candy, or a small toy. If considering candy or any type of food as a prize, the therapist should discuss this with the parents first to inquire about any allergies or special diets the child may have.

Divide and Conquer

Therapy Goals: Social navigation, connection, and executive functioning

Level: Child and adolescent

Materials: Balloon

Modality: Individual, family, and group

Introduction

This play therapy intervention focuses on goals of working together with another person to accomplish a task, connection, and executive functioning. This play intervention provides and fun and engaging game to help children and adolescents notice others and work with other people in a cooperative format. It incorporates a teamwork concept and gives the child choices and control.

Instructions

1 The therapist explains to the child that they are going to play a game and they have to focus on working together as a team.

2 The therapist and child each choose an area to stand in the playroom.
3 The therapist explains to the child that they can position themselves and their feet anywhere in the playroom but once in place, they have to pretend that their feet are stuck to the floor, and they cannot move their feet.
4 The therapist and child hit a balloon in the air back and forth and try to keep it from touching the ground without moving their feet.
5 The therapist and child should spend time discussing and strategizing how they will work together to keep the balloon in the air and that the only way to succeed at the game is by paying attention to each other and working as a team.
6 The therapist and child can also strategize and develop a plan deciding where each person will stand to cover the most playroom space. If the balloon hits the ground, the therapist and child can stop and re-strategize on different places to stand and start over seeing if they can keep the balloon in the air longer. The therapist should empower the child to lead out in creating a plan.

Rationale

This play therapy technique helps with social navigation related to working as a team and working with another person to accomplish a task. It further promotes body awareness, connection, and executive functioning. The therapist and child will try to work together to keep the balloon from hitting the ground. The therapist and child should focus on coordinating where they are going to stand to try and cover as much space as possible in the playroom and discuss how they are going to keep the balloon from touching the ground. This play intervention can also be implemented in group format and can be taught to parents to play at home with their child and other family members can also participate.

Pose

Therapy Needs: Social navigation, emotion expression, sensory processing, and connection

Level: Child and adolescent

Materials: Mirror

Modality: Individual

Introduction

Autistic and neurodivergent children and adolescents can have sensory issues in understanding their own bodies and the body language of others especially when they are in various social situations. This play therapy intervention focuses on helping children and adolescents learn how to notice their affect, body language, and body responses. It also helps children understand how to better recognize other people's body language.

Instructions

1 The therapist explains to the child that they are going to be working on body awareness.
2 The therapist creates a list of various poses that the therapist and child are going to perform.
3 Each pose demonstrates a different type of body expression.
4 The therapist and child will each perform a pose from the list and perform it in front of a mirror so they can see themselves.
5 As the child performs the pose, the therapist will point out the different components of the child's body language and what the pose could mean or represent and examples of when that type of body language could be helpful. The therapist should also encourage the child to notice how their body feels in each pose.
6 The therapist can make the intervention more engaging by including props such as wigs, hats, and dress up clothes.
7 The therapist should go through several poses with the child and this intervention can be repeated from session to session. Some example poses might include happy pose, sad pose, unfriendly pose, friendly pose, leave me alone pose, I want to play pose, tired pose, confused pose, proud pose, excited pose, normal pose, scared pose, out of control pose, feeling calm pose, etc.
8 The child should be encouraged to create poses the therapist and child can complete.

Rationale

Pose play therapy intervention helps children and adolescents work on improving social navigation, connection, sensory processing, and emotion expression. Many children and adolescents may present "flat" and have a difficult time understanding and being aware of their body presentations and recognizing other people's body signs. This play intervention provides the opportunity to practice awareness. Parents can be taught this intervention to implement at home and encouraged to play with their child regularly and note any gains when the child is able to display a variety of body understanding and awareness components in real situations.

References

Bailin, A. (2019). Clearing up some misconceptions about neurodiversity. *Scientific American*. https://blogs.scientificamerican.com/observations/clearing-up-some-misconceptions-about-neurodiversity/

Grant, R. J. (2017). *Play based interventions for autism spectrum disorder and other developmental disabilities*. Routledge.

15
Emotion Identification and Expression Interventions

Identifying and Expressing Emotions

Emotion identification and expression can be a helpful awareness for any child. A lack of awareness can often lead to additional issues and/or struggles both interpersonally and in relationships. A child who struggles to understand emotional presence, may become overly emotional, may not display emotions, may lack appropriate emotional expression, may not understand or be able to differentiate emotions, may not recognize emotions in others, or may not be able to regulate their emotional states which can lead to dysregulation. If children cannot regulate their emotions, it can be a very frightening experience for the child. Being able to regulate, begins with identification and awareness.

Autistic and neurodivergent children and adolescents may struggle with identifying their emotions and with being able to express their emotions. Some children may have Alexithymia – an inability to identify and describe emotions that one is experiencing. Some of the signs of Alexithymia include a lack of impulse control, dysregulated or disruptive outbursts, indifference towards other people, difficulties with articulating emotions, difficulties with naming different kinds of emotions, struggling to identify emotions expressed by others, and heightened sensitivity to sights, sounds, or physical touch.

Identifying and expressing both positive and negative emotions can be a challenge, and often without affirming and supportive help, these children and adolescents will produce negative, unwanted behaviors when they become dysregulated. Some of the signs of emotional dysregulation include mouthing or chewing on objects or fingers, holding or needing comforting objects, increases in stimming – tip toe walking, rocking back and forth, hand flapping, humming and making random noises, becoming aggressive, becoming withdrawn, attempting to remove themselves from a stressful

DOI: 10.4324/9781003207610-16

situation, and seeking out extra routine and/or predictability. Adults will need to pay close attention and recognize the signs that a child is struggling with emotional regulation needs and move quickly to provide affirming support instead of accusations, consequences, and threating with punishments if the behavior does not change.

In AutPlay Therapy, there are six categories of emotion identification and expression that are loosely conceptualized. The categories include identifying emotions, understanding and expression of emotions, emotion/situation recognition, recognizing emotions in others, sharing emotional experiences, and overall awareness and managing of emotions. The categories are not sequential in development and can mix and overlap at any time. Further, each neurodivergent child may display and possess identification and expression in their own way that does not look the way a neurotypical child may display emotion identification and expression. There is not one right way, neurodivergent children can possess identification and expression in the ways that make sense for them.

The six emotion identification and expression categories are defined below:

1 *Identifying Emotions* refers to a child's ability to identify emotions, accurately label emotions, and reference several emotions as age-appropriate.
2 *Understanding and Expression of Emotions* refers to a child's ability to understand specific emotions they may be experiencing, such as frustration versus anger, and being able to express the emotion they are feeling in a way that is adaptive and helps process the emotion, such as communicating their feelings to others.
3 *Emotion/Situation Recognition* refers to a child's ability to recognize that certain emotions would typically correspond to certain situations such as a woman attends a funeral, this would likely make her feel sad.
4 *Recognizing Emotions in Others* refers to a child's ability to recognize emotions and emotional expression in other people such as recognizing when a parent is sad or angry, or when another child at school is feeling lonely. This often works in conjunction with relationship development.
5 *Sharing Emotional Experiences* refers to a child's ability to mutually participate in sharing emotion with another person, such as connecting with another in excitement while participating in a mutual activity.
6 *Overall Awareness and Managing Emotions* refers to a child's overall ability to be aware of and process their emotions, such as identifying feelings and being able to express them in an adaptive way and understanding how to handle negative emotions they may experience.

In AutPlay Therapy, play therapy interventions that focus on emotion identification and expression can be individualized to each child and adolescent to help address their specific needs. Play therapy interventions should be natural, playful, and engaging to children. Play therapy interventions should also align with the child's play preferences and interests. Many play therapy interventions can be implemented repeatedly with the therapist in session and at home with parents if it is something the child wants to continue to play. During the intake and assessment phase, a child's emotion identification and expression strengths and needs should be assessed using the AutPlay Emotional Regulation Inventory, parent and child feedback, and therapist observations. It is critical that emotion identification and expression needs are thoroughly assessed during the intake and assessment phase. Remember that neurodivergent children can possess identification and expression in the ways that make sense for them which may not look that same as it does in neurotypical children. Proper assessment will help identify the strengths and needs of the child and the play preferences of the child, which would all be considered in selecting structured play therapy interventions.

Feeling Face Fans

Therapy Needs: Emotion identification and expression, regulation, and connection

Level: Child and adolescent

Materials: White paper, construction paper (or paper plates), wood sticks, glue, and markers

Modality: Individual, group, and family

Introduction

Neurodivergent children may have needs and difficulty identifying and expressing their feelings. Some children may need help with regulating their feelings which may begin with recognizing a feeling and being able to name it and connect their feelings to real life situations. This play intervention creates a strong visual aid that children can keep and help them remember, identify, and connect their feelings to applicable experiences. The fan design provides children the ability to express in a manner that does not rely on verbal expression.

Instructions

1 The child is instructed to cut two round circles (or any shape) out of white pieces of paper (white paper plates can also be used).
2 On one of the circles, the child draws a feeling face and writes the feeling word on the piece of paper that corresponds with the feeling face.
3 On the other piece of paper, the child draws a different feeling face and writes the feeling word. The therapist should instruct the child to try and think of opposite feelings like mad and happy for their feeling fans.
4 The child glues both sides together with a wooden stick in the middle.
5 The child can make several feeling face fans representing several different opposite feelings.
6 The therapist and child talk about the feelings the child has chosen and the concept of opposite feelings.
7 The therapist and child practice making faces that match the feeling face fans the child drew initially and talk about a time or situation when the child has experienced the feeling.
8 If the child is having a difficult time thinking of an experience, the therapist can ask some helpful questions like "What do you feel in school during PE class?" or "How does your brother make you feel?" These types of questions may help the child connect the emotion with a real experience.

Rationale

This play therapy technique helps the child work on identifying emotions and understanding and expressing emotions (especially the concept of opposite emotions and connecting emotions to real experiences). This play technique may also help with recognizing emotions in others. The child may have difficulty identifying feelings and identifying opposites. The therapist can participate, model, and work with the child to identify feelings and construct the feeling face fans.

Me and My Feelings

Therapy Needs: Emotion identification and expression, and regulation

Level: Child and adolescent

Materials: White paper, construction paper, markers, scissors, and glue

Modality: Individual and group

Introduction

Me and My Feelings is designed to help children and adolescents identify and make a connection with the emotions that they experience. It incorporates a strong visual element to help the child recognize their emotional self and begin to talk about and process their emotions.

Instructions

1 The therapist explains to the child that they will be working on identifying emotions.
2 The child draws an outline of a person on a white piece of paper.
3 The therapist explains that the person is going to represent the child. The child makes the person look like themselves (they draw their own face and hair on the person).
4 The child is instructed to think about different feelings they have had (for some children it might be helpful to give them a specific topic to connect their feelings to such as school, their family, or going on vacation). Using construction paper, the child cuts out different colors to represent different feelings the child has felt. The construction paper should be cut in different sizes to represent different levels of feelings; small pieces are feelings that are not felt as often, while larger pieces are feelings the child has more often.
5 The child glues the pieces on their paper person, placing them wherever they want.
6 The child then writes the feeling on the piece of construction paper that they have glued onto their person.
7 Once the child has finished their feeling person, The therapist discusses with the child the feelings that they selected and talks about situations or experiences when they have felt that way.

Rationale

Me and My Feelings helps children and adolescents work on identifying emotions and understanding and expressing emotions. The child also works on fine motor skills and verbal communication with this technique. The child's feelings may change day-to-day, and the level that the child is feeling will also change from day-to-day. This is a concept that can be discussed with the child along with helping the child understand that all people experience various emotions at different times. Parents can be taught to implement this intervention at home with their child and encouraged to complete a *Me and My Feelings* person periodically to help their child gain more practice in identifying and discussing emotions. Figure 15.1 provides an example of a completed *Me and My Feelings* intervention.

Feelings Scenarios

Therapy Needs: Emotion identification and expression, and social navigation

Level: Child and adolescent

Materials: Index cards, and a pencil

Modality: Individual

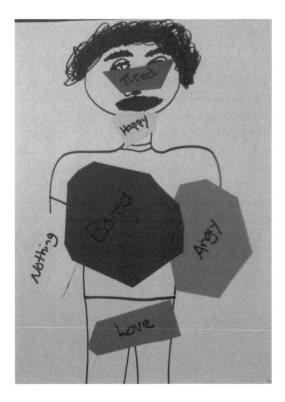

Figure 15.1 Me and My Feelings Example.

Introduction

Autistic and neurodivergent children and adolescents may struggle with being able to express their emotions. This play therapy intervention helps children and adolescents make a connection between emotions they may experience, specific scenarios that trigger those emotions, and how to express their emotions. This play intervention can be tailored to cover real life scenarios that the child has struggled with in the past.

Instructions

1 Before the session, the therapist writes down different situations or scenarios that would evoke different feelings (typically the therapist will write down on index cards, situations the child has experienced in the past or is experiencing in the present).
2 The therapist should try to think of situations that would be relevant for the specific child.
3 The therapist explains they are going to read scenarios that could cause someone to have one or more feelings.
4 The therapist and child take turns reading the situations and showing what feeling(s) would be appropriate in the situation using their body and facial expressions or saying the feelings.
5 Once the feeling(s) has been expressed, the therapist and child can discuss the feeling(s) appropriate for the situation and discuss if the child has ever been in that situation and felt that way.
6 The therapist can further discuss with the child ideas for how to appropriately express the emotions that might be felt in the situation.
7 Once all of the scenarios have been completed, the therapist can ask the child if they have any scenarios they would like to practice.

Rationale

This play therapy technique helps with identifying emotions, expressing emotions, recognizing emotions in others, and understanding emotion/ situation recognition. This play technique also helps the child become more comfortable talking about feelings. This play intervention can be used to talk about specific situations that are difficult for the child to handle in terms of their emotional self. If the child is comfortable, a further process question could be to ask the child what they could do to help with uncomfortable emotions in the situation. Parents can be taught this intervention and they can continue to practice with their child at home.

Examples of Possible Feelings Scenarios

- A student at your school tells you that you are stupid.
- You are playing your favorite video game and your mom tells you that you have to stop and go to the grocery store with her.
- Your mom and dad tell you that you are going on a trip to Disney World.
- Your sister breaks your favorite toy.
- You win an award at school for best behavior.
- You have an excellent school report card.
- You are playing at home and accidently break one of your parent's pictures.
- You are at the mall with your parents and get lost from them.
- Your teacher gives you a surprise math test, and you do not know how to do it.
- When you get home from school, you want to play on your computer but discover it is broken.
- Your dad tells you that you must go watch a school play that your brother is participating in.
- Your teacher tells you that you will not have any homework for a whole week.
- You are playing at recess and some other students ask you to play with them.
- You are playing at recess and no one else will play with you.
- You are riding in your car and your brother and sister are being extremely loud.
- Some other students at school start making fun of you.
- Your parents buy you a present that is your favorite new toy.

Feelings Detective

Therapy Needs: Emotion identification and expression, regulation, and social awareness

Level: Child and adolescent

Materials: Paper, and a pencil

Modality: Individual and group

Introduction

Autistic and neurodivergent children and adolescents may have challenges in recognizing their own emotions and have a difficult time recognizing emotions in others. This play therapy intervention helps children and adolescents learn to identify emotions in others and in themselves. It also helps children with social awareness in noticing what other people are doing and how they are behaving.

Instructions

1 The therapist will type or write on a piece of paper a list of feelings the child will try to find during the week before their next session (an example can be found in the appendix).
2 The therapist explains to the child that they will be the therapist's feelings detective, and the child is to take the list home to observe people and try to identify each feeling on the list.
3 If the child thinks they observe a person displaying one of the feelings, they will write it down on their feeling's detective sheet. If they cannot write, their parent can help them. If they are not sure about the feeling they observe, they can ask their parent for help.
4 The child brings the list back to the next session, and the therapist and child go over the list together and talk about the feelings that the child found.
5 This is usually followed by creating another feelings list and sending it home, this time with the instructions being that the child has to try and find the feelings in themselves.
6 When they notice they are having one of the feelings, they write it down on their feeling's detective sheet.
7 The child is instructed to bring the list back to the next counseling session to discuss with the therapist. New lists can be created with different feelings if the intervention is something the child would like to continue to play.

Rationale

Feelings Detective helps work on identifying emotions and recognizing emotions in others. This play technique also works on social awareness in the areas of observing others and paying attention to what they are doing. The therapist can create a list of basic feelings to begin with such as happy, sad, mad, etc. or create the list with the client. More lists can be created at a later session with more advanced feelings. Parents should be instructed to assist their child in completing the list by helping the child verify feelings and providing opportunities for the child to observe other people.

An Emotional Story

Therapy Needs: Emotion identification and expression, regulation, and executive functioning

Level: Child and adolescent

Materials: Paper and a pencil

Modality: Individual and group

Introduction

This play therapy intervention helps children work on identifying and expressing feelings. It also helps with executive functioning struggles in the areas of maintaining attention and listening for key words or phrases. It can also help children recognize when someone is experiencing an emotion and why another person might be experiencing a certain emotion.

Instructions

1 Before the session, the therapist writes one to three short stories that reference people feeling various emotions (some examples are provided at the end of the intervention description).
2 The therapist reads one of the emotion stories to the child.
3 As the therapist is reading the story, the child is instructed to listen to the story, stop the therapist at any point, and identify every time an emotion is expressed in the story.
4 The child is asked to share what emotion is expressed, who in the story is expressing the emotion, why the person in the story is expressing the emotion, and if they would feel that way in the same situation.
5 These are questions that can be asked by the therapist each time the child stops the story to identify an emotion.
6 After the story is finished, the therapist can read another story or ask the child if they want to write their own emotion story.

7 If the child writes their own emotion story, they can then read the story and have the therapist identify the emotions.

8 When reading the story to the child, it is likely the child will miss some emotions. The therapist can stop the story and mention to the child that there was an emotion that the child missed and re-read that section of the story to provide the child an opportunity to identify the emotion.

Rationale

This play therapy technique works on sharing emotional experiences as well as several other emotional regulation categories. The difficulty and length of the story could vary depending on the child's age. Several different stories can be written referencing many different situations and stories can be written that reflect the child's life. Children who struggle recognizing the emotions in the story may need to start by reading the story themselves, circling all the emotions they find in the story, then discussing the emotions.

Example Emotional Story 1 – Sam's First Day of School

Sam was awakened by his alarm clock. It was 7:00 am and time to get up and get ready for the first day of school. Sam was feeling tired and really didn't want to get out of bed. Sam's mother told him he had to get out of bed and get dressed; she was worried he would miss the school bus. Sam got out of bed and started getting dressed. Sam was excited to see some friends he had not seen all summer but anxious that there might be a bully at school. Sam got dressed and ate his breakfast which gave him a sick feeling in his stomach. Sam continued to feel anxious as he got on the school bus. There was a lot of noise on the bus, and Sam was getting irritated by all the loudness. The bus finally got to school, and Sam went into his classroom. Sam was feeling relieved to finally be at school. Sally, one of Sam's best friends, came and sat beside him; this made Sam happy, and he thought maybe school was not so bad. Sam started to feel excited about going to school this year even if it meant he had to get up at 7:00 am every morning.

Example Emotional Story 2 – Sally's Brother

Sally walked into her room ready to play with all her toys and have a lot of fun! As she walked into her room, her mood changed from excited to angry!

Sally's little brother Michael was in her room, and he had broken several of her toys. Sally was so angry that she yelled at the top of her lungs for Michael to get out of her room! Michael seemed surprised and scared at the same time. Michael quickly ran out of Sally's room. As Sally looked around her room, she felt sad, many of her favorite toys were broken. Sally's mother heard Sally yell at Michael and came into Sally's room. She saw Sally looking sad and upset and realized what had happened. Sally's mother told Sally that everything would be OK; they would replace all the toys that had gotten broken. Sally started to feel happy. Sally's mother also told Sally that they would get a special lock for her door so her brother could not get in. Sally was excited to get some new toys and relieved that her brother would not be able to get in her room.

Example Emotional Story 3 – Video Game

Liam was so excited! Today was the day his new video game would arrive at his home. He had pre-ordered it a month ago and had been waiting anxiously and patiently and was ready to get this game in his hands. He saw the van pull into his driveway and the delivery person drop a package off on his porch. He could hardly control himself; he was so elated! He was sure this would be the happiest day of his life. He retrieved the package from the porch, opened it and saw it – Warp Racing 3. He was about to escape into peaceful fun when suddenly he heard his mom say, "No video game until your room is cleaned." Liam was devastated, he felt a mix of sadness and frustration. He wanted to play his game now, he felt so impatient he couldn't wait. Luckily, Liam was able to calm himself down and created a plan to clean his room quickly. Liam moved faster than he had ever moved and got his room cleaned in 10 minutes – a new record! He felt pretty proud of his plan and effort. He then settled into his favorite chair for a long, pleasing, play time of Warp Racing 3.

Alphabet Feelings

Therapy Needs: Emotion identification and expression, and regulation

Level: Child and adolescent

Materials: *Alphabet Feelings* list, feeling face cards, poster, or pictures

Modality: Individual

Introduction

Autistic and neurodivergent children and adolescents may benefit from having a visual aid or accommodation to help them identify their feelings. This play therapy intervention covers identifying emotions, noticing emotion in others, talking about emotion producing situations, and how to handle negative emotions. It also incorporates social awareness of noticing others, specifically in regard to emotional expression.

Instructions

1   The therapist explains to the child that they will be talking about feelings using the letters of the alphabet.
2   The therapist instructs the child to pick one letter from the alphabet and turn it into a feeling word such as A=Angry (see example list at the end of this intervention description).
3   If needed, the therapist can help the child identify a feeling.
4   The therapist then shows a picture of someone expressing that feeling (pictures can be cut out from a magazine or presented from a deck of feeling face cards).
5   The therapist asks the child to show what they might do or look like if they were having that feeling.
6   The therapist then asks the child to think of a time when they have felt that way.
7   The therapist then asks how they might express the feeling if they needed another person to know how they were feeling.
8   If it is a negative feeling, the child can be asked to try and identify something that helps them feel better.
9   After the feeling has been completed, the therapist and child can pick another letter and complete the process with another feeling. It is not necessary to get through the whole alphabet and not necessary to go in alphabetical order.

Rationale

Alphabet Feelings is an intervention that focuses on a full range of possible emotional regulation needs. This play therapy technique helps work on overall awareness of emotions as well as several other emotional regulation categories. Depending on the age of the child, the therapist may do a great deal of assisting in this play technique. This play intervention is also easily adapted to address whatever components the therapist and child want to address. This play technique can be completed multiple times using all the letters of the alphabet and identifying multiple feelings for each letter. Parents can be taught how to implement this intervention at home and work on completing the entire alphabet addressing a variety of different feelings. The child can also be given a copy if the *Alphabet Feeling* list to take home and use as an aid to help them identify feelings.

Alphabet Feelings List

A – angry, annoyed, amused, anxious, awkward, abandoned, afraid, affectionate, aggressive, arrogant, admired, adventurous, ashamed.

B – brave, bold, blissful, bitter, bored, battered.

C – calm, caring, cheerful, confident, confused, comfortable, cooperative, curious, considerate, combative.

D – defiant, discouraged, disappointed, dedicated, dejected, daring, delighted, depressed, devoted, dumb, distracted, different, destructive.

E – excited, enraged, envious, energetic, encouraged, eager, ecstatic, embarrassed, empty, excluded, enthusiastic.

F – fearful, fearless, frightened, free, fierce, fragile, fun, funny, furious, frustrated, frail, friendly

G – genuine, glad, grateful, guilty.

H – happy, hateful, healthy, helpless, honest, hopeless, hopeful, horrible, hostile, humiliated, hurt.

I – Impatient, inconsiderate, insecure, inspired, insulted, interested, intense, intrigued, irritated, isolated.

J – jealous, joyful.

K – kind.

L – lonely, loving, loved, lousy, lovely, livid.

M – mad, mean, miserable, moody, mournful, manic, malicious.

N – nice, nasty, needy, nervous, negative, neglected.

O – optimistic, outraged, overjoyed, overwhelmed.

P – peaceful, proud, panicked, patient, pathetic, peaceful, pessimistic, pleased, polite.

Q – quiet.

R – rejected, rebellious, rage, regretful, rejected, relieved, rotten, ruined, resentful.

S – sad, satisfied, scared, secure, sensitive, shy, spontaneous, strong, surprised, sweet, sympathetic, stressed, sleepy, smart, stupid.

T – terrified, terrific, tender, tense, thoughtful, threatened, thrilled, tough, trustworthy, tired.

U – uncomfortable, understanding, unappreciated, uncertain, unloved, unworthy, useless, unusual.

V – vulnerable, violent, violated, vivacious.

W – weird, weak, warm, wild, worried, worthless, worthy.

X – can you think of a feeling or create a new one?

Y – young, youthful, yucky.

Z – zany, zealous.

Worry Tree

Therapy Needs: Emotion identification and expression, regulation, and anxiety reduction

Level: Child and adolescent

Materials: Construction paper, markers, scissors, and glue

Modality: Individual and group

Introduction

Neurodivergent children and adolescents may be strong visual learners and presenting information in a visual format can help increase understanding. *Worry Tree* creates an expressive art visual aid that children can keep at home to help them remember approaches and ideas for calming and regulating – various strategies to decrease their worry and anxiety.

Instructions

1 The therapist tells the child they will be working on ways to help the child calm and regulate when they are feeling anxious and dysregulated.

2 The therapist instructs the child to draw a tree on a piece of construction paper.

3 The child then makes several leaves out of construction paper and tapes them on the tree.

4 The therapist and child write different things the child worries about on the leaves. The therapist and child talk about the different worries and

if each worry is a legitimate thing to worry about or something that is not realistic (this is a good time to talk about realistic versus unrealistic worries, as children can have several unrealistic worries).

5 The therapist and child then talk about a calming technique that can be done for each worry.

6 The calming techniques are then written anywhere on the tree. The therapist and child role play through scenarios that create anxiety and practice a calming strategy.

7 The child takes the tree home and is encouraged to reference it to help them remember the calming techniques when they are feeling worried.

8 If the child discovers that there is something on a leaf that they no longer worry about, they can remove that leaf from the tree and they can also add leaves if they discover something new that creates anxiety.

Rationale

This play therapy technique helps children and adolescents work on understanding and expressing emotions and regulating negative emotions of worry and anxiety. The tree can be modified to represent any emotion the child might need help with such as an angry tree or a scared tree. Younger children may require assistance from the therapist in terms of identification of situations that create dysregulation and calming techniques to help regulate the child. This intervention would be a good option for children who prefer more expressive play interventions. Figure 15.2 provides an example of a completed *Worry Tree*.

Schedule Party

Therapy Needs: Emotion identification and expression, regulation, anxiety reduction, and executive functioning

Level: Child

Materials: Various party toys, and schedule-making materials

Modality: Individual and family

Introduction

Many autistic and neurodivergent children are visual learners and they often use and benefit from a variety of visual schedules. These schedules can

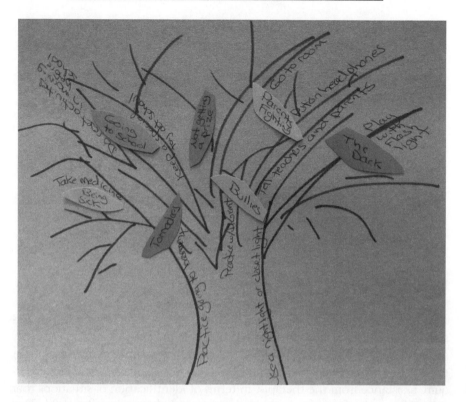

Figure 15.2 Worry Tree Example.

also be appealing for providing routine and predictability. One type of visual schedule that is helpful for regulation and helping to stay calm during transitions is a weekly visual schedule. This play intervention describes a fun and engaging way for children and parents to create a weekly visual schedule.

Instructions

1 The therapist works with the parents to teach them how to create a visual schedule displaying the child's weekly activities.

2 There are a variety of ways to present the schedule and parents should choose the method they feel will work best. A dry erase board works well but other examples would be a paper schedule, one made with a computer program, one displayed on the child's tablet, or a homemade Velcro schedule.

3 The therapist teaches the parents how to have a "Scheduling Party." Parents should establish a time each week to create the next week's schedule and have the child participate (the parent and child work on it together).

4 This should be called a scheduling party and the parents should have party hats to wear, noise makers, balloons, etc. Parent and child should go through each day and after each day has been scheduled, the child should get a piece of candy, blow a noise maker, hits some balloons, etc.

5 The idea is to have a small celebration after each day has been scheduled.

6 The parents are encouraged to keep the atmosphere fun and engaging for the child.

7 Weekly schedules typically include each day of the week, and each day is broken down hourly from the time the child wakes until they go to sleep.

8 The parent explains to the child they can look at the schedule regularly and see what is happening each day. The "party" format is designed to help engage the child toward the schedule and view it as something positive. The child can look forward to the fun time with their parent each week.

Rationale

This play therapy technique helps children work on general regulation and feeling positive and comfortable with the use of a weekly visual schedule. The scheduling party presents the opportunity for the parent and child to have a playful interaction and for the child to feel positively about their visual schedule. Visual schedules in general are helpful for decreasing dysregulation and helping children transition. The format of the schedule will depend on the child's age (words vs pictures) and interests (it could be a Minecraft themed schedule). Several weekly visual schedule examples can be found online by searching for visual schedule examples.

New Plan/Same Plan

Therapy Needs: Regulation, and anxiety reduction

Level: Child

Materials: Foam or cardboard pieces, markers, various art decorations, and glue

Modality: Individual

Introduction

Neurodivergent children may have a difficult time with transitions, spontaneous happenings, and changes to the original plan the child was expecting. This expressive play therapy intervention provides parents with an aid to help children handle changes to the plan or schedule and produce a more calm and regulated response from the child.

Instructions

1 Using card stock, cardboard, or foam pieces, the therapist and child will create two cards.
2 One card will have a large S (same) drawn on it and the other will have a large N (new) drawn on it.
3 The child will decorate both cards anyway they like. The therapist will talk about how sometimes there is a plan, and something happens, and it changes (the N card) and sometimes the plan stays the same (the S card). The therapist and child will practice several situations where the plan has changed unexpectedly and the child is given the N card and given some regulation affirmations – "The plan has changed, you are going to hear a new plan, and this is okay."
4 The child will take the cards home and give them to the parents. The parents will use the cards to help the child understand when there is a new plan.
5 The child and parents are both instructed that the parents will keep the cards and when there is a new plan (a change has happened), the parents will present the N card to the child and wait a few seconds to let the child process that they are about to hear a new plan. Then, the parents will tell the child what the new plan is.
6 The S card is used when the child asks if there is a new plan or if things are the same. The parent can present the S card to the child if the plan is the same.
7 These cards give the child a visual and tactile aid that is designed to help them regulate when there is a change from what they were expecting.
8 Some parents have found it helpful to make more than one set of cards to have in different locations.

Rationale

This play therapy technique helps children with managing dysregulation in regard to transitions and spontaneous or unplanned changes. The therapist should emphasize to the child that the N card represents a new plan, and the S card represents the same plan. It is important that the child understand when they receive the N card that a new plan, different from what the child was expecting, is about to be presented and this will be ok. This helps the child make an association that it is ok to hear a change and begin to prepare themselves. Parents are taught the approach so they know when the child brings home cards, what the cards are for. Parents may want to make more than one set of cards to carry one in their car and keep one at home. Figure 15.3 provides an example of completed N and S cards.

Potato Head Feelings

Therapy Needs: Emotion identification and expression, regulation, and connection

Level: Child

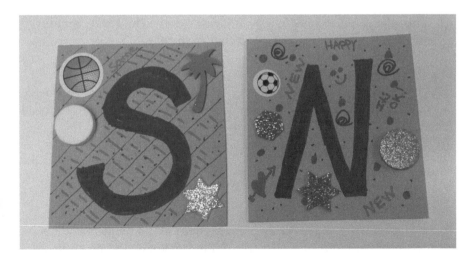

Figure 15.3 Same Plan New Plan Cards Example.

Materials: Mr. and Ms. Potato Head toys

Modality: Individual, family, and group

Introduction

Autistic and neurodivergent children may struggle with identifying emotions. This play therapy intervention involves constructive play and creates a playful way to engage children in identifying emotions. Several different emotion expressions can be made with potato head accessory pieces. It is best for the therapist and child to each have their own potato head and both be making feeling faces and expressions.

Instructions

1 Using Mr. or Ms. Potato Head (Hasbro Toys) and various accessory pieces, the child will create as many potato head faces as they can showing as many feeling face expressions as they can think of to create.
2 The therapist also participates and creates potato head feeling faces.
3 Once a face has been created, it is shown to the other person and the other person has to try and identify the feeling face.
4 Once the correct feeling has been identified, the child and therapist try to make the feeling expression on their own faces.
5 The therapist can also ask the child to share about a time that they have felt that way.
6 The therapist and child should try to create as many potato head feeling faces as they can think of. The process should be fun and silly, using all kinds of parts that may not even make sense.
7 It is helpful if the therapist has collected several accessory pieces.

Rationale

Potato Head Feelings works on identifying emotions and understanding and expression of emotions. It also works on fine motor skills and connection related to the playful interaction between the therapist and child. The therapist will need to purchase a Mr. or Ms. Potato Head; the more accessory pieces the better for more options in creating various feeling faces. *Potato Head Feelings* is a positive and playful way to engage children through a popular toy and it works well for children who prefer constructive play. This intervention can be implemented in a group setting and taught to parents to implement at home with the whole family participating and playing with the child.

What Are They Feeling?

Therapy Needs: Emotion identification and expression, regulation, and social awareness

Level: Child and adolescent

Materials: Magazines, index cards, pen, and glue

Modality: Individual, and group

Introduction

Neurodivergent children and adolescents may have a difficult time recognizing and understanding emotions in other people and being aware of what is possibly happening with another person. This play therapy intervention helps children think about and identify what another person might be feeling, why they might be feeling that way, and noticing the actions of another person for possible caution or safety concerns.

Instructions

1 Using magazines, the child is instructed to cut out pictures of people showing different emotions, actions, or states of being. The therapist can participate and help the child with cutting out examples and help the child with any of the processes in the intervention.
2 Once the child has gathered several different examples, the child glues the pictures on index cards and writes on the pictures the emotion(s) they think the person is showing. The therapist could also use the pictures to discuss if the person seems safe or unsafe or do they seem suspicious.
3 On the back of the index card, the child writes all the things they believe could make the person feel that way.
4 If the emotion(s) identified is a negative one, an additional question for the child might be "What would help that person feel better?"

5 Instead of making the cards from magazines, therapists may want to buy cards that display people in different situations showing different emotions. These cards can usually be found at education supply stores.

6 Depending on the child's emotional regulation needs, they may need help in identifying emotions. The child may also need help in thinking of reasons a person may be feeling the emotion. The therapist should guide and help the child through each step of this play intervention taking advantage of opportunities to help the child gain information about emotions.

Rationale

This play therapy technique helps children and adolescents work on identifying emotions, understanding and expressing emotions, and recognizing emotions in others. Children also work on fine motor skills and social safety related issues. Children and adolescents can create a whole deck of different feelings and reasons why someone would feel the emotions. Children can also be continually adding to their deck; when a child identifies a new feeling, they can create a new card and add it to their card deck. These cards should be created and sent home with the child. The child can use the card deck to reference emotions they might identify in themselves, or emotions identified in other people. Parents can also be taught to create new cards at home with their child.

Feelings Paint Swatch Key Ring

Therapy Needs: Emotion identification and expression, regulation, and anxiety reduction

Level: Child and adolescent

Materials: Paint chips (swatch), hole punch, markers, and a key ring

Modality: Individual, family, and group

Introduction

Autistic and neurodivergent children may struggle to communicate to others what they are feeling, especially when they are very dysregulated. This intervention provides children and adolescents with an aid they can use to help communicate what they are feeling and gives adults a better understanding of what is happening with the child.

Instructions

1   The therapist explains to the child that they are going to use paint sample swatches to make a feelings swatch key ring.
2   The therapist gives the child several paint chip samples that have been cut into smaller sizes.
3   There should be a variety of colors available for the child to choose from.
4   The child thinks of different feelings they experience sometimes and chooses a different paint chip color to go with each feeling.
5   The child writes the feelings on the paint chips.
6   Once all the paint chips are completed, the child uses a hole punch on each chip and then places the chips on a key ring.
7   The child has created a feelings swatch key ring that they can carry around and use to show others what they are feeling.
8   Once the feelings swatch key ring is complete, the therapist and child review each feeling together and talk about times the child has felt each feeling.
9   The therapist and child can also practice scenarios where the child might use their key ring.
10 It is recommended to begin with 8–10 feelings. More feelings can be added at any time. The therapist will want to make sure that feelings the child typically struggles with are included on the key ring.

Rationale

This play therapy technique helps work on identifying emotions, emotion expression, communicating feelings, and regulation. This play technique represents an accommodation aid that the child can use at home or school to help communicate to others what they are feeling. The child can add feelings any time. When creating the feelings swatch key ring, it will likely be necessary for the therapist to add some feelings that the child leaves out. It is important to make sure that feelings the child often has are represented on the swatch. Parents are taught about the swatch key ring and instructed to encourage their child to use the swatch. Parents can also help the child add feelings to the swatch key ring. Figure 15.4 provides an example of a completed *Feelings Paint Swatch Key Ring*.

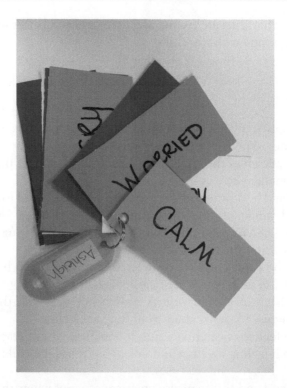

Figure 15.4 Feelings Paint Swatch Key Ring Example.

Feeling Face Cards

Therapy Needs: Emotion identification and expressions, regulation, social navigation, and connection

Level: Child and adolescent

Materials: Deck of feeling face cards

Modality: Individual, family, and group

Introduction

Using a deck of feeling face cards (which can be purchased from several education and therapy stores), the therapist and child will play various popular card games with an emotion focus twist. Example games might include Feelings Go Fish, Feelings Memory, or Feelings Bingo.

Instructions

1 Feelings Bingo is played by separating all the feeling matching cards into two piles. From one pile, lay two rows of five cards face up so each player has two rows of five cards (this creates the bingo card showing the feeling faces the player is trying to match). Take the remaining cards and shuffle them in with the other pile. Place the pile down between the players, each player draws a card and tries to find a match. All the matches must be drawn for someone to win. Each time there is a match, that person has to share the definition of the feeling.
2 In Feelings Go Fish and Feelings Memory, each time a match is found, the person has to share a time that they have felt that way.
3 All three of these games can have multiple variations and multiple games can be created with a deck of feeling face cards.
4 The therapist may also develop several ways to add an emotion focus to other popular card games.
5 The Feelings Playing Cards by Jim Borgman contain instructions for several popular card games that can be adapted to address emotion identification and expression elements.

Rationale

Feeling Face Cards play intervention can potentially address any emotion expression or regulation need depending on the variation of the games. The therapist will want to consider the age of the child when selecting a card game. Parents can easily be taught the games and are encouraged to purchase a deck of feeling face cards and periodically play the card games with their child. This play intervention provides an opportunity for the whole family to participate. Several different games can be played and repeated.

Perspective Puppets

Therapy Needs: Emotion identification and expression, regulation, executive functioning, and social navigation

Level: Child

Materials: Puppets

Modality: Individual

Introduction

This play therapy intervention works on helping children learn about how their feelings can be different from someone else's feelings – understanding that others can have beliefs, desires, and thoughts that are different from our own. Children sometimes need help with perspective taking and how to manage differences.

Instructions

1 The therapist explains to the child that they will be using puppets (miniature people or animals could also be used) to talk about how people have different opinions and can feel differently about the same thing.
2 The therapist chooses three puppets (people puppets are preferable) and creates a simple story.
3 Each puppet has a different thought and/or feeling about the same thing. For example, each puppet tastes an apple pie; one puppet loves it; one puppet hates it; and one puppet says the pie is okay.
4 Then the puppets taste a different kind of pie such as a chocolate, and again, each one expresses a different thought and feeling about liking or disliking the pie.
5 This type of story should be presented three to four times.
6 The therapist should then try to get the child to participate in the story by pretending to taste a pie and giving their thoughts and feelings.
7 If the child is successfully engaging, then the therapist should try to get the child to create a similar puppet story, or the therapist and child can create one together.
8 The therapist can practice this intervention several times implementing several different stories all with the same theme of each puppet having a different perspective.

Rationale

This play therapy technique works primarily on helping children understand others can have a different feeling or thought about something and this is okay. When a child can understand that other people can have different thoughts and feelings from themselves, it aids in social relationships and better awareness of emotions. The story can be about anything, as long as each puppet expresses a different thought and feeling. The puppet story should be animated and fun and the therapist should look for opportunities to get the child involved in the story and practicing taking different perspectives.

My Emotions Cards

Therapy Needs: Emotion identification and expression, and regulation

Level: Child and adolescent

Materials: Blank deck of cards, and markers

Modality: Individual

Introduction

My Emotion Cards provides the opportunity for children and adolescents to create their own feelings card deck. The finished card deck can be used to play several games that help the child identify and share emotions. The therapist can work with the child and the parents to establish several games that can be played with the card deck.

Instructions

1 The therapist explains to the child that they are going to create their own card deck that focuses on feelings.
2 Using a blank deck of cards (which can be purchased at most educational supply stores), the child is instructed to draw feeling faces on the cards and write the feeling word on the card as well.
3 The child should make two of each feeling card so there is a matching card.
4 The therapist may have to help the child with writing and spelling and even identifying several feelings.
5 The therapist can also provide a feeling chart for the child to look at.
6 The child should try to create as many feeling faces cards as they can think of and draw the faces as best as they can. The child can decorate the cards any way they like.
7 It is also appropriate for the therapist to make some cards and add them to the child's deck, especially if they are emotions that the therapist knows that the child needs help with.

8 After the child has finished the card deck, the therapist and child play some feeling card games together. Some examples would include Feelings Go Fish and Feeling Matching. The therapist and child should try to think of other games that they could play with the feelings card deck, maybe even creating a new game.

Rationale

This play therapy technique can potentially address any emotional regulation need depending on the variation of the games. The child can take the card deck home and play games with their parents. Several different games can be played, and the games can be played repeatedly. The child will likely not use all the blank cards, so they can take them home and add to the card deck as they discover new feelings. The therapist will likely have to share card game ideas with the parents and encourage them to think of new games to play.

16

Connection (Relationship Development) Interventions

Connecting and Engaging

Autistic and neurodivergent children and adolescents possess a sense of connection, engagement, and desire for relationship development. Many children would likely do poorly if they were suddenly removed from their caregivers and those important to them. A great myth has existed that autistic and neurodivergent children do not form relationships, connect with others, or care about these processes. This could not be further from the truth. These children, like all children, have a desire, longing, and an importance regarding relationship development. Many autistic and neurodivergent children are misunderstood and neurotypical individuals often do not recognize the relationship development processes of neurodivergent children.

Neurodivergent children (like all children) may have difficulty displaying and expressing connection in meaningful ways and they may have a difficult time expressing connection in a neurotypical socially constructed "acceptable" way. Also, it is possible that other needs (issues) are interfering with the child being able to engage in relationship in the ways they would like. This might include social anxiety issues, trauma responses, sensory challenges, etc. Therapy goals for addressing connection and relationship development may mean addressing the issues that are creating blocks to the natural experience of relationship and connection.

Connection and relationship development cannot be considered without a focus on the parent–

child relationship. This is the beginning and essence of the development of these constructs. What is happening between child and parent cannot be undervalued. Parent and child need to feel connection between themselves as the child utilizes the healthy parent–child connection to reach out and

DOI: 10.4324/9781003207610-17

explore connection in other ways with other people. Often neurodivergent children establish closeness with others in which they feel safe. In this relationship, they will seek support from adults with whom they are comfortable and show enjoyment in their close relationships. In AutPlay Therapy connection related goals may be established more for the parent than the child. It may be that the parent needs help with connection and relationship work, and the parent and child will participate in the AutPlay family play therapy process together with this therapy goal in mind.

The connection and relationship development play interventions in this chapter are designed to increase connection between child and caregiver, increase relationship development between child and other significant relationships, teach children and adolescents how to be more successful in achieving their connection and relationship development goals, and provide a fun, natural, playful atmosphere for children and adolescents to explore, heal, and grow regarding relationship and connection needs.

The connection and relationship development play interventions in this chapter range from simple to more complex by design. Therapists should be mindful of the age of the child they are working with and choose interventions that are most appropriate. Therapists should also be mindful of the parent/child relationship and the parents own mental health needs. The therapist would not want to engage or entrust the parent to be a safe and reliable partner in the process if the parent is not in a healthy space to produce this type of attunement with their child. Forcing a child or parent to participate in a connection based play intervention in which they are uncomfortable with, or that is beyond their current relationship processes, will likely result in a myriad of poor outcomes. It may also result in the parent and child becoming resistant to participating in future connection based interventions and/or therapy in general.

It must be understood that autistic and neurodivergent children universally have a desire for greater connection with others and a longing to have deeper relationship experiences at least to a level that they feel comfortable with. Consequently, children dealing with these issues are not experiencing the level of connection and relationship which they desire and seem to struggle with how to attain the level of connection they would like to have. Through consistent and mindful introduction and implementation of play therapy interventions designed to increase a child's opportunities for creating and maintaining meaningful connection and relationships at their desired comfort level, children can feel fulfilled and content in this area of their lives.

It is likely that each child and adolescent will present with different goals/ needs in terms of how much connection they develop, what level of relationship each child and adolescent is seeking, and what they are comfortable with. It is not necessary for every person, neurotypical or neurodivergent, to possess the same desire and level in relationship development. There is some subjectivity that should be implemented in determining what level of connection each child and adolescent may need and what level they may want to achieve in terms of greater connection and relationship development with others.

AutPlay Therapy connection focused play interventions provide for structured, or directive play therapy techniques that the parent and child can do together that helps foster relationship development and connection. Parents can complete the AutPlay Connection Inventory during the Intake and Assessment Phase to better identify any connection related needs. These play techniques are designed to be fun and connecting for both the parent and child. It is important to note that there is connection (relationship development) work happening throughout the AutPlay Therapy protocol. Relationship development is considered a core change agent and is implemented, and role modeled by the therapist from the beginning of therapy to the end. Regardless of the therapy goals and/or the specific focus of play approach or intervention, relationship development and connection are happening.

Make My Moves

Therapy Needs: Connection (relationship development), sensory processing, social engagement, and anxiety reduction

Level: Child

Materials: None

Modality: Individual, family, and group

Introduction

Make My Moves is a movement-based play intervention. It is designed to help increase awareness of another person, increase connection with others, improve relaxation ability (anxiety reduction), turn taking, work on sensory related issues (specifically vestibular and proprioceptive), and help with regulation. This intervention is simple yet fun and engaging and can incorporate many different elements. It can also be played repeatedly and easily taught to others.

Instructions

1 The therapist explains to the child that they will be playing a game where they have to follow each other's movements.
2 The child and therapist stand facing each other. One person is designated the leader. The leader makes various movements such as moving arms up and down, moving legs, moving head back and forth, and moving around the room in various ways.
3 The follower must mimic or follow the moves that the leader is doing. The follower should try to observe closely what the leader is doing and do the same thing, If the leader is moving around the room, the follower should move around the room in the same pattern.
4 Whoever begins as the leader, should lead for a few minutes, and then switch the leader. The therapist and child can continue to switch back and forth in the leader role until the game is over.
5 The moves can vary in complexity and in speed (slow down and speed up). For decreasing anxiety and helping the child to regulate, the therapist should incorporate mid-line crossing moves – moves that activate the whole brain and cross the right and left hemispheres. Several mid-line crossing moves can be found in the book *Brain Gym* by Paul and Gail Dennison.
6 The child and therapist continue to play the game until the child is no longer interested.

Rationale

This play therapy intervention is designed to work on connection and relationship development. It also has additional social and regulation benefits such as turn taking, following another's' lead, whole body movement, and midline crossing moves. The technique can be played individually with the child or including the parent with each person rotating roles as the leader. The therapist will likely want to begin with slow and simple movements and progress as the child gets used to the technique. The therapist should be mindful of the child's comfort level and any possible physical challenges. This intervention works best with children who enjoy movement play and is facilitated in a space that is large enough for engaging movement around the room.

Where Am I Going?

Therapy Needs: Connection (relationship development), social engagement, and executive functioning skills.

Level: Child

Materials: None

Modality: Individual, and group

Introduction

This play intervention involves moving around a room. There will need to be enough space so the child and therapist can easily navigate around a room in different directions. This intervention helps children address and work on developing connection, social engagement, discernment, focus, and calculations in a fun and engaging manner. It also involves turn taking and can be easy modified for younger or older children.

Instructions

1 The therapist explains to the child that they will be playing a game that involves moving around the room.
2 The therapist and child hold hands and stand facing each other.
3 One person is designated the leader (ideally the therapist would be the leader first to help model how the game is played).
4 The therapist explains that no words will be spoken, and the leader will move around the room in different directions (forward, backward, left, and right) and the follower must follow the leader and maintain holding hands.
5 The child and therapist will create signals to indicate which direction the leader will be moving. For example, a squeeze of the right hand for moving to the right, a squeeze of the left hand for moving to the left, stomping the right foot to move forward, and stomping the left foot to move backward. Both players will have to remember what each signal

means or they may get their "signals crossed!" This can be challenging for executive functioning processing as the leaders forward would be the followers backward and vice versa.

6 After about five minutes of play, the roles can be switched, and the child can become the leader.
7 The child and therapist can play the game repeatedly switching back and forth in the leader role until the child is no longer interested in playing.

Rationale

This play therapy technique can help children feel more comfortable in connection and relationship development with others. It can also help improve executive functioning skills and confidence in social engagement. The game is often fun and silly as someone usually forgets a signal and the two players may be moving in opposite directions. If someone forgets or gets the signals crossed. It should be laughed off and the game restarted. The therapist should start as leader and begin with simple and slow moves, giving the child plenty of time to process the signal. The speed and complexity can increase as the child gets used to the technique. The therapist should be mindful of any frustration from the child and aware of any motor or physical movement issues. The therapist may need to remind the child what the signals mean and to continue to hold hands. Parents can be taught the intervention and instructed to play at home with their child. This intervention can also be implanted in a group format.

Body Part Bubble Pop

Therapy Needs: Connection (relationship development), social engagement, anxiety reduction, and regulation

Level: Child

Materials: Bubbles

Modality: Individual

Introduction

Body Part Bubble Pop utilizes bubbles in a simple, playful game. Many children enjoy bubble play and find bubble blowing and popping regulating. This play technique helps address connection and relationship development needs. It also provides a level of social engagement and interaction and can help reduce anxiety and serve as a regulation intervention. This intervention might be especially beneficial for children with higher needs or children who do not do well attuning to another person or following structured interventions.

Instructions

1 The therapist explains to the child that they will be playing a game together using bubbles.
2 The therapist instructs to the child that they will start blowing bubbles and the child has to try to pop the bubbles before the bubbles hit the ground.
3 After a few minutes of play, the therapist tells the child that they must try to pop all the bubbles before they hit the ground using a specific body part. For example, the therapist might instruct the child that they must try to pop the bubbles using their thumbs only.
4 After a few minutes of popping the bubbles this way, the therapist might instruct the child that they will switch and now try to pop the bubbles using only their elbows.
5 This continues for several rounds. Other body part examples include fingers, ear, nose, feet, shoulders, knees, head, and butt (a favorite of many children).
6 The child and therapist can also switch roles with the therapist popping the bubbles however the child decides.
7 Play should continue with the child and therapist switching roles periodically until the child is no longer interested in playing the game.

Rationale

Body Part Bubble Pop helps children increase comfort in connecting with others and increasing relationship development. It also helps address attunement and social engagement (in a fun and anxiety reducing manner) with another person. An added (advanced) element to this technique would be to have the child say positive things about themselves or a family member while they are trying to pop all the bubbles. This advanced element would help with whole brain activation, regulation, and executive functioning skills. This play intervention should start very basic with simply blowing the bubbles and having the child pop them, as the child is capable, more specific instructions can be added. This play technique can easily be taught to parents and parents can play the intervention with their child at home. The therapist should be mindful of space and make sure there is enough space to move without running into something. The therapist should also be mindful of any physical limitations the child may have.

Family Name

Therapy Needs: Connection (relationship development), assessment, and family issues

Level: Child and adolescent

Materials: Paper, markers, art decorations, and glue

Modality: Individual, and family

Introduction

This play therapy intervention provides the opportunity to connect with and learn more about the child and their family. It also gives the child and parent (if they are participating) practice thinking about, understanding, and expressing connection with their family members. This technique can provide a positive interaction between parent and child if therapy goals include addressing parent/child strained relationship. This is an expressive activity; the child can be as creative as they like or as simple as they like in their creation. The therapist may assist the child if needed. Figure 16.1 shows a completed example of the *Family Name* activity.

Instructions

1 The therapist explains to the child that they will be creating an art project that describes the child's family.
2 The child draws the child's last name in bubble letters on a piece of paper (for younger children or children with higher support needs, the therapist will likely assist the child in drawing their last name). If the parent is participating, they can create their own family name or the child and parent can work on one together.
3 The child's last name is then decorated by the child with things that remind the child of their family.

4 Once the child is finished, the therapist processes with the child what they created and how it reminds them of their family.

5 The child takes the finished name home and keeps it in their room or hangs it up somewhere in the home. If the parent does not participate in the play intervention, the child is encouraged to share what they made with their parent.

6 This can also be done as a family play therapy intervention with the whole family participating. Each family member can create their own and then share with each other or they can all work together to create one.

Rationale

Family Name works on connection and relationship development specifically with parents and other family members. It can also serve as an assessment play therapy intervention providing information for the therapist about the child's family and the child's relationship with their family. It is designed to help the child think about their family and create something that shows the child's feelings of connection with their family. It also has the potential to reveal strain or relationship needs in the family. The child will be creating something that is a concrete representation of a connection with their family which can be positive for other family members to see. The therapist can process with the child helping them express positive emotions and/or unmet needs or concerns. Figure 16.1 provides an example of a completed *Family Name*.

Construction Paper Decoration

Therapy Needs: Connection (relationship development)

Level: Child and adolescents

Materials: Construction paper, string, art decorations, scissors, and glue

Modality: Individual, family, and group

Introduction

Construction Paper Decoration helps the therapist increase connection and relationship development with the child. It also helps children feel more

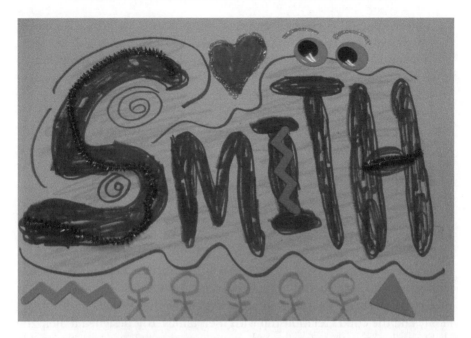

Figure 16.1 Family Name Example.

comfortable and less anxious in interacting with others. The child and the therapist participate in a constructive and expressive play intervention designed to focus on thinking about another person and doing something nice for that person. It also presents the opportunity to work on fine motor and executive functioning skills.

Instructions

1 The therapist explains to the child that they will be creating things for each other out of construction paper and other materials.
2 Construction paper, string, aluminum foil, or any other appropriate materials can be used in this intervention.
3 The child and therapist make items out of the chosen materials to give to the other person. The items are decorative items the other person can wear such as rings, hats, necklaces, bracelets, glasses, crowns, ties, belts, pins, etc.
4 Once an object has been made, the person who made it physically places it on the other person as a gift.

5 The child and therapist can make several things for each other and completely decorate the other person.
6 The play intervention continues until the child and therapist have finished making everything they want to create for the other person.
7 It is recommended to have a mirror present so the child can see themselves wearing the different items the therapist has placed on them.

Rationale

This play therapy technique provides an opportunity to work on connection and relationship development with the child. It involves components of thinking about another person, attuning to that person, and doing something nice for another person. It is important that the process be reciprocal; the therapist should make items and physically place them on the child, and the child should make items and physically place them on the therapist. If the child is uncomfortable with the therapist physically placing the items on the child, the therapist can hand the items to the child. This play technique can also be taught to parents to complete with their child at home. It can also be implemented by the therapist as a family play intervention.

All Around Me

Therapy Needs: Connection (relationship development), assessment, and family issues

Level: Child and adolescent

Materials: Miniatures

Modality: Individual

Introduction

All Around Me is designed to help increase connection and relationship development and help children think about and express positive sentiment about their family members. It also serves as an assessment intervention that helps the therapist learn more about the child and the child's family members and relationships. There is a symbolic component in this intervention where the child is asked to select miniatures to represent each person in their family. It is important to note that some children may struggle with symbolism. The therapist should try to be aware of this before implementing this intervention.

Instructions

1 The therapist explains to the child that they are going to play a game using miniatures.
2 The child picks a miniature to represent each person in their family.
3 The child sits on the floor and places the miniatures around themselves, so the miniatures are surrounding the child with each miniature facing the child.
4 The child then turns and faces each miniature one at a time and tells the therapist who the miniature represents and tells the therapist something positive about that family member. If the child cannot think of anything positive, they can say anything they like about the family member.
5 The therapist can also ask questions about each family member trying to help the child expand on talking about each family member.
6 The play intervention ends once the child has discussed each family member.

Rationale

This play technique works on connection and relationship development specifically in regard to family relationships. It is important that the therapist listen to the child and provide the child space to share whatever they want about each of their family members. The therapist can also ask questions about each family member as the child is sharing about that particular family member. Many children will likely not share much information about their family members, so the therapist can look for opportunities to ask questions. This play technique can be repeated several times in several different sessions with the therapist. Parents can participate in this play technique with their child in session but are not expected to complete the intervention at home. Most parents will not have a miniature collection to be able to conduct this technique at home. One variation that parents could do at home is to have the child draw something to represent each person in their family.

Guess Touches

Therapy Needs: Connection (relationship development) and sensory processing

Level: Child

Materials: Several tactile objects

Modality: Individual

Introduction

This play therapy intervention works on improving connection and relationship development and addresses sensory processing needs. *Guess Touches* works on helping children become more comfortable with connection through physical touch. It also addresses sensory processing issues related to touch (tactile) needs. Therapists should fully explain this play intervention to the child before beginning, especially to confirm that the child is comfortable with closing their eyes and experiencing touch/tactile sensation. It is essential to acquire the child's consent before implementing any intervention that includes touch. The therapist should explain and demonstrate on themselves so the child understands what will be happening.

Instructions

1 The therapist explains to the child that they will be playing a game using several different items and touching them to each other's skin.
2 The therapist displays all of the objects that may be used (typically around ten objects). The child should look at the objects and touch each one to see how it feels. The therapist should ask the child which of the objects feels the best (most satisfying).
3 The therapist instructs the child to close their eyes and the therapist is going to touch some part of the child's skin with one of the objects. This is done very quickly, and the therapist should touch the child on an arm, nose, ear, etc. nothing that would be too invasive or personal.
4 The therapist will then tell the child to open their eyes and the child has to tell the therapist which object was used and where the object touched them on the skin.

5 The therapist will go through approximately 5–6 objects. Once the therapist has used the objects, the child and therapist can switch roles. They can keep playing the game switching back and forth until the child is no longer interested.

6 Some examples of objects that can be used include a feather, a cotton ball, a Kleenex, a piece of material, ribbon, sandpaper, buttons, a pipe cleaner, a paint brush, a stuffed animal, a LEGO, etc.

Rationale

This play therapy technique focuses on connection and relationship development and sensory needs, especially in regard to becoming comfortable with touch sensation. This play technique can be played repeatedly with new objects being selected. The therapist should try to think of as many objects as they can to use in the game (the more variety, the more interesting the game will be). If the child is not comfortable with the game concept or becomes uncomfortable at any point, the therapist should not continue with the intervention. The play technique can be taught to parents and parents can play the technique at home with their child. Whether in session with the therapist or at home with parents, it is important to be sensitive to the sensory comfort level of the child with implementing this intervention.

Here Comes the Candy

Therapy Needs: Connection (relationship development), social engagement, and anxiety reduction

Level: Child

Materials: Candy

Modality: Individual, and group

Introduction

Here Comes the Candy works on connection and relationship development as well as sensory processing issues especially related to helping children become more aware of themselves, the space around them, and others. Candy is used as a guide for completing sensory based (proprioceptive and vestibular) activities. The therapist should make sure the child eats candy and discover some favorite candies. The therapist should also make sure the child is not on any special restriction or diet. If the child does not eat candy, then many things can be substituted such as stickers or small toys as long as it is something the child enjoys.

Instructions

1 The therapist explains to the child that they will be playing several games and the child will have a chance to receive a piece of candy as each activity is finished.
2 The therapist should pick one of the child's favorite candies, such as M&Ms (it is best to use a candy that has multiple pieces).
3 The therapist will explain they are going to do various activities and at the end of each activity the child will get a piece of candy.
4 Activities are short and focused on connecting with another person and addressing sensory related needs.
5 The therapist introduces an activity and explains how it is done. The therapist and child both complete the activity and then the child receives a piece of candy. The therapist then introduces the next activity. The therapist will want several activities to compete, approximately 10–12.

Rationale

This technique works on connection, relationship development, body awareness, and vestibular and proprioceptive sensory processing. The child and therapist are connecting in a playful way through the activities. The child is also working on proprioceptive and vestibular sensory processing needs though the activities which are selected for this purpose. Candy is used but an alternative can also be implemented. If candy is used, it is important to select a candy such as M&Ms or Skittles, so one piece can be given after each activity. Some of the activities will go quickly. The therapist can also repeat activities if it is something the child enjoys. The play technique can be taught to parents to do at home.

Example Activities for Here Comes the Candy

- Spin around in a circle
- Give yourself a tight hug

- Do some jumping jacks
- Act like you are flying around the room
- Make your body into your favorite animal
- Hold hands and spin around the room
- Play patty cake
- Skip around the room
- Roll yourself in to a ball
- Hit a balloon back and forth
- Do some wall roles
- Hop around the room
- Bend down and touch your toes
- Balance on one foot
- Play the hand stack game
- Dance together

Hats and Masks

Therapy Needs: Connection (relationship development) and social engagement

Level: Child

Materials: Various hats and masks

Modality: Individual

Introduction

Hats and Masks is a fun and interactive play therapy intervention for children that can be easily implemented for autistic and neurodivergent children. It includes a reciprocal element that helps children improve relationship and connection with others. It also involves paying attention to others and having fun together. The implementation is typically non-invasive, and children respond positively.

Instructions

1 The therapist explains to the child they are going to play a game using several different hats and masks.

2 This play intervention is usually done in a play therapy room but can be implemented in any setting if the therapist provides several hats and masks and has access to a mirror.
3 The therapist presents several different hats and masks to choose from and the therapist and child take turns placing different hats and masks on each other (creating a "look" for each other) and then looking in a mirror to see how they look.
4 The therapist and child each choose the hat and mask they want the other person to wear and place that hat and mask on the other person. It is important that each person put the hat and mask on the other person, this process works on improving connection.
5 It is also important to have a mirror close by so when the hats and masks are put on, the child can see themselves.
6 The child and therapist can play this intervention several times choosing several different hat and mask combinations for each other.
7 The play technique can be expanded by seeing what other objects in the playroom can be turned into hats or masks and/or using other dress up items.

Rationale

This play therapy technique works primarily on connection and relationship development, especially in the areas of attuning to another person and interacting with others. It is important that the intervention is reciprocal; the therapist should place hats and masks on the child, and the child should place hats and masks on the therapist. This provides opportunity for the child to pay attention and be aware of others. It also provides opportunity for both child and therapist to join together in the fun and silliness of the intervention. The play technique can be taught to parents and parents are instructed to play the technique with their child at home several times throughout the week. If parents do not have a hat/mask collection, they can vary the intervention using other objects around the house that could be used as hats or masks.

Tell Me About Your Family

Therapy Needs: Connection (relationship development) and assessment

Level: Child and adolescent

Materials: Sand tray, and miniatures

Modality: Individual

Introduction

Autistic and neurodivergent children and adolescents may have a difficult time connecting with others even in their family relationships. *Tell Me About your Family* works on increasing positive expression and connection with a child's family members. The therapist should be aware of the symbolism involved in this intervention (miniatures are chosen by the child to represent members of their family) and the sensory element of the sand (sand trays are typically used) and make sure the child is comfortable with both before beginning.

Instructions

1 The therapist explains to the child that they will be completing an activity using a sand tray and miniatures.
2 The therapist should make sure the child is comfortable working in the sand. The child may not like the sand, have a sensory issue, or may have an allergy. If the sand will not work, an alternative tray can be used such as beans, rice, or confetti. It is also possible to simply use the miniatures and no trays.
3 The therapist instructs the child to select a miniature to represent each person in their family and place the miniatures in the sand tray (wherever and however they want to place them in the sand tray).
4 After the child is finished, the therapist asks the child to share who each miniature represents and tell something about that family member.
5 The therapist can also ask questions about the family members.
6 The therapist may have to help the child choose miniatures and help the child talk about their family members. If a child is having trouble selecting miniatures, then the therapist could ask questions such as "What does your mom like to do?" or "Does your brother like computers?" The therapist could help the child select a miniature based on the child's answer.
7 After the child has finished the sand tray and the sand tray has been discussed, the therapist can take a picture (with the child's permission) of the sand tray and the child can take the picture home and share the picture with their family.

Rationale

This play therapy technique works on connection and relationship development especially related to family relationships. It also serves as an assessment intervention providing opportunity for the therapist to learn more about the child and their family. The play technique can be done several times in several different sessions with the therapist (the child may have new things to share each time). It is unlikely that this play intervention will be taught to parents and implemented at home, as most parents will not have a sand tray or a collection of miniatures. The child is able to take a picture home and can share the picture with their family.

Write and Move

Therapy Needs: Connection (relationship development), regulation, and sensory processing

Level: Child and adolescent

Materials: Paper, and markers

Modality: Individual

Introduction

Write and Move is a play therapy intervention that incorporates sensory processing with relationship development. This play intervention is designed to work on physical connection between the child and another person as well as potentially address one or more of the eight sensory processing areas: sight, smell, taste, hearing, touch, vestibular, proprioceptive, and interoceptive.

Instructions

1 The therapist explains to the child that they will be creating and acting out a poem together.
2 The poem will focus on the eight sensory areas. The therapist may begin by briefly explaining the eight sensory processing areas.
3 The therapist and child work together to create an eight line poem.
4 Each line represents a different sensory area.

5 The therapist and child write the poem and create a movement to go with each line of the poem.

6 The movements should try to connect the child and therapist physically.

7 After the poem has been written and the movements have been decided, the therapist and child will read the poem and act out the movements together.

The poem should follow the following script:

> I see... I hear... I smell... I taste... I feel... I Move... I Also Move... My body...

Rationale

This play therapy technique works on connection and relationship development by having the child work with the therapist in creating a poem and movements. This play technique also works on regulation and sensory processing needs in one or all of the eight sensory areas. It can be easily taught to parents to complete at home. The parent and child can be encouraged to create several different sensory poems at home and during the next session, show the therapist some they have created. It is important that the movements that are created be sensitive to what the child can do physically. Ideally the movements would connect the child with the therapist and/or parent. If this level of contact is not comfortable for the child and/or a physically connecting movement cannot be thought of, the movement can be anything the child and therapist do at the same time. This play intervention involves a level of physical touch. The therapist will want to make sure the child is comfortable with the physical touch (demonstrate) before implementing the intervention.

Sample Poem with Movement Idea

I see the light through these glasses (put glasses on each other and look at the light together)

I hear the drum (one person holds the drum, the other person beats the drum)

I smell the essential oil spray (one person sprays in the air and they both hop up in the air to smell it)

I taste this piece of candy (each person hands the other person a piece of candy to eat)

I feel this flow ring (the two people holds hands and let a flow ring move up and down their arms)

I Move around with other people (both people holds hands and spin around the room)

I Also Move up and down (each person bends down to touch their toes and comes back up and gives each other a high five)

My body feels a lot of ways (each person takes a turn giving the other person a hand massage)

You, Me, and LEGO

Therapy Needs: Connection (relationship development) and social navigation

Level: Child and adolescent

Materials: Several LEGO bricks (regular or Duplo depending on the age of the child). Off brand of bricks can also be used.

Modality: Individual, and group

Introduction

Many autistic and neurodivergent children and adolescents respond positively to playing with LEGO bricks. This play therapy intervention incorporates brick play (a form of constructive play) and provides the opportunity for children to focus on their family members and practice working with another person to complete a task.

Instructions

1 The therapist explains to the child that they will be completing an activity that involves working with LEGO bricks.
2 The therapist and child begin by each one building something out of the bricks.
3 The therapist instructs the child that they can build anything they want but whatever they build, it has to be something that would be in a family.
4 The therapist also builds something that would be in a family.

5 Once the therapist and child are finished, each one should share what they built and how it can be found in a family.
6 The therapist then instructs the child that they must work together and combine what each one has created and make one object
7 The new combined object also must be something that would be found in a family.
8 More bricks can be added in the joining together phase, and after the therapist and child are finished, each one can talk about what they made together and discuss the process of working together to create something.

Rationale

You, Me, and LEGO works on connection, relationship development, and social navigation related to cooperation and working with others to complete a task. The therapist should have a significant LEGO brick supply available to complete this play therapy technique and the therapist may want to limit the individual creation time to 10–15 minutes. It is important that the therapist and child work together to combine their creations. The therapist should not do all the work, nor should the therapist let the child do all the work; it should be a collaborative approach. The therapist should spend some time talking to the child about what it feels like to work with someone else and have someone else share and implement their own ideas. The therapist might ask the child about how they felt when they had to work with others to accomplish something.

Family Bubbles

Therapy Needs: Connection (relationship development) and social navigation

Level: Child and adolescent

Materials: None

Modality: Family, and group

Introduction

Children and adolescents and their family members may need to work on better relationship connection and developing positive interactions. *Family*

Bubbles is a play intervention that works on increasing relationship development. In addition, there are some social navigation elements which include having the family participate together in a playful and interacting game.

Instructions

1 The therapist explains to the family that they will be playing a game together to work on connection.
2 The therapist explains that the family members are going to pair up and hold both hands with their partner. For example, if there were six family members, there would be three pairs.
3 The therapist will ask the family members to begin walking around the room while holding hands with their partner.
4 The pair cannot touch any other family pair, if they do touch another family pair then they both "pop" and they have to sit out until only one or no family pair remains.
5 The therapist should periodically change the instructions for the family pairs such as instructing them to hop around the room, skip around the room, walk in slow motion around the room, or move quickly around the room.
6 This intervention works best when there are enough family members to for at least three pairs. The therapist can also participate if needed (if there is an odd number of family members).
7 If there is only a couple of family pairs, the therapist can participate by moving around and trying to run into the pairs while the pairs work together to try and avoid the therapist.

Rationale

This play therapy intervention works on improving connection and relationship development as well as social navigation awareness related to working with another person and joint attention. It is designed as a family intervention but can also be used in groups, especially social/relational focused groups. The therapist will want to make the play intervention fun and positive and focus on the experience not a competition to see who can win. The intervention can be played repeatedly with the pairs switching to another family member so the child experiences being in a pair with each of their family members. Parents can implement this game at home with their family and play periodically between sessions.

Hula Hoop Exchange

Therapy Needs: Connection (relationship development), social awareness, and sensory processing

Level: Child and adolescent

Materials: Two hula hoops

Modality: Individual, family, and group

Introduction

Autistic and neurodivergent children and adolescents may have needs related to participating in a reciprocal way with others whether through an activity, a conversation, or in play. This play therapy intervention addresses increasing relationship with another person, working with another person in a reciprocal capacity, and sensory processing in the areas of vestibular and proprioceptive experience.

Instructions

1 The therapist explains to the child that they will be playing several interactive games using hula hoops.
2 The therapist and child stand about 4–5 feet from each other facing each other.
3 The therapist and child each hold a hula hoop in their right hands. When the therapist says "Go" the therapist and child will roll their hula hoops to the other person to catch. This goes back and for the several times.
4 Another play intervention involves the therapist and child each holding a hula hoop on their right hand and when the therapist says "Go" the therapist and child will each gently toss their hula hoop to the other person to catch. This goes back and forth several times.
5 An additional intervention involves the hula hoops being placed on the floor beside each other.
6 The therapist and child each stand in one of the hula hoops.
7 When the therapist says "Switch" the therapist and child will jump into the other persons hula hoop. This goes back and forth several times.
8 The therapist should demonstrate each hula hoop game before implementing with the child. Each hula hoop game can be played several

minutes, and the child can be given an opportunity to think of other connecting hula hoop games.

Rationale

Hula Hoop Exchange works on increasing relationship connection, social awareness, and sensory processing in the areas of vestibular and proprioceptive. The therapist should be aware of the child's physical abilities and adjust each hula hoop game accordingly. The therapist will also want to make sure that nothing is attempted at a level that could injure the child. This play therapy intervention can be taught to parents to play at home with their child. *Hula Hoop Exchange* can also be implemented in a group format.

Let's Stick Together

Therapy Needs: Connection (relationship development), social awareness, and sensory processing

Level: Child and adolescent

Materials: None

Modality: Family, and group

Introduction

Autistic and neurodivergent children and adolescents may need help in working on sensory processing issues, body awareness, interactions with others, as well as connection skills. *Let's Stick Together* is a fun and engaging play therapy intervention that incorporates movement to work on the above mentioned needs. It is mainly designed to be implemented in a family setting but is also applicable to group work, especially social/relational focused groups.

Instructions

1 The therapist explains to the family that they will be playing a game together that works on increasing relationship connection.

2 The therapist explains that each person in the family will begin by moving around the room in a certain way that the therapist decides. After a few minutes the therapist will state a new way to move around the room. The moving around the room can be things like walk around the room, skip around the room, hop around the room, walk backward around the room, act silly as you walk around the room, etc.

3 Each family member moves around the room as instructed and tries to avoid the other family members.

4 If two people touch in any way then they are now stuck together and they continue moving around the room together, pretending they are physically stuck to each other.

5 Once two family members have gotten stuck together, they will purposefully try to catch (stick to) other family members.

6 Moving around the room in different ways continues until the whole family (or group) is stuck together.

7 Once the whole family is stuck together, the therapist can spend a few minutes having the whole family try to move around the room in different ways with them all stuck together. The therapist can also participate if more people are needed.

Rationale

This play intervention helps children work on strengthening relationship connection especially with their family members. It also works on social awareness and sensory processing in the areas of vestibular, proprioceptive, and tactile (touch). This game can be played repeatedly with family members taking turns deciding what the movements will be. It is important to keep the intervention fun and noncompetitive. The therapist should emphasis that the family focus on being playful and enjoying the game together.

17
Anxiety Reduction, Sensory Integration, and Regulation Interventions

AutPlay Model of Dysregulation

In AutPlay Therapy, regulation is broadly defined and applied to the self. It is considered the pursuit of a desired system state that provides for emotions, behavior, cognitions, sensory areas, and body movement to be aligned and manageable when faced with a challenging situation which is creating a dysregulated reaction. Regulation must be understood in conjunction with dysregulation, which is defined as a state of being where a person's system has become overwhelmed with an inability to organize and navigate their emotions, sensory areas, behavior, cognitions, and reactions. It is not premeditated and is usually a very upsetting experience for the individual.

The following presents the AutPlay Therapy model of dysregulation. The child's dysregulation can be visualized like water in a glass, the water can rise (increase in dysregulation) or decline (decrease in dysregulation or regulation increasing). Many things can cause dysregulation to increase in a child – social struggles, sensory struggles, unexpected changes, anxiety, new situations, physical issues, inability to modulate emotions, etc. When the water (dysregulation) gets to the top of the glass and overflows, this is the stereotypical dysregulation meltdown.

Dysregulation creates inconsistent behavior – a child may accomplish something one day that seems very challenging and have a negative behavior reaction to something the next day that seems very easy. These "behavior reactions" (which is what usually gets the attention of others) will depend on the level of dysregulation in the child (water in the glass). Some level of dysregulation is usually present in a neurodivergent child. When it reaches a level the child can no longer contain, outward behavior happens, and the child feels like they are in an out of control state with little to no ability to regulate. The dysregulated state and accompanying behavior is often

DOI: 10.4324/9781003207610-18

mislabeled and misunderstood. The dysregulated behavior is not pre-planned or pre-meditated on the part of the child. It is not the child trying to get attention, trying to get out of something, or personally trying to "get" an adult. The child is likely feeling extremely unsettled, scared, and out of control.

When a child is in a full dysregulated state, the best approach is to let the child calm down in a quiet, safe, private place. Consequences will not change dysregulated behavior. A preventative approach needs to be implemented. Identifying, addressing, and improving the areas that are creating the dysregulation is critical. Helping children learn about their own regulatory system is one of the most beneficial and empowering things that an adult can do for a neurodivergent child.

Many interventions and activities can help children regulate, understand their body's regulation and dysregulation processes, and build up their regulatory system. Most involve sensory and movement interventions, expressive art techniques, and traditional relaxation but each child will be different regarding what helps them regulate their system. It is important for the adults around the child to understand what is happing to the child, do not label it as misbehavior, recognize the discomfort and often fear the child is experiencing, do not punish a dysregulated state, apply co-regulation, support and empower the child, and work to prevent dysregulation through sustainable processes. The key is the child's ability to regulate. This is something that often takes time, self-understanding, support, co-facilitation and regulation, and caring adults who are willing to walk through the process with the child.

Movement and Whole Brain Activation

In AutPlay Therapy many regulation and sensory processing interventions are movement play based. It is well understood that children are not biologically designed to sit in one place and think critically. Children like to move, explore, and play. Often children will engage with the world through playful action and movement. The play therapy process should be a space for movement expression with age-appropriate, action-oriented techniques or the ability for non-directive movement in the playroom. Having movement tools in the playroom communicates that movement play preferences are valued and supported and for those children who prefer this type of play, it gives them their play outlet for addressing their needs.

Some children may seek or prefer movement more than other children. This can take on many "looks" from bouncing on an exercise ball while they talk, to playing an animal movement game, to large full body sensory focused movements. Movement strengthens both the prefrontal cortex (which is involved in executive functioning) and the hippocampus (which plays a key role in memory and learning). In this way, movement supports a child's ability to regulate, think creatively, make decisions, focus, understand their body system, and retrieve key information.

Physical activity also increases levels of serotonin, norepinephrine, dopamine, and endorphins that support emotional well-being, motivation and response to stress. Strong evidence supports the connection between movement, regulation, and learning. Evidence from imaging sources, anatomical studies, and clinical data shows that moderate movement activities can enhance cognitive processing. Whole brain movement means activating both the left and right side of the brain to function as a whole. When we use both sides of our brain instead of just the left or right, we are able to apply both logical thinking and creative thinking to the same problem. There are numerous benefits to implementing whole brain movement-based play interventions. Some of the benefits include higher levels of thinking, increased creativity, better understanding of emotions, decreased anxiety, regulation, and the ability to utilize all processes of thought.

Malher-Moran (2018) stated that the right side of the brain is generally responsible for nonverbal (bodily) communication and for creative processes. It is also responsible for play and autobiographical expression. The left side of the brain is connected to logic, language, and organization. Children, especially young children, are generally right-brain dominant. They express through play and creative processes. By allowing the right side of the brain to be active in therapy through movement, play, and action, a therapist can meet the child at the developmentally appropriate level. Furthering the process with age-appropriate verbal reflection assists in integrating both sides of the brain.

Malher-Moran (2018) furthered that the lower part of the brain governs automatic responses, including the fight, flight, or freeze response to danger. The higher, outer part of the brain is involved with judgment, problem-solving, and thinking through situations. The higher, thinking part of the brain has limited capacity when the lower brain is activated. Not feeling safe, experiencing new situations, and/or having a history of trauma are just a few ways the lower brain may be activated. Regulation of the lower brain generally comes from interventions involving the senses. Smell, sound, body movements, grounding, play, expressive art, and breathwork might all be used to assist a child with lower brain regulation.

Before implementing any structured play therapy interventions to address regulation and sensory goals, the therapist should have a clear understanding of the child's therapy needs and the child's play preferences. Interventions should be chosen that address the therapy needs and align with the child's play preferences. In AutPlay Therapy, typical regulation and sensory related play interventions are simple brain based, sensory, and movement interventions which focus on one or more of the following: understanding of the self and internal systems, whole brain activation, midline crossing, "resetting" thoughts, decreasing anxiety and dysregulation, creating a calm and relaxed state, processing sensory areas, and executive functioning.

Midline Mirror Moves

Therapy Needs: Regulation, sensory integration, anxiety reduction, executive functioning, and connection

Level: Child and adolescent

Materials: None

Modality: Individual, group, and family

Introduction

Autistic and neurodivergent children and adolescents often need help with regulating their system. There is a whole myriad of things that can accompany each day that dysregulates the child's system. This play therapy intervention is a simple game that helps children regulate, reduce anxiety, and increase connection and relationship development. This play intervention involves movement play and it requires no materials. It can be easily implemented in any setting.

Instruction

1 The therapist explains to the child that they will be playing a game where they mirror each other's movements.
2 The therapist and child stand across from each other.
3 Typically the therapist will go first, and the child will mirror the therapist.
4 The therapist instructs the child that they will do all the moves the therapist does like a mirror.

5 The therapist begins moving their hands, arms, legs, body in different ways and the child mimics the moves. The therapist should be sure to move slow enough that the child can keep up with the moves.

6 The therapist is purposeful in making several midline crossing moves. These are moves that cross the right and left hemispheres of the brain and thus activate the whole brain. Any move that is crossing over body parts from one side to the other is usually an effective midline crossing move. If the therapist is unsure what a midline crossing move would be, they can do a quick internet search.

7 The therapist will lead for a few minutes and then the child can have a turn leading and the therapist follows the child's moves.

8 The therapist and child can switch back and forth every few minutes.

9 The game continues until the child is no longer interested in playing.

Rationale

A common therapy goal involves helping children regulate and reduce anxiety levels. *Midline Mirror Moves* is a play therapy intervention that addresses these needs. Midline crossing movements have also been shown to help with sensory processing and increasing focus and attention. The intervention is implemented in a playful and engagement way that also helps increase connection between the therapist and child. This play intervention can be easily taught to parents and the parent and child can play the game at home.

Running All Ways

Therapy Needs: Regulation, sensory integration, and anxiety reduction

Level: Child and adolescent

Materials: None

Modality: Individual, family, and group

Introduction

This play therapy intervention is designed to help children regulate their system, improve sensory processing needs (proprioceptive and vestibular), and reduce anxiety. It is a simple game that can be played in any setting and requires no materials. It is a movement-based play activity that asks the child to run in different ways. The therapist should be mindful of any physical needs the child may have that would prevent them from engaging in this intervention.

Instruction

1 The therapist explains to the child that they are going to do an activity together that involves running in a variety of ways.
2 The therapist and child each pick a spot on the floor where they are going to try and stay while they are running (running in place). Once the spot is decided, a piece of tape can be put on the floor to mark the spot.
3 The therapist will begin by calling out different types of styles of running and both the therapist and child will do that type of running. For example, the therapist might say, "Run fast." The therapist and child would both run in place fast (trying to stay in their spot) until the therapist called out a different style.
4 The therapist will call out a different style of running after about 10–20 seconds, styles can also be repeated.
5 The therapist will be the lead for a few minutes, then the child can have a turn at being the lead and calling out different running styles.
6 Some examples of running styles include running fast, in slow motion, easy jog, like an animal (a specific animal can be named), like you are scared, silly, on your tippy toes, bending over, with your hands on your head, etc.
7 The therapist and child switch back and forth on who calls out the running styles and continue to play the game until the child is no longer interested.

Rationale

Running All Ways is a simple play therapy intervention but can help address a variety of therapy needs. The primary focus would be on giving the child an activity they could do to help regulate their system, reduce anxiety, and address sensory processing needs. The running styles can and should be fun, silly, and constantly changing to keep the activity engaging. For an added element, the therapist could include props like trying to bounce a ball while you are running or holding a balloon on your head while you are running. This play intervention can be easily taught to parents and implemented at home.

Backward Moves

Therapy Needs: Regulation, sensory integration, and anxiety reduction

Level: Child and adolescent

Materials: None

Modality: Individual, family, and group

Introduction

Backward moves is a movement-based play therapy intervention that asks the child to do several different moves with all of them being done backwards. This play intervention activates the whole brain and helps address needs related to regulating, sensory processing, and anxiety reduction. It requires no materials and can be implemented in a variety of settings.

Instruction

1 The therapist explains to the child they will be doing a game together where they have to do several different moves, but they all have to be done backwards.
2 The therapist should have prepared a list of moves that they and the child can do such as walk, hop, dance, etc. backwards.
3 The therapist will begin by saying "let's walk around the room backwards." After around a minute the therapist will switch the move to something else such as "let's hop backwards around the room." The therapist will switch the move periodically.
4 After a few minutes, the child can lead out and suggest moves to do backwards.
5 The intervention does not have to be just movements. The therapist and child can also try to think about how to say a word backwards and how to write or draw something backwards.
6 Additional moves could include act like you are swimming backwards, act silly moving backwards, move in slow motion backwards, and crawl backwards.
7 The therapist and child keep playing the game until the child is no longer interested.

Rationale

This play therapy intervention is a simple movement-based game that can help children with regulation needs, sensory issues related to proprioceptive and vestibular areas, and anxiety reduction. It provides the child with a tool they can use to help them that is executed in a fun playful experience. The intervention can be done with music playing in the background if the child would prefer music. This intervention can be taught to parents and played at home.

Fast and Slow Balloons

Therapy Needs: Regulation, sensory integration, and anxiety reduction

Level: Child and adolescent

Materials: Balloon

Modality: Individual and group

Introduction

Many children have issues with regulating their system and understanding the concepts of how their system feels regulated versus dysregulated. Fast and slow or up and down play interventions can help children better understand their body systems and how regulated/dysregulated feels. This play therapy intervention utilizes balloons in a game format that helps address regulation and sensory needs and helps children learn about regulation processes.

Instruction

1 The therapist explains to the child that they will be playing a game using balloons.
2 The therapist or child blows up a balloon and ties it off.
3 The therapist and child position themselves across from each other with about 5–10 feet between them.
4 The therapist explains that they are going to be hitting the balloon back and forth and they are going to change the speed periodically. The

therapist will say "fast" or "slow" and both of them will hit the balloon as instructed.

5 The therapist begins by saying "slow" and the therapist and child hit the balloon back and forth slowly. If the balloon gets out of control, the person will slowly go get the balloon and continue to hit is slowly.

6 After a bit of time the therapist will say "fast" and immediately the therapist and child begin hitting the balloon fast. If the balloon gets out of control (and it will), the person gets the balloon as fast as they can and continues to hit it.

7 Periodically the therapist will change the speed, the speed changes can even happen quickly back and forth.

8 After some time, the therapist can ask the child if they want to be the one who calls out the speed changes. The therapist and child can take turns calling out the speeds.

9 If appropriate, the therapist can process with the child how it feels to shift from slow to fast and how it feels in their body (system). The therapist can make the connection to how their body shifts from regulated to dysregulated.

10 The therapist and child continue to play until the child is no longer interested.

Rationale

Fast and Slow Balloons utilizes a common fast/slow up/down process in helping children regulate and better understand their regulatory system. The process can also be done utilizing musical instruments or simply running in place. Therapists should be aware of any balloon related allergies and/or any fears a child might have about balloons before introducing this intervention. It can be taught to parents to play at home with their child.

Bubble Pop Brain Blast

Therapy Needs: Regulation, sensory integration, anxiety reduction, and executive functioning

Level: Child and adolescent

Materials: Bubbles

Modality: Individual, family, and group

Introduction

This play therapy intervention uses bubble blowing in a fun, fast, and silly game that helps address dysregulation issues, sensory processing (proprioception), and anxiety reduction. It should be implemented in a space that provides for some movement.

Instruction

1 The therapist explains to the child that they are going to play a game that involves blowing and popping bubbles.
2 The therapist will begin as the bubble blower and will blow bubbles while the child tries to pop them before they touch the ground.
3 There is an added twist – while the child is trying to pop the bubbles, they must also be naming off things from a pre-chosen subject like animals, fruits, sports, feelings, etc. The popping and naming should be happening concurrently.
4 The therapist's role is to keep popping the bubbles and encouraging the child to pop and name.
5 This is a challenging whole brain activation activity. It would be highly unlikely that someone would be able to pop all the bubbles before they hit the floor and be consistently naming off different things from a chosen subject. It ultimately becomes silly and that is the goal.
6 The therapist will want to clarify that it is not competitive and is just for fun.
7 After a few minutes the therapist and child can switch roles. The pre-chosen category can keep changing to whatever the therapist and child want it to be.
8 The therapist and child continue taking turns blowing the bubbles until the child no longer wants to play the intervention.

Rationale

This play therapy intervention helps address regulation needs, sensory processing work, and anxiety reduction. There is also an element of executive functioning involved. It is a playful interactive game and is easy to implement in any setting. The intervention can be taught to parents to play with their child at home.

Pool Noodle Sword Battle

Therapy Needs: Regulation, sensory integration, anxiety reduction, and executive functioning

Level: Child

Materials: Pool noodles

Modality: Individual

Introduction

Pool Noodle Sword Battle is a play therapy intervention that involves using pool noodles as swords. It also requires enough space to safely move around. This play intervention is designed to help children with dysregulation struggles, sensory processing needs, and anxiety reduction. It is a movement-based play intervention so the therapist should be mindful of the child's physical needs before implementing this intervention.

Instruction

1 The therapist shares with the child that they will be playing a game that involves using pool noodles as swords and they will be having a pool noodle sword battle (it is easiest to buy one pool noodle and cut it in half to make two swords).
2 The therapist and child each pick a pool noodle sword and the therapist explains that the child is going to learn some battle moves.
3 The therapist introduces simply hitting each other's sword back and forth in a typical sword battle fashion. The therapist then introduces the child to dunk and jump moves.
4 For the dunk move, the therapist will say "Dunk" and the child dunks down as the therapist moves their sword swiping toward the child's head (the therapist is deliberate to not actually hit the child in the head). For the jump move, the therapist says "Jump" and the child jumps as the therapist moves their sword swiping at the child's feet (again the therapist is deliberate to not actually hit the child's feet).
5 The therapist and child practice the dunk and jump moves for a few minutes.

6 The therapist then introduces the spin around move – spin to the left or spin to the right. The therapist will say the direction and spin and the child spins around and then keeps participating in the sword battle.

7 The therapist and child practice the spin move for a few minutes.

8 The therapist and child are now ready for a full battle. They will sword fight and periodically the therapist will call out one of the moves and the child will do the move. The therapist can even call out moves in a sequence.

9 For regulation purposes, it is important that the therapist call out different moves or combinations of moves regularly. The therapist and the child can also think of additional moves to add to the battle.

10 The therapist and child continue to play the intervention until the child is no longer interested.

Rationale

Pool Noodle Sword Battle is a fun and interactive game that helps children regulate, process sensory needs (proprioception), and reduce anxiety. The game can take many looks with different moves being added to the game. It is important that moves help activate the whole brain in order to get the regulation benefit. Pool noodles should be used as they are soft in case someone accidently gets hit. This play intervention can be taught to parents to implement at home with their child.

Punching Bag Moves

Therapy Needs: Regulation, sensory integration, anxiety reduction, and executive functioning

Level: Child

Materials: Punching bag

Modality: Individual

Introduction

This play therapy intervention utilizes some type of punching bag. It can be a standard punching bag or some type of bop bag. The punching bag is used to deliver a variety of movements that help regulate a child's system. This intervention focuses on helping children regulate, process sensory needs, and reduce anxiety levels. It is a movement-based intervention so the therapist should be mindful of any physical needs the child has and provide plenty of space to implement the intervention.

Instruction

1   The therapist explains to the child they will be doing an activity that uses a punching bag. It is helpful for the therapist to have some type of punching gloves available for children to wear if they desire this.
2   The therapist states they are going to be learning some punching bag moves.
3   The therapist begins by having the child punch the bag with their fists in a typical punching movement.
4   The therapist then introduces kicking the punching bag alternating the right and left feet.
5   The therapist then introduces kneeing the bag, again alternating between the right and left knees.
6   Finally, the therapist introduces a right or left spin around and then a punch or kick move.
7   The child practices each of the moves to become more familiar with them. Once the child is ready, the therapist will begin calling out different moves for the child to do. Th therapist can combine moves and can slow down or speed up the action.
8   The therapist and child can create additional moves and come up with unique moves.
9   The therapist and child continue to play the intervention until the child is no longer interested.

Rationale

Punching Bag Moves is designed to provide a fun activity children can do to help them regulate their system, address sensory processing needs, and reduce anxiety. Once the child learns the activity (if they have access to a punching bag), they can complete the intervention on their own anytime they feel it would benefit them. The intervention can be shared with parents so they can support the process at home.

Sensory Mandala

Therapy Needs: Sensory processing, regulation, and anxiety reduction

Level: Child and adolescent

Materials: Card stock or cardboard, markers, tape or glue, and a variety of sensory materials (tactile and olfactory).

Modality: Individual, family, and group

Introduction

Sensory Mandala play intervention provides children and adolescents the opportunity to engage in an expressive play activity that can help regulate their system, reduce anxiety, and address sensory processing needs. The child can create a sensory mandala on their own, as part of a group process, or in family work. The sensory element of a sensory mandala provides a unique blending of Jungian mandala creation with sensory processing technique.

Instruction

1　The therapist communicates to the child that they will be creating a sensory mandala
2　The therapist gives the child a copy of a mandala template (drawn circle) on a piece of card stock or cardboard. The child can also draw their own mandala circle outline.
3　Using a card stock instead of paper may be preferred, as some sensory mandalas become too heavy for regular paper.
4　The therapist displays several sensory related materials that the child can use in creating the mandala. The child is instructed to examine, touch, and smell all the items and choose the ones that feel the best to them. Sample sensory items include the following: Velcro, ribbon, sandpaper, buttons, beads, glitter, glitter glue, puffy stickers, pot pourri, feathers, burlap, cotton balls, pom poms, pipe cleaners, denim, material (various textures), essential oils, spices, dried pasta, and popsicle sticks.
5　The child is instructed that they can use markers or crayons and design and/or color anything in the mandala that they want, and they also need to use the sensory items selected and place them in the mandala. The sensory items can be glued or taped onto the mandala.

6 Before the child begins to create their sensory mandala, the therapist has the child position themselves in a comfortable way, take three deep breathes, and begin to relax. The child can then construct the sensory mandala as they choose.

7 The child creates the sensory mandala while the therapist observes.

8 Once the child has finished, the therapist can ask the child to share about their mandala, specifically what sensory items the child chose and why they chose those items. The child can spend time looking at the mandala and touching the different tactile items the child chose for their mandala. If the child chose any scented items, they can also spend time smelling the different items.

9 The therapist can discuss with the child that they can create mandalas anytime they would like to help with feeling calm or relaxed, and the child can keep all the mandalas that they create as regulation reminders.

Rationale

Mandala work, from a Jungian perspective, can be a calming, reflective, and relaxing experience. Adding the sensory component enhances the sensory processing element for the child. The *Sensory Mandala* play therapy intervention offers an activity that is more expressive for children who respond to and enjoy expressive play and activities. Children can create a sensory mandala anytime on their own when they feel like they need a regulating activity, or it can be part of a sensory processing break that has been established for the child. Parents can learn about the intervention and support the process at home.

Sensory Rock Play

Therapy Needs: Sensory processing and regulation

Level: Child and adolescent

Materials: Rocks, tub or soapy water, and sharpies or paint

Modality: Individual and group

Introduction

This play therapy intervention incorporates art and creation with sensory processing and regulation. This intervention is especially beneficial for children and adolescents who need tactile, visual, and olfactory sensory experiences. The therapist should prepare a tube of soapy water. The therapist can have several small-to-medium sized rocks prepared for the activity, or the therapist and the child can collect the rocks together. This intervention can be a little messy. The therapist should prepare an appropriate space for water and paint.

Instruction

1 The therapist will explain to the child that they will be painting rocks.
2 The therapist will have a tub of soapy water, a few rocks (5–6), and paints or sharpies ready to go.
3 The therapist explains they will begin by washing the rocks to remove any dirt. The child should wash the rocks and then place them on a dry towel (it may take a while for the rocks to dry enough to paint. If there is little time available for this activity, the therapist could provide a hair dryer to blow dry the rocks).
4 Once the rocks are dry, the child should make sure their hands are clean and dry and they can begin decorating and painting the rocks.
5 The child is instructed that they can use the sharpies or paints to design the rocks however they want. The theme of the rocks is what feels good, calm, and relaxing, so the painting of the rocks should reflect these ideas for the child.
6 Once the child has finished designing the rocks, they can take the rocks home and keep them to use as regulation reminders.

Rationale

Sensory Rock Play provides the child or adolescent with a tactile experience of washing the rocks in soapy water. The therapist can experiment with different scents for the soap. The therapist can also provide scented markers or paints for a more olfactory experience. The coloring of the rocks provides a visual experience and a regulating experience. The therapist will want to make sure the child associates the whole activity and especially the painted rocks with feeling good and regulated. This play intervention can be repeated multiple times with the child creating and collecting several rocks.

Ways We Cross the Room

Therapy Needs: Regulation, sensory processing, and anxiety reduction

Level: Child and adolescent

Materials: None

Modality: Individual and group

Introduction

Ways We Cross the Room is a simple interactive and playful intervention. It is designed to help children address regulation needs and sensory processing challenges. It is a movement-based play therapy intervention. The therapist will want to make sure there is plenty of space to complete the intervention.

Instruction

1 The therapist explains to the child that they are going to play a game where they cross the room in various ways.
2 The therapist and child position themselves on each side of the room.
3 The therapist begins by saying a way they both have to cross the room. For example, the therapist says. "We have to cross the room acting like our favorite animal." Both the therapist and child then cross the room moving like their favorite animal.
4 Once they are across the room, the child goes next and says a way they have to cross the room.
5 If the child cannot think of any way to cross the room, the therapist can provide options.
6 This continues several times until the child is no longer interested in playing the game.
7 The therapist should choose moves that cross the midline and activate the whole body to help address regulation and sensory needs. Some examples include hop on one foot, skip, crawl backwards, act silly, swinging your arms back and forth, with your body twisted like a pretzel, with your hands on your head, etc.

Rationale

This play therapy intervention provides children with a fun and interactive game that can help regulate their system and address sensory needs related to proprioceptive and vestibular needs. It can be played in any setting where there is enough space to do the movement. No materials are needed but props can be used such as balls to carry or bean bags to balance, etc. Parents can be taught the intervention to implement at home with their child.

One Color Picture

Therapy Needs: Regulation and anxiety reduction

Level: Child and adolescent

Materials: Paper and markers or crayons

Modality: Individual and group

Introduction

One Color Picture play intervention implements a traditional relaxation technique using a picture drawing concept. The intervention helps children regulate their system and reduce anxiety levels. It involves a level of progressive relaxation that might be challenging for some children. The therapist will want to monitor for this when implementing this intervention.

Instruction

1 The therapist explains to the child that they will be creating a picture that helps with regulating and relaxation.
2 The therapist gives the child a white piece of paper that they will draw on. The therapist also gives the child a box of markers or crayons.
3 The therapist explains to the child that the child is going to close their eyes and the therapist is going to have them imagine doing something that feels relaxing, calming, or fun.
4 Many children may not understand the feeling of calm or relaxed and may respond better to thinking about what they like to do, what feels good, and what feels fun.
5 The child closes their eyes and the therapist asks them to image something that makes them feel or think of being calm or relaxed or having fun. The therapist tells the child to think about the thing or place or situation and focus on doing that thing or being in that place. The therapist

tells the child to focus on the feeling of calm or having fun. Lastly, the therapist tells the child to image one color that goes with the place or situation and to visualize that color with the place and the feeling.

6 After the child has been in the visualization for a while (it should not take long), the therapist tells the child to open their eyes and find the color they saw and draw whatever comes to mind on their paper.

7 Once the child is done with the drawing, the therapist can ask the child to share about their experience and drawing.

8 The child can take the picture home and make a one color picture any time they want.

Rationale

This play therapy intervention uses a traditional relaxation technique (guided visualization) combined with an expressive art intervention. It is implemented to help children regulate their system and decrease anxiety. Some children may find this type of activity regulating while others may not like it. The therapist should monitor for the child's preferences and reaction. This play intervention can be taught to parents and implemented at home.

Hula Hoop Walk

Therapy Needs: Regulation and sensory processing

Level: Child

Materials: Large hula hoop

Modality: Individual and group

Introduction

Autistic and neurodivergent child may have issues with regulation and sensory needs and may respond positively to movement-based play. *Hula Hoop Walk* is a play therapy intervention that utilizes movement in a game play format. The intervention helps address regulation and sensory processing needs. The therapist will need to make sure there is a space big enough to place a large hula hoop on the floor and to be able to move around it. The therapist will need to make sure the child does not have any physical needs that would prevent them from participating.

Instruction

1 The therapist explains to the child that they will be playing a game using a hula hoop.
2 The therapist places a large hula hoop on the floor.
3 The therapist explains they are going to be doing different moves around and inside the hula hoop.
4 The therapist begins by saying they must walk around the hula hoop in a circle. Both the therapist and child then walk around the hula hoop and keep circling it until a new instruction is given.
5 After a short amount of time, the therapist might say, "now we must jump in and out of the hula hoop." Both the therapist and child then start jumping in and out of the hula hoop until a new move is stated.
6 The therapist should share a few moves and then ask the child if they want to give the moves. If the child does not want to or cannot think of anything then the therapist can continue.
7 Some additional moves include hopping around the hula hoop, holding hands while facing each other and walking around the hula hoop, walking backwards around the hula hoop. Walking around in slow motion, standing still in the hula hoop for 20 seconds, etc.
8 The intervention can continue to be played until the child is no longer interested.

Rationale

This play therapy intervention uses a hula hoop and movement-based play in a game format. It provides children with a playful way to help regulate their system and address sensory needs related to proprioception and vestibular areas. The instructions use one large hula hoop that the therapist and child share, but the therapist can use two hula hoops with each person having their own to use. Parents can be taught the intervention and play the game at home with their child.

10 Cloud Relaxation

Therapy Needs: Regulation and anxiety reduction

Level: Child and adolescent

Materials: Paper and a pencil

Modality: Individual and group

Introduction

10 Could Relaxation play intervention presents a simple visual guide for helping children and adolescents practice deep breathing. This process helps address regulating the system and reducing anxiety through deep breathing. Many children can benefit from deep breathing but often do not implement the practice in real application. Incorporating a visual guide helps ensure utilization and application.

Instruction

1 The therapist explains to the child they are going to practice some deep breathing by creating a guide on a piece of paper.
2 The therapist gives the child a piece of paper and instructs them to draw 10 clouds randomly on the paper.
3 The therapist then instructs the child to number the clouds randomly 1–10.
4 Once the 10 cloud paper is completed. The therapist will demonstrate the deep breathing guide.
5 The child is instructed to place their pencil on cloud one and take one deep breath.
6 The child then draws a line to cloud two and then takes two deep breathes. The child then draws a line to cloud three and takes three deep breathes. This continues until the child gets to cloud ten and takes ten deep breaths. At this point the child has completed the guide.
7 The therapist may need to explain the concept of taking a deep breath – inhale through the nose, hold for a couple of seconds, and then exhale through the mouth.
8 Once the guide has been completed, the therapist can ask the child how they feel and if they notice anything different after the deep breathing.
9 The therapist can emphasize with the child that they can create a 10 cloud guide anytime and do some deep breathing if they feel it will help them regulate.

Rationale

This play therapy intervention is basically teaching the child how to do deep breathing. It provides the child with a guide from start to finish for completing deep breathing. The guide is simple and can be completed by the child anytime – they only need access to a piece of paper and a pencil. This intervention can be taught to parents and they can support the process at home.

Sensory Likes and Dislikes

Therapy Needs: Sensory processing and regulation

Level: Individual and adolescent

Materials: Paper and a pencil

Modality: Individual and group

Introduction

Sensory Likes and Dislikes is a play therapy intervention that helps children and adolescents better identify what sensory needs they are experiencing and what sensory input can be comforting or pleasing to the child. This play intervention creates a visual reminder of positive techniques the child can implement when they are experiencing sensory dysregulation.

Instruction

1　On a piece of white paper, the child draws a picture of each of the following: a hand, a pair of lips, eyes, a nose, an ear, and the outline of a body.
2　On each one of the drawings, the child writes or draws things they like and do not like that correspond with each sense – touch (hand), taste (lips), sight (eyes), smell (nose), sound (ear), proprioceptive, vestibular, interception (body). If the child does not like to write or draw, they can tell the therapist and the therapist can write them down.
3　Once the child has finished, the therapist and child take each area, one at a time, and on the back side of the paper, write ideas, strategies, activities the child could do whenever they experience something related to that sense that feels uncomfortable or dysregulating. For example, in the eyes, bright sun is bothersome, and putting on sunglasses helps.
4　The therapist and child then role play and the child practices experiencing the sensory discomfort and implementing some of the activities that were written down for that area.
5　The therapist and child can discuss, and role play all six drawings.

Rationale

This play therapy intervention provides a playful and visual way for children to work on decreasing anxiety and dysregulation that is caused by sensory processing challenges. The therapist should have a basic understanding of what sensory challenges the child struggles with prior to completing this intervention. The therapist should be mindful of helping the child identify positive coping skills that they can implement when experiencing a sensory processing problem.

Coffee Filter Mandala (adapted from *Finding Meaning with Mandalas* by Tracy Turner-Bumberry, LPC, RPT-S)

Therapy Needs: Regulation and sensory processing

Level: Child and adolescent

Materials: Coffee filter, washable markers, small spray bottle of essential oil (preferably a scent the child likes), cardboard, table cloth or protective covering, black and white construction paper, and paper towels (for cleanup).

Modality: Individual and group

Introduction

This play therapy intervention incorporates an expressive art intervention with regulation and sensory processing. Children and adolescents with olfactory (smell) processing needs will enjoy this play intervention. The therapist should explore with the child or adolescent what scents they typically like before introducing this play intervention. The essential oil used should be a scent that is appealing to the child.

Instruction

1 The therapist explains to the child they will be making a mandala using coffee filters.
2 The therapist will place the coffee filter on top of a white piece of paper, which is on top of a piece of cardboard or card stock for extra support,

3 The therapist hands the child some washable markers and instructs them to create any type of design on the coffee filter. The therapist may want to remind the child that this picture will change quite a bit from its original form, so it may be better to create colors and shapes rather than an actual picture.
4 Once the child has finished, the therapist will hand the child a spray bottle of a selected essential oil.
5 The child is instructed to spray the coffee filter as little or as much as they desire. The therapist may want to suggest to the child to begin by spraying just a little and notice how the design begins to transform.
6 The therapist watches with the child as the coffee filter changes into an abstract creation and they notice the aroma of the essential oil.
7 If desired, the child can make additional coffee filter mandalas.
8 The therapist may follow up with some processing questions such as, "How did you notice your drawing changing while you were spraying it?" "How did you notice the spray scent as it was being sprayed on your drawing?" "How did it feel as you noticed the scent?" "Are there areas in your life you would like to spray away and start clean?" "Did you notice any feelings of calmness or relaxation while completing this activity?" and "When and where in your life could you complete more coffee filter mandalas?"

Rationale

Coffee Filter Mandala intervention provides a non-threatening process to explore regulation and sensory processing needs. The child or adolescent can make several mandalas using multiple essential oil sprays. If the child finds this intervention helpful, it can be repeated regularly, and the child can learn to implement it on their own. Parents can be made aware of the intervention and support the process at home.

Reference

Malher-Moran, M. S. (2018). Why is engaging a child's brain and body in therapy important? *Good Therapy*. https://www.goodtherapy.org/blog/why-is-engaging-childs-brain-body-in-therapy-important-0725184

Conclusion

Neurodiversity defines a more balanced and accurate perspective of what is really going on in human neurotypes. Instead of regarding traditionally pathologized populations as less than, devalued, problematic, needing a cure or fix, the emphasis in neurodiversity is placed on differences (Armstrong, 2010). There is no argument that neurodivergent children can have mental health needs and those needs should be addressed. The goal of the play therapist is to realize that the mental health needs exist somewhat independently of the neurodivergence. The neurodivergence is more of an operating system so the therapy may shift or adjust to best fit the neurodivergent child in order to help them with their therapy goals. Think of this scenario, if you were working with a neurotypical child who had a therapy need of decreasing anxiety. Would you conceptualize that the child was too neurotypical and this was creating the anxiety, thus we need to make the child less neurotypical and then the anxiety will go away?

Children are people, they are not projects. I fundamentally believe that play therapy is the best therapeutic approach for working with children. Nothing else values children, empowers them, and addresses their self-worth, while simultaneously addressing their mental health needs. For the neurodivergent child, play therapy, and the therapeutic powers of play are a welcome reprieve from the historically devaluing processes and systems these children have been subjected. AutPlay Therapy is the aggregation of not only my lived experience but also the fulfillment and realization of a neurodiversity affirming mental health approach that can be implemented with children and families.

You do not have to be neurodivergent to work with neurodivergent children. You do not have to be neurodivergent to support, value, build relationship, and affirm neurodivergent children. But you do have to commit to deconstructing ableist practices, you do have to believe in the neurodiversity

DOI: 10.4324/9781003207610-19

paradigm, and you do have to apply neurodiversity affirming constructs. And why wouldn't you want to? It's the better way. It is the heart of the play therapy – for children to leave our playrooms, leave our presence feeling better than when they came in. The only way to truly do this with neurodivergent clients is to commit to being an affirming professional.

Reference

Armstrong, T. (2010). *Neurodiversity: Discovering the extraordinary gifts of autism, ADHD, dyslexia, and other brain differences*. Da Capo Press.

Common Terms Related to Neurodivergence

Ableism: the discrimination against people with disabilities; devaluing and limiting the potential of people with physical, intellectual, or mental disorders and disabilities. The belief (consciously aware or conditioned) that those without disability are superior. Ableism practices can sometimes be conditioned, with individuals participating in ableist behaviors without realizing.

Actual Autistic: a term that refers to individuals who are autistic and who speak from their perspective of being autistic.

Alexithymia: is a personality trait characterized by the subclinical inability to identify and describe emotions experienced by oneself.

Aphantasia: is a phenomenon in which people are unable to visualize imagery.

Atypical: is not typical, or not conforming to the common type: irregular or abnormal.

Code Switching: trying to act like others, or act in a way that gains acceptance from the people or group a person is around so as not to draw negative attention to oneself.

Compulsions: are deliberate repetitive behaviors that follow specific rules, such as pertaining to cleaning, checking, or counting.

Developmental Delay: is when a child does not reach their developmental milestones at the expected times. It is an ongoing major or minor delay in the process of development.

Dysregulation: is a term used in the mental health community to refer to an emotional response that is poorly modulated and does not fall within the conventionally accepted range of emotive response. It can be looked at as a child's inability to manage or regulate their emotions which typically results in various negative behaviors.

Echolalia: is a child's automatic repetition of vocalizations made by another person. It is closely related to echopraxia, the automatic repetition of movements made by another person. Echolalia can be present with autism and other developmental disabilities. A typical pediatric presentation of echolalia might be as follows: a child is asked "Do you want dinner?"; the child echoes back "Do you want dinner?", followed by a pause, and then a response, "Yes. What's for dinner?" In delayed echolalia, a phrase is repeated after a delay, such as a person with autism who repeats TV commercials, favorite movie scripts, or parental reprimands.

Expressive Language: is the use of verbal behavior, or speech, to communicate thoughts, ideas, and feelings with others.

Hyperarousal: a state of increased psychological and physiological tension marked by such effects as reduced pain tolerance, anxiety, exaggerated startle responses, insomnia, and fatigue.

Hyperlexia: is characterized by having an average or above-average IQ and word-reading ability well above what would be expected at a given age. It can be viewed as a super ability in which word recognition ability goes far above expected levels of skill.

Hypoarousal: a physiological state where your body slows down. It may include feelings of sadness, irritability, and nervousness.

Identity-First Language: Using language that places a person's identity first such as saying, "autistic child" or "autistic person." Research supports that the majority of autistic adults prefer identity-first language over person-first language (child with autism).

Individualized Education Program (IEP): is an educational plan designed to meet the unique education needs of one child, who may have a disability, as defined by federal regulations. An IEP is intended to help children reach targeted educational goals. IEPs are mandated by the Individuals with Disabilities Education Act (IDEA).

Masking: The act of hiding autism/neurodivergent features and/or characteristics. Also, hiding one's identity as being autistic/neurodivergent. This is typically done in response to neurotypical expectations to act a certain way. Over time, this process can become psychologically distressing to autistic individuals.

Medical Model of Disability: Regarding autism, this model views autism as a disorder, something that is a problem that needs to be fixed, treated, or cured.

Neurodivergent: Refers to a mind that functions in ways that diverge significantly from the dominant societal standards of what is normal and expected. This often includes diagnoses such as autism, sensory challenges, ADHD, and learning disorders.

Neurodiversity: In the 1990s, an autistic sociologist named Judy Singer coined the term "neurodiversity." Neurodiversity is an approach to learning and disability that argues diverse neurological conditions are a result of normal variations in the human genome. Every person is part of neurodiversity; we all have a unique way that our brain is wired to operate and navigate.

Neurodiversity Affirming: A belief and commitment in approach, which means valuing and respecting the different ways an autistic or neurodivergent client may process, feel, respond, communicate, and play. It means allowing the child to be themself and not trying to change them to fit a neurotypical standard. Further, it means giving the client a voice in the decision-making process regarding their therapy.

Neurodiversity Movement: A social justice movement that seeks civil rights, equality, respect, and full societal inclusion for the neurodivergent.

Neurodiversity Paradigm: A perspective on neurodiversity that includes the belief that all humans are diverse in their neurocognitive functioning; there is no one normal standard for neurocognitive functioning.

Neurotypical: A term used to describe individuals who are not neurodivergent and of societal-viewed typical development, intellect, and cognitive abilities.

Non-Autistic: Anyone who does not have autism. This can include neurodivergent individuals who are not autistic but have some other neurodivergence.

Obsessions: are the domination of one's thoughts or feelings by a persistent idea, image, desire, etc. Obsessions are thoughts that recur and persist despite efforts to ignore or confront them.

Perseveration: refers to repeating or "getting stuck" carrying out a behavior (e.g., putting in and taking out a puzzle piece) when it is no longer appropriate.

Person First Language: referring to and using person before a diagnosis such as person with autism.

Pragmatic Speech: is language used to communicate and socialize.

Receptive Language: is the comprehension of language; listening, and understanding what is communicated. It is the receiving aspect of language. Sometimes, reading is included when referring to receptive language, but some use the term for spoken communication only. It involves being attentive to what is said, the ability to comprehend the message, the speed of processing the message, and concentrating on the message. Receptive language also includes understanding figurative language, as well as literal language. Receptive language includes being able to follow a series of commands.

Regulation: is a child's ability to notice and respond to internal and external sensory input, and then adjust his emotions and behavior to the demands of his surroundings.

Sensory Processing: the way the nervous system receives messages from the senses and turns them into appropriate motor and behavioral responses. Processing issues exist when sensory signals do not get organized into appropriate responses which create challenges in performing everyday tasks and may manifest in motor clumsiness, behavioral problems, anxiety, depression, and school failure. The eight sensory areas are sight, smell, taste, hearing, touch, vestibular, and proprioception.

Social Model of Disability: Regarding autism, this model views autism as a person's identity and not what makes a person disabled. Rather, it is society's views of autism that makes an autistic person disabled.

Social Reciprocity: Social reciprocity is the back-and-forth flow of social interaction. The term "reciprocity" refers to how the behavior of one person influences and is influenced by the behavior of another person and vice versa.

Spectrum Disorder: is a term that refers to three disorders that previously using DSM-IV criteria, fell under the umbrella of autism spectrum disorders: Autism, Asperger's, and Pervasive Developmental Disorder NOS.

Stimming: is a repetitive body movement, such as hand flapping, that is hypothesized to stimulate one or more senses. The term is shorthand for self-stimulation. Repetitive movement, or stereotypy, is often referred to as stimming under the hypothesis that it has a function related to sensory input.

Parent Guide for Implementing the AutPlay Follow Me Approach (FMA)

1 Set the stage for your play times by choosing a day and time to have your play time and a location in your home for the play time. Be mindful to choose times and locations that will be the least distracting for you and your child. Avoid times and locations where you or your child may be distracted by other people, tasks, or objects in your surroundings.

2 Begin the play time with an introductory statement such as "This is our special play time, you can play anything you want and I will be in here with you."

3 Let your child lead the play time. He or she can choose to play with what he or she wants and how he or she wants. Follow your child as he or she transitions from one toy or activity to another. Try to stay physically close to your child.

4 Periodically make tracking and reflective statements.

5 Periodically ask your child questions.

6 Periodically try to engage with your child in what he or she is playing with. Look for opportunities to inset yourself into the play and notice instances where your child is accepting your attempts to engage and playing back with you.

7 Try to engage your child in ways that promote attunement and acknowledgement skills.

8 Be mindful of your child's limits. Do not push your child to engage with you to the point of dysregulating your child. If you feel that your child has reached his or her limit, then end the play time.

9 Make note of instances where your child demonstrates any of the basics skills that have been targeted and any advances in reciprocal play or interaction that your child produces.

10 End the play time with a closing statement such as "In 5 minutes out play time with be over." After 5 minutes, "Our play time is over; we will play again next time."

11 Complete the In Home Play Times Summary Sheet and bring it with you to discuss with the therapist during your next appointment.

Follow Me Approach (FMA) Skills

Starting and Ending the Play Times – The parent begins by introducing the child to the play space. The parent explains to the child that, "This is our special play space, and you can do whatever you like in here, and I will be in here with you." The parent gives a five-minute verbal and visual warning that the play session is almost over and again at the one-minute mark. The verbal statement can be "We have five minutes left of our special play time and then it will be over for today," and again at the one minute, "We have one minute left of our special play time today and then it will be over." The visual can be as simple as the parent holding up their hand with five fingers and then one finger as they are giving the verbal warnings. When the session is over, the parent states, "Our time is up for today."

Nondirective Play Skill – The child leads the play in the session. The child is allowed to maneuver around the play time and play with or attend to anything they like. The child is also allowed to switch from toy or types of play as they like. The child leads the time, and the parent follows the child figuratively and literally in the play time. The parent stays present and attuned with the child, paying attention to the child, and observing the child closely. The parent does not try to lead the play or direct the child to participate in play the parent wants to do.

Reflective and Tracking Statements Skill – The parent periodically provides a reflective and/or tracking statement. These statements communicate to the child that the parent is present with them, sees them, and is attuning to them.

Example Reflective Statement would be a child struggling to get a cap off a marker. The child is looking frustrated with their effort. The parent might say "That cap is frustrating you," or "You are frustrated that the cap will not come off." Another example would be if the child says "This is my favorite" while tightly hugging a stuffed animal. The parent might reflect "You really like that one," or "That one makes you feel happy."

Example Tracking Statement would be if the child is scooping up sand and putting it into a bucket, the parent might say "You are putting the sand in the bucket," or "You are doing what you want with the sand." Another example would be if the child paints a picture and holds it up to show the parent, the parent might say "You finished the whole painting," or "You finished that and now you are showing me."

Asking Questions Skill – The parent periodically will ask the child a question. The questions are designed to communicate to the child that the parent is present, to begin developing social navigation, and to help the parent assess for engagement improvement. The questions asked should be in the moment and related to what is happening in the play time. An example would be the child painting blue on a piece of paper and the parent asking, "Do you like the color blue?"

Engage with the Child Skill – The parent is periodically trying to engage with the child in whatever the child is doing (the child's play). Remember that the child leads and chooses whatever the child wants to play with, and the parent follows the child and tries to get involved with what the child is doing. The parent should make attempts throughout the play time. How many attempts, in what ways, and at what time is left to the parent's discretion. The following provides examples of engaging with the child:

- The child starts playing with the play dishes. The parent sits beside the child and takes a bowl and puts it on the parent's head and says to the child, "Look at my silly bowl hat." The parent is trying to engage the child by having the child look at the parent and notice the bowl on the parent's head. The parent might take a bowl or plate and put it on the child's head and say, "Look at the plate on your head." The parent might ask the child to put a bowl or plate on the parent's head and see if they can begin to engage in this activity back and forth.
- The child starts playing with the sand tray building a sandcastle. The parent moves beside the child and starts adding sand to the castle or asks the child where to put the sand. The parent might try pushing sand to the child to use for their castle. The parent might also try building their own castle in a separate area in the sand tray.
- The child is shooting a basketball into the basketball hoop. The parent moves beside the child and helps get the ball and hand it back to the child after they shoot a basket. The parent might also try getting another basketball and also shooting the ball in the basket. The parent could try getting the child to take turns shooting the basketball or allow the parent to pass the basketball to the child and then the child shoots it.

Being Mindful of Limits Skill – The parent should be sensitive to the child's comfort, feelings of safety, and regulation level. Some play times may be mostly tracking and reflecting statements if the child is displaying discomfort with the parent's attempts to engage. The parent should not engage or try to get involved with what the child is doing to the point where the child becomes fully dysregulated and has a meltdown.

Setting Limits – The limit-setting approach in the FMA is fairly simple. Many of the children that will be participating in the FMA may not understand limit-setting models that are too verbal or too cognitive and they may need a more basic redirection. For most limit setting needs, the parent should simply redirect the child or remove the limit causing toy or material.

In Home Follow Me Approach (FMA) Play Times Summary Sheet

Child's Name _____ Parent's Name _____

Date of Play Time _____

Description of Play Time

_____

_____

_____

_____

_____

_____

Issues or Questions about the Play Time

_____

_____

_____

_____

_____

_____

Observations Related to Improvements in Engagement or Therapy Goals

_____

_____

_____

_____

_____

_____

Limit-Setting Guide in the AutPlay Follow Me Approach

The three R's limit-setting model stands for redirect, replacement, and removal.

Redirect – If the child begins to or is breaking a limit. The therapist could begin with redirection which means redirecting the child's focus and energy away from a problematic situation to something that is allowed. For example, away from throwing sand all over the playroom to shooting baskets in the basketball hoop. The therapist would simply try to redirect the child to another activity, toy, or object to transition their attention off the limit violation. There does not need to be any dialogue about a limit being broken or that the child needs to stop. In this situation, the therapist realizes the limit is being broken and moves to see if redirecting will suffice.

Replacement – If the child begins or is in process of breaking a limit, the therapist could begin with implementing a replacement activity. Redirecting and replacing are two processes can be used interchangeably. Replacement means literally replacing what is happening (something that is likely meeting a need for the child) with something new or different that is acceptable (continues to meet the need for the child). For example, the child is smashing a toy truck into the floor which is breaking the truck. The therapist or parent would quickly select another object such as a rubber hammer and play doh and put it in the child's free hand showing them how to smash the play doh while taking the truck away from the child. Replacement can also be replacing a game that is being played with the child with a different game. Where redirection is the act of transitioning the child's attention or trying to distract the child away, replacement is giving the child a tangible, acceptable alternative that continues to meet their need. As with redirecting, there does not need to be any dialogue about the limit being broken when using the replacement strategy.

Removal – If a child is beginning to or in the process of breaking a limit, redirecting and replacement should be implemented first. If these processes do not work, then removal is the final option. The first step in removal is verbally explaining to the child that they need to discontinue a limit-setting behavior, or a toy/material may be removed from the playroom or the play session may end. In situations where a toy or material can be removed, the therapist might say "Michael in here you cannot cut the dolls hair, if you keep trying to cut the hair, I will take the doll and scissors out of the playroom." If the verbal prompt does not stop the behavior, then removal is implemented.

The therapist would remove the doll and scissors from the playroom and continue with the session. If removal involves the child needing to leave the playroom (usually due to unsafe behavior), the therapist could try guiding the child into another location, possibly where the child can be alone or minimally supervised while the child calms down. In an extreme case, removal might involve ending the session and physically taking the child out of the clinic. If physical removal is necessary, then a parent should be the one to physically remove the child. This is done in extreme cases where the child or others are in danger due to the child's behavior, and action is needed to keep everyone safe (Table A.1).

Feeling List

Accepted	Afraid	Affectionate	Loyal
Angry	Miserable	Anxious	Misunderstood
Peaceful	Beautiful	Playful	Ashamed
Brave	Awkward	Calm	Proud
Capable	Quiet	Bored	Overwhelmed
Caring	Relaxed	Confused	Cheerful
Relieved	Defeated	Comfortable	Safe
Competent	Satisfied	Concerned	Mad
Depressed	Pressured	Confident	Provoked
Content	Desperate	Regretful	Courageous
Silly	Lonely	Rejected	Curious
Special	Disappointed	Remorseful	Strong
Discouraged	Disgusted	Sad	Sympathetic
Excited	Embarrassed	Shy	Forgiving
Thankful	Sorry	Friendly	Thrilled

Fearful	Stubborn	Nervous	Stupid
Glad	Understood	Frustrated	Good
Unique	Furious	Tired	Grateful
Valuable	Guilty	Touchy	Great
Hateful	Happy	Helpless	Hopeful
Wonderful	Hopeless	Humorous	Worthwhile
Unattractive	Joyful	Uncertain	Lovable
Humiliated	Uncomfortable	Loved	Hurt
Ignored	Impatient	Indecisive	Inferior
Insecure	Irritated	Jealous	Worried

Table A.1 Suggested Toys and Materials ListToys

Human miniatures/figures	Animal miniatures
Car, plane, and boat miniatures	Sand tray
Toy food, dishes, and kitchen area	Water tray
Set of building blocks	Set of LEGO bricks
An assortment of various fidgets	Sensory balls and toys
Hula Hoop	Rope
An assortment of hats & masks	Mirror
Balloons	Bubbles
Toy phone	Toy computer
Basketball	Basketball goal

(*Continued*)

Table A.1 Continued Suggested Toys and Materials ListToys

Doctors' kit	Cash register
Large cardboard bricks	Toy money
Toy musical instruments	Nerf guns
Foam swords (pool noodles)	Beach ball
Mr. Potato Head Game	Feeling Face Cards
iPad	Nintendo Switch

Expressive Materials

White paper	Construction paper
Paints/markers/crayons	Blank puzzles
An assortment of art (decoration) supplies	Stickers
Clay/Play Doh	Magazines
Dry erase board	Dry erase markers
An assortment of art (construction) supplies	Buddha Board

Social Needs Cross Off Sheet

Flip a coin or chip onto the sheet and wherever it lands is the social need that will be discussed and/or practiced. Once it is finished, cross it off (Tables A.2, A.3, Figures A.1–A.3).

Table A.2 Four Square Grid

Table A.3 Nine Square Grid

Social Navigation Pick Up Sticks Examples

RED

Name two things that make a good friend

Name three fun things you could do with other people

Ask someone in the room a question

What is your favorite feeling

BLUE

Say some ways kids get bullied at school

Name two things you can do to feel less nervous

Talk about something you did with a friend

Act like you are playing your favorite sport

YELLOW

What is a feeling you don't like

What is a fun memory you have

Talk about a time you felt uncomfortable at school

What would you do if you could do anything you wanted

GREEN

Tell a story about something you did

Ask someone in the room a question

Say two things that make you feel nervous

Talk about something fun you do at school

BLACK

What is something that makes you uncomfortable

What is one of your favorite things to do

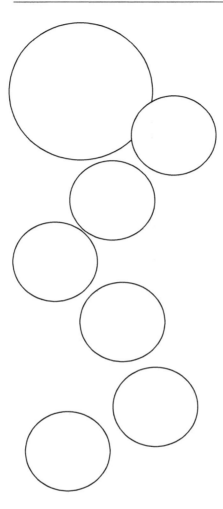

Figure A.1 Friendship Universe Worksheet.

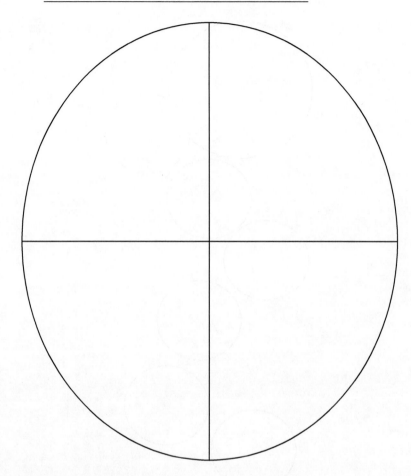

Figure A.2 My Safety Wheel Worksheet.

Figure A.3 Conversation Bubbles Worksheet.

Feelings Detective Worksheet

Name:_____

Find These Feelings:

Happy

Lonely

Excited

Mad

Proud

Nervous

Loved

Shy

Jealous

AutPlay Autism Checklist-R

Child's Name _____Age____Gender____Date_____

The AutPlay Autism Checklist-Revised is a strengths-based autism screening instrument to help assess the possibility of autism and need for further evaluation. Place a check by each statement that describes your child. If you are unsure, leave the statement blank.

_____ Seems to have their own way of communicating and interacting

_____ Shows or seems to have strong reactions to sensory experiences

_____ Seems to do things in a way that might not be expected

_____ Views relationships and interactions with peers differently than what might be expected

_____ Prefers constructive play (Legos, blocks, train track)

_____ Does not seem interested in and does not display pretend play

_____ Spends time playing alone or seems to prefer to play alone

_____ Prefers solitary activities

_____ Prefers or displays nonverbal communication

_____ Displays stimming (hand or finger flapping, twisting, or spinning)

_____ Displays stimming while talking or looking away while talking

_____ Seems bored when talking with others

_____ Seems drawn to or prefers technology play (electronics)

_____ Seems to prefer sensory based play

_____ Has an intense focus on specific things or subjects

_____ Preoccupation with one or more interests

_____ Prefers a routine, schedule, or planned activity

_____ Displays a special interest and seems not interested in things outside of the special interest

_____ Not as interested in social processes that may be common with peers

About the AutPlay Autism Checklist-R

The checklist is based in a reframe of the DMS-V diagnostic criteria for Autism Spectrum Disorder and focuses on viewing the child from a more strength-based description. It is valid for children ages 4–11. The checklist is designed to be completed by a parent or other caregiver who is familiar or involved enough with the child to provide accurate feedback. Therapists should use the checklist in the following ways:

1   As part of an autism screening procedure to determine if further evaluation is needed.
2   As an assessment tool to gain further information about a child's strengths and needs.
3   As an aid in developing therapy goals.

Instructions for completing the AutPlay Autism Checklist-R

Therapists should give the checklist to parents and/or caregivers who are familiar with the child (this might include foster parents, school teachers, nannies, or other relatives). Parents and/or caregivers are instructed to complete the checklist by placing a check next to any statement they feel describes the child. Parents and/or caregivers are not given a copy of the About the AutPlay Autism Checklist-R (page 2). Therapists should review and share results with parents and/or caregivers and provide recommendations.

Scoring

The AutPlay Autism Checklist-R is not a diagnostic tool. When completing the AutPlay Autism Checklist-R as part of an autism screening, therapists should compare results on the checklist with other screening inventories or procedures as part of a comprehensive screening protocol and consider additional factors to determine if further evaluation is warranted. The checklist should not be the sole instrument used for an autism screening.

The following scoring guide is designed to help inform further recommendations:

0–1 – Not indicative of further evaluation
2–5 – Possible referral for further evaluation
6 or above – Indicative of further evaluation

Therapists looking for more resources for conducting autism screenings should consider conducting a child observation, a parent–child observation, and implementing additional inventories.

Therapists should refer parents and/or caregivers for a full evaluation if there is an indication of autism.

Child Name _____ Score _____ Date _____

AutPlay Child Observation Form

Child's Name_____ Age____ Gender_____ Date_____

Communication (does child make any verbal comments, are comments relevant/understandable, does child exchange in conversation, answer questions, is there other (nonverbal) communication?)

Play (what does the child play with, do they play with any toys, do they play with other materials or non-toy objects, what seems to be their play interests/preferences?)

Relation (how does the child seem to navigate relationally, any social interaction with the therapist, what social strengths are observed, are there any observed social/relational navigation needs?)

Attention/Focus/Impulsivity (does the child seem to maintain attention for an amount of time, do they wander around the room continuously, does the child keep focus on any toys, complete tasks, do they appear impulsive?)

Interaction (does the child interact with the therapist, does the child seem to want to be alone, does child seem to notice or respond to the therapist being in the room, do they attempt to connect with the therapist?)

AutPlay Child/Parent Observation Form

Child's Name_____ Age____ Gender_____ Date_____

General Child and Parent Interaction (describe the interaction between the parent and child, do the interactions occur smoothly or forced, does the parent and child seem to listen to, respond to, or engage with each other?) Joint Play, Child and Parent Together (does the child and parent play together, describe type, quality, and quantity of play together, does play together seem forced or natural?)

Verbal and Nonverbal Communication (does the child and parent engage in verbal reciprocal communication, do child and parent exchange nonverbal communication, do they notice each other's nonverbal communication, what is the parent and child communication style?)

Parent Initiations Toward Child (does the parent initiate interaction with the child, how does the parent attempt to initiate with the child, how does the child respond to the parents' initiations?)

Limits (If any limits occur during the observation, how are they handled by the parent, what is the response of the child?)

AutPlay Assessment of Play–Page One

Child's Name_____ Age____ Gender_____ Date_____

Read the following play categories and definitions and rate where you feel your child is at in terms of possessing and demonstrating this type of play.

Functional Play is a term also used for relational play, it means denoting use of objects in play for the purposes for which they were intended, e.g., using simple objects correctly, combining related objects, and making objects do
what they are made to do (setting up a bowling set and bowling).
NO–1   2   3   4   5   6   7   8   9   10–YES

Symbolic Play refers to symbolic, or pretend play which occurs when children begin to substitute one object for another. For example, using a hairbrush to represent a microphone. The child may pretend to do something (with or without the object present or with an object representing another object) or be someone.
NO–1   2   3   4   5   6   7   8   9   10–YES

Cooperative Play refers to a play where children plan, assign roles, and play together. Cooperative play is goal-oriented and children play in an organized manner toward a common end. Moreover, Cooperative play is a "true social play" in which children cooperate or assume reciprocal roles.
NO–1   2   3   4   5   6   7   8   9   10–YES

Sociodramatic Play refers to play involving acting out scripts, scenes, and plays adopted from cartoons, books. Children take/assume roles using themselves and/or characters like dolls, figures, and puppets as they interact together on common themes.
NO–1   2   3   4   5   6   7   8   9   10–YES

Peer play refers to interactions with one's peers, which provide opportunities for physical, cognitive, social, and emotional development.
NO–1   2   3   4   5   6   7   8   9   10–YES

Constructive Play characterized as manipulation of objects for the purpose of constructing or creating something. Children use materials to achieve a specific goal in mind that requires transformation of objects into a new configuration. Lego pieces turned to cars or houses are an example of this play.
NO–1   2   3   4   5   6   7   8   9   10–YES

Sensory Play involves playing with toys or items for the purpose of sensory sensations or sensory seeking. Enjoying the toy or object because of how it feels or what it produces for the senses. Sensory balls, putty, and exercise balls are examples.
NO–1   2   3   4   5   6   7   8   9   10–YES

Technology Play characterized by playing online and video games alone or with others. This might involve a tablet, a game station, or playing games on a computer.
NO–1   2   3   4   5   6   7   8   9   10–YES

AutPlay Assessment of Play – Page Two

Child's Name_____ Age____ Gender_____ Date_____

Please answer the following questions regarding your child's play. Try to think about specific times you have observed or played with your child and answer the questions as completely as possible.

Does your child play with toys?

Does your child play independently?

Does your child play with other children?

Does your child initial play with other children or adults?

Do you have play times with your child?

Does your child interact with you during play times?

Does your child do pretend play or metaphor play?

Does your child play with objects that would not be considered toys?

If someone (child or adult) asks your child to play, what does your child usually do?

Does your child seem to want to play?

Does your child seem to like technology-based play?

Describe your child's play.

AutPlay Connection Inventory–Child (3–11)

Child's Name_____ Age____ Gender_____ Date_____

Rate the following connection related statements on the continuum from does not display to displays, with a 1 being does not display at all and a 5 being fully displays. A does not display selection does not mean an issue or problem. This inventory is designed to better understand the child.

My child gives hugs and/or other physical touch.

1   2   3   4   5

My child communicates, "I love you" and/or makes other endearing statements.

1   2   3   4

My child receives hugs and/or other physical touch.

1   2   3   4   5

My child seems to want comfort from me or others when distressed.

1   2   3   4   5

My child displays interest and a desire to be with me or others.

1   2   3   4   5

My child indicates awareness of me or others.

1   2   3   4   5

My child appears to struggle with giving or receiving nurture/love from me.

1   2   3   4   5

My child appears to avoid physical closeness and touch.

1   2   3   4   5

My child initiates games and play with others.

1   2   3   4   5

My child will participate if games or play are initiated by others.

1   2   3   4   5

My child responds appropriately when others engage them.

1   2   3   4   5

My child seems inconsistent in their affection toward family members.

1   2   3   4   5

My child talks about or seems interested in being with me, other family members, or peers.

1   2   3   4   5

AutPlay Connection Inventory–Adolescent (12–18)

Child's Name_____ Age____ Gender_____ Date_____

Rate the following connection related statements on the continuum from does not display to displays, with a 1 being does not display at all and a 5 being fully displays. A does not display selection does not mean an issue or problem. This inventory is designed to better understand the adolescent.

My adolescent engages in, seeks, seems comfortable with physical affection (hugs, touch, etc.).
1   2   3   4   5

My adolescent communicates, "I love you" and/or makes other endearing statements.
1   2   3   4   5

My adolescent seems comfortable receiving hugs and/or other physical touch.
1   2   3   4   5

My adolescent will display sad, hurt, or vulnerable emotions if the situation warrants such a response.
1   2   3   4   5

My adolescent displays empathy toward others.
1   2   3   4   5

My adolescent makes appropriate acknowledgment of others.
1   2   3   4   5

My adolescent seems inconsistent in their affection toward me, family members, and others.
1   2   3   4   5

My adolescent appears unable to give or receive love.
1   2   3   4   5

My adolescent appears to avoid physical closeness and touch.
1   2   3   4   5

My adolescent initiates games or "hang out" time with others.
1   2   3   4   5

My adolescent will participate if others initiate games or "hang out" time.
1   2   3   4   5

My adolescent participates in or seems to want to participate in family activities.
1   2   3   4   5

My adolescent seems to have an appropriate parent/adolescent connection.
1   2   3   4   5

AutPlay Emotional Regulation Inventory–Child (3–11)–Page One

Child's Name_____ Age_____ Gender_____ Date_____

Rate the following emotional regulation statements on the continuum from does not display to displays, with a 1 being does not display at all and a 5 being fully displays. A does not display selection does not mean an issue or problem. This inventory is designed to better understand the child.

My child verbalizes positive emotions.

1   2   3   4   5

My child verbalizes negative emotions.

1   2   3   4   5

My child shows appropriate body language to match an emotion.

1   2   3   4   5

My child can differentiate between at least 5 emotions (as age appropriate).

1   2   3   4   5

My child recognizes when another person is feeling something.

1   2   3   4   5

My child can accurately identify an emotion in another person.

1   2   3   4   5

My child understands anxiety and can self-calm.

1   2   3   4   5

My child understands anger and knows anger reducing strategies.

1   2   3   4   5

My child can verbalize when they feel angry or anxious.

1   2   3   4   5

My child shows emotions in pretend or symbolic play.

1   2   3   4   5

My child can verbalize when they feel confused.

1   2   3   4   5

My child can identify an emotion that goes with a certain situation such as what someone would feel when they are at a funeral.

1   2   3   4   5

AutPlay Emotional Regulation Inventory–Child (3–11)–Page Two

Please answer the following questions regarding your child's emotional regulation. Try to think about specific times you have observed with your child and answer the questions as completely as possible.

1 Describe a situation in which your child expressed an emotion.

2 Describe a situation where your child was expressing a negative emotion and was able to self-calm.

3 Describe a situation when your child accurately identified an emotion in another person.

4 Describe how emotions are shown and expressed in your family.

5 Describe how emotions are currently taught and/or modeled for your child.

AutPlay Emotional Regulation Inventory–Adolescent (12–18)– Page One

Child's Name_____ Age____ Gender_____ Date_____

Rate the following emotional regulation statements on the continuum from does not display to displays, with a 1 being does not display at all and a 5 being fully displays. A does not display selection does not mean an issue or problem. This inventory is designed to better understand the adolescent.

My adolescent indicates positive emotions.

1   2   3   4   5

My adolescent indicates negative emotions.

1   2   3   4   5

My adolescent shows appropriate body language to match an emotion.

1   2   3   4   5

My adolescent can differentiate between at least ten emotions.

1   2   3   4   5

My adolescent recognizes emotions in others.

1   2   3   4   5

My adolescent can accurately identify an emotion in another person.

1   2   3   4   5

My adolescent understands anxiety and can self-calm when anxious.

1   2   3   4   5

My adolescent understands anger and knows anger reducing strategies.

1   2   3   4   5

My adolescent can indicate when they feel angry or anxious.

1   2   3   4   5

My adolescent shows emotion regarding peer and family relationships.

1   2   3   4   5

My adolescent seems to understand and express empathy.

1   2   3   4   5

My adolescent can identify an emotion that goes with a certain situation such as what someone would feel when they are at a funeral.

1   2   3   4   5

AutPlay Emotional Regulation Inventory–Adolescent (12–18)– Page Two

Please answer the following questions regarding your adolescent's emotional regulation. Try to think about specific times you have observed with your adolescent and answer the questions as completely as possible.

1 Describe a situation in which your adolescent expressed an emotion.

2 Describe a situation where your adolescent was expressing a negative emotion and was able to self-calm.

3 Describe a situation when your adolescent accurately identified an emotion in another person.

4 Describe how emotions are show and expressed in your family.

5 Describe how emotions are currently taught and/or modeled for your adolescent.

AutPlay Social Navigation Inventory

Name_____Age_____Gender_____Date_____

How would you describe your child's social navigation?

_____

_____

_____

Does your child play with or hang out with others? Please describe.

_____

_____

_____

Please describe any of the following possible needs your child may be having–experiencing bulling, peer rejection, safety awareness concerns, social anxiety, misunderstood by others, self-esteem struggles, self-awareness, unhappy with current peer/friendship situations.

_____

_____

_____

What is your child's social and other strengths?

_____

_____

_____

What does social navigation look like in your family?

_____

_____

_____

AutPlay Special Interests Inventory

Child's Name_____Age_____Gender_____Date_____

What do you like to do for fun?

If you could wake up tomorrow and do whatever you wanted, what would you do?

What do you talk about a lot?

What do you think about a lot?

Do you have a favorite game?

What do you do that feels good to you?

What things are you interested in?

How do you spend your free time?

AutPlay Dysregulated Behaviors Assessment—Page One

Child's Name_____ Age____ Gender_____ Date_____

Please answer the following open-ended questions regarding your child's behavior. Try to recall specific situations and behaviors. If you are unsure, leave the question blank.

1 Does your child seem to have sensory issues? If so, what type?

2 Do you understand the difference between a dysregulated "meltdown" vs. a more intentional behavior response?

3 What does your child's unwanted behaviors look like? Please describe context, actions, words, etc.

4 Are there specific times and or situations when you child is more likely to have unwanted behaviors? Please describe.

5 Do you notice specific triggers that seem to create/precede unwanted behaviors?

6 What is the typical intensity and duration of unwanted behaviors?

7 How frequently, in a week's time, does your child have an unwanted behavior?

8 Does your child have unwanted behaviors at school? If so, describe.

9 How do you currently address or manage your child's unwanted behaviors?

10 Does your child seem particularly dysregulated or "edgy" right after school?

11 Have you discovered anything that seems to help your child calm when they are having unwanted behaviors?

AutPlay Behavior Communication Assessment

Child's Name _____ Age_____ Gender_____ Date_____

Reporting Source for Assessment:

Parent Observation _____ Teacher Observation _____ Therapist Observation _____ Other _____

Describe the behavior, the intensity of the behavior, the frequency of the behavior, the duration of the behavior.

_____
_____
_____
_____

Describe where the behavior occurred, the place, the time, the people involved.

_____
_____
_____
_____

Describe what preceded the behavior, what is happening before the behavior occurs, what is happening in the environment, what are other people doing?

_____
_____
_____
_____

Describe what the observed response to the behavior is, how do other people respond, how does the child's caregiver (adult) respond?

_____
_____
_____
_____

What appears to be the purpose of the behavior? What could the child be communicating?

_____
_____
_____
_____

What could be adjusted or modified that might help prevent future behavior?

_____
_____
_____
_____

AutPlay Parent Self Care Inventory

Please complete the following questions. Try to reflect on and think about each question and answer as thoroughly as possible. If you are unsure, leave blank.

1 Do you have support people in your life? If so, who and in what ways do they provide support for you or your family?

2 Are you involved with any community agencies or programs that provide support services? If so, what type of support are you receiving?

3 Do you have any leisure time that is child free? If yes, describe the leisure time.

4 What do you do for relaxation?

5 What does self care mean to you? Describe your current level of self care.

6 What would be your ideal balance of child care and self care? (Table A.4).

Table A.4 Play Therapy Intervention Tracking Sheet

Therapy Goal/Need Addressed (Emotional, Social, Connection, etc.)	AutPlay Therapy Intervention	Session Date

Index